Therapeutic Medicinal Plants in Traditional Persian Medicine

Traditional Persian Medicine (TPM) is one of the oldest medical doctrines, globally known due to pioneering physicians and scientists. The greatest source of natural medicines in TPM originates from medicinal plants. *Therapeutic Medicinal Plants in Traditional Persian Medicine* provides a background on the history of TPM, as well as an introduction to 40 of the most popular medicinal plants used in TPM. It is a practical guide for readers interested in medicinal plants used in the prevention, management, and treatment of different diseases.

Features:

- Includes both traditional therapeutic applications and modern evidence/uses
- Makes a comparison between preclinical and clinical studies
- Provides information on major chemical constituents, therapeutic uses, adverse reactions, and safety for each plant species.

A volume in the Exploring Medicinal Plants series, this book is a valuable resource for researchers, students, academicians, and scientists dealing with medicinal plants, as well as for those interested in the fields of pharmacognosy, naturopathy, phytotherapy, and traditional medicines.

Exploring Medicinal Plants
Series Editor: Azamal Husen, *Wolaita Sodo University, Ethiopia*

Medicinal plants render a rich source of bioactive compounds used in drug formulation and development; they play a key role in traditional or indigenous health systems. As the demand for herbal medicines increases worldwide, supply is declining as most of the harvest is derived from naturally growing vegetation. Considering global interests and covering several important aspects associated with medicinal plants, the Exploring Medicinal Plants series comprises volumes valuable to academia, practitioners, and researchers interested in medicinal plants. Topics provide information on a range of subjects including diversity, conservation, propagation, cultivation, physiology, molecular biology, growth response under extreme environment, handling, storage, bioactive compounds, secondary metabolites, extraction, therapeutics, mode of action, and healthcare practices.

Led by Azamal Husen, PhD, this series is directed to a broad range of researchers and professionals consisting of topical books exploring information related to medicinal plants. It includes edited volumes, references, and textbooks available for individual print and electronic purchases.

Aquatic Medicinal Plants
Edited by Archana Bachheti, Rakesh Kumar Bachheti, and Azamal Husen

Antidiabetic Medicinal Plants and Herbal Treatments
Edited by Azamal Husen

Ethnobotany and Ethnopharmacology of Medicinal and Aromatic Plants
Steps Towards Drugs Discovery
Edited by Mohd Adnan, Mitesh Patel and Mejdi Snoussi

Wild Mushrooms and Health
Diversity, Phytochemistry, Medicinal Benefits, and Cultivation
Edited by Kamal Ch. Semwal, Steve L. Stephenson, and Azamal Husen

Medicinal Roots and Tubers for Pharmaceutical and Commercial Applications
Edited by Rakesh Kumar Bachheti and Archana Bachheti

Pharmacological Aspects of Essential Oils
Current and Future Trends
Edited by Sunita Singh, Pankaj Kumar Chaurasia and Shashi Lata Bharati

Promising Antiviral Herbal and Medicinal Plants
Edited by Nadeem Akhtar, Azamal Husen, Vagish Dwibedi, and Santosh Kumar Rath

Antimalarial Medicinal Plants
Edited by Azamal Husen

Medicinal Spice and Condiment Crops
Edited by Azamal Husen

Therapeutic Medicinal Plants in Traditional Persian Medicine
Edited by Roja Rahimi and Roodabeh Bahramsoltani

Medicinal Plants for the Management of Neurodegenerative Diseases
Edited by Jamal Akhtar, Maryam Sarwat and Fouzia Bashir

For more information about this series, please visit: www.routledge.com/Exploring-Medicinal-Plants/book-series/CRCEMP

Therapeutic Medicinal Plants in Traditional Persian Medicine

Edited by
Roja Rahimi and Roodabeh Bahramsoltani

CRC Press
Taylor & Francis Group
Boca Raton London New York

CRC Press is an imprint of the
Taylor & Francis Group, an **informa** business

Cover image: Mr. Mehdi Keyhan

First edition published 2024
by CRC Press
2385 NW Executive Center Drive, Suite 320, Boca Raton FL 33431

and by CRC Press
4 Park Square, Milton Park, Abingdon, Oxon, OX14 4RN

CRC Press is an imprint of Taylor & Francis Group, LLC

ISBN: 9781032295466 (hbk)
ISBN: 9781032295503 (pbk)
ISBN: 9781003302100 (ebk)

DOI: 10.1201/b22971

Typeset in Times
by Newgen Publishing UK

Dedication

In loving memory of
Professor Gholamreza Amin
and
Professor Abolghasem Soltani
who devoted their lives to developing the knowledge of medicinal plants.

Foreword

Traditional medicine has a long history and is the sum total of the knowledge, skill, and practices based on the theories, beliefs, and experiences indigenous to different cultures. It is used in the maintenance of health as well as in the prevention, diagnosis, improvement, or treatment of physical and mental illness. Traditional medicine is an important and often underestimated health resource with many applications, especially in the prevention and management of lifestyle-related chronic diseases.

In the current global health landscape, traditional and complementary medicine is gaining more and more recognition and importance. International health policy-making organizations such as the World Health Organization are acknowledging the potential of these alternative treatments. The global community is beginning to recognize the importance of these alternative treatments, not only for their potential to reduce the side effects and costs associated with conventional medicine, but also for their therapeutic benefits.

In an era where the world is increasingly turning to traditional and complementary medicine, one of the challenges that we face is the lack of accessible and accurate information. Misinformation and misconceptions about herbal medicine are widespread, leading to confusion and mistrust. This is where the current book, introducing 40 herbs in Traditional Persian Medicine, fills a much-needed gap.

The information presented in this book is not just accurate; it is meticulously researched and compiled. The outstanding team behind this book has worked tirelessly to ensure that the data you find here is both reliable and comprehensive. Knowledge is power, and with this book, the readers are empowered to make informed decisions about their own health, and their patients' health.

The editors of this book are renowned and are among the top 1% scientists in the field of pharmacology and toxicology in 2022 according to Essential Science Indicators. Their expertise and cutting-edge knowledge have been instrumental in bringing this book to life. They are trusted figures in the scientific community, distinguished scientists from Tehran University of Medical Sciences (TUMS), and their commitment to spreading awareness about the benefits of herbal medicine is truly commendable so readers can trust the information presented, knowing it comes from some of the most respected minds in the field.

TUMS is the oldest and most prestigious medical university in Iran, with a history of more than 170 years and a leading position in research and education, which offers various programs in medicine, dentistry, pharmacy, and all other allied fields, with more than 250 majors, 18 hospitals, and 1,900 faculty members.

TUMS is a pioneer in traditional and herbal medicine, with a dedicated school and research center for this field with strong collaboration with international institutions. So, this book is more than just a compilation of data; it is a testament to the potential of herbal medicine and a valuable resource for anyone interested in exploring its benefits. It is my sincere hope that this book will serve as a stepping stone for readers to embark on their journey into the world of Traditional Medicine.

With best regards,
Mohammad H. Ayati, MD, PhD
Associate Professor
Vice-Chancellor for International Affairs
Tehran University of Medical Sciences

Foreword

Preface

Traditional Persian Medicine (TPM) is one of the oldest medical doctrines dating back thousands of years and mostly associated with the names of pioneer physicians and pharmacists (the so-called *Hakim*) such as Avicenna and Rhazes. This medical doctrine is now part of the academic educational system in medical universities of Iran, and numerous research papers have been published based on the investigations related to the therapeutic claims, natural medicines, and historical aspects of TPM.

This book is devoted to the introduction of the most popular medicinal plants used in TPM for therapeutic purposes. The main audience of this book are clinicians and health practitioners who are interested in managing their patients with natural medicines, as well as researchers interested in developing new drugs based on the ideas obtained from traditional medicines, including TPM. Also, all researchers, students, and academicians dealing with medicinal plants, pharmacognosy, naturopathy, traditional medicines, phytotherapy, phytopharmacology, complementary and alternative medicine, and especially TPM would find this book of great value to them.

This book contains two introductory chapters providing some background information on TPM, followed by 40 plant monographs on the most popular medicinal plants used in TPM. In each monograph, a brief explanation of the plant names and phytochemical profile is provided first, followed by the therapeutic applications mentioned in TPM textbooks. For this purpose, we idenified two TPM textbooks, namely, *Al-Qānūn fi-ṭ-Ṭibb* (*The canon of medicine*) written by Avicenna in 1025 AD, which is one of the most important TPM books, and *Makhzan al-Adwiya* (*Treasury of drugs*) written by Aghili Khorasani (1771 AD), which is one of the most recent and greatest books of *Materia medica* in TPM. In the next parts of each monograph, we review the clinical and preclinical studies published on the chosen plant. We have attempted to mention all related clinical trials, systematic reviews, and meta-analyses since these studies provide a high level of evidence for the clinical application of these plants and are of a great significance to clinicians. Regarding preclinical studies, we discuss only pharmacological activities in line with the therapeutic claims of TPM for that plant, so that researchers might be motivated to undertake further mechanistic and clinical studies to confirm the safety and efficacy of these herbs in future studies. As safety is always a major concern for natural medicines, sections regarding possible adverse effects, use during pregnancy and lactation, herb–drug interactions, and precautions are provided under each monograph. In the final part of each monograph, the method of administration as well as the recommended dosage are provided with reference to both published studies and phytotherapy textbooks.

This book is one of the first of its kind serving as an introductory text on TPM medicinal plants for the international audience and has resulted from a collaboration of 40 specialists in TPM, traditional pharmacy, and history of medicine. We would like to express our deepest gratitude to all the contributors without whom this book would not have been possible.

The editors would also like to thank Dr. Mehdi Sabet Jahromi for his technical assistance during the preparation of this book and offer special thanks to Mr. Mehdi Keyhan for preparing the photos of plant samples.

Roja Rahimi, Pharm.D., PhD,
Professor of Traditional Pharmacy

Roodabeh Bahramsoltani, Pharm.D., PhD,
Assistant Professor of Traditional Pharmacy
Tehran, Iran
October 2023

About the Editors

Roja Rahimi, PhD, graduated with a PharmD degree from Shiraz University of Medical Sciences, Shiraz, Iran, and continued her education to receive a PhD in traditional pharmacy from Tehran University of Medical Sciences, Tehran, Iran. She also holds a postdoc in Pharmacology of Medicinal Plants Used in Gastrointestinal Disorders in Persian Medicine. She is now a professor of traditional pharmacy at the School of Persian Medicine, Tehran University of Medical Sciences. She has been listed among the Top 1% of highly cited scientists according to the Essential Science Indicator (ESI) in 2015–2017 and 2022. She has contributed to more than 200 articles and several book chapters for international publishers. Her field of expertise focuses on the evaluation of safety and efficacy of Traditional Persian Medicine formulations in preclinical and clinical settings.

Roodabeh Bahramsoltani, PhD, graduated with a PharmD degree and then a PhD degree in traditional pharmacy from Tehran University of Medical Sciences, Tehran, Iran. She is now an assistant professor of traditional pharmacy at the School of Persian Medicine, Tehran University of Medical Sciences. She has been listed among the Top 1% of highly cited scientists in 2022 based on the Essential Science Indicator (ESI) and has authored more than 60 papers and several book chapters. She is interested in the development of natural medicinal preparations based on Traditional Persian Medicine textbooks and the evaluation of their pharmacological activities in animal/cellular models.

About the editors

Contributors

Zohreh Abolhassanzadeh
Medical Plants Research Center, Basic Health Sciences Institute, Shahrekord University of Medical Sciences, Shahr-e Kord, Iran.

Hananeh Aliakbarzadeh
Department of Traditional Persian Medicine, School of Persian Medicine, Tehran University of Medical Sciences, Tehran, Iran.

Ehsan Amiri-Ardekani
Department of Phytopharmaceuticals (Traditional Pharmacy), Faculty of Pharmacy, Shiraz University of Medical Sciences, Shiraz, Iran; and Research Center for Traditional Medicine and History of Medicine, Shiraz University of Medical Sciences, Shiraz, Iran.

Parmis Badr
Pharmaceutical Sciences Research Centre, Shiraz University of Medical Sciences, Shiraz, Iran; and Phytopharmaceutical Technology and Traditional Medicine Incubator, Shiraz University of Medical Sciences, Shiraz, Iran.

Roodabeh Bahramsoltani
Department of Traditional Pharmacy, School of Persian Medicine, Tehran University of Medical Sciences, Tehran, Iran; and PhytoPharmacology Interest Group (PPIG), Universal Scientific Education and Research Network (USERN), Tehran, Iran.

Mahbubeh Bozorgi
Department of Traditional Pharmacy, School of Persian Medicine, Shahed University, Tehran, Iran.

Babak Daneshfard
Chronic Respiratory Diseases Research Center, National Research Institute of Tuberculosis and Lung Diseases (NRITLD), Shahid Beheshti University of Medical Sciences, Tehran, Iran; and Persian Medicine Network (PMN), Universal Scientific Education and Research Network (USERN), Tehran, Iran.

Fatemeh Etemadpour
Department of Phytopharmaceuticals (Traditional Pharmacy), School of Pharmacy, Shiraz University of Medical Sciences, Shiraz, Iran.

Sajad Fakhri
Pharmaceutical Sciences Research Center, Health Institute, Kermanshah University of Medical Sciences, Kermanshah, Iran.

Mohammad Hosein Farzaei
Pharmaceutical Sciences Research Center, Health Institute, Kermanshah University of Medical Sciences, Kermanshah, Iran.

Nafiseh Hosseini Yekta
Department of Traditional Medicine, Faculty of Traditional Medicine, Shahid Beheshti University of Medical Sciences, Tehran, Iran.

Rezvan Ghaderpanah
Students Research Committee, School of Medicine, Shiraz University of Medical Sciences, Shiraz, Iran.

Mohammad Hashem Hashempur
Research Center for Traditional Medicine and History of Medicine, Department of Persian Medicine, School of Medicine, Shiraz University of Medical Sciences, Shiraz, Iran.

Shahrzad Irannejad
Institute of the History of Pharmacy and Medicine, Philipps University of Marburg, Germany.

Mehdi Sabet Jahromi
Department of Agriculture, Medicinal Plants and Drugs Research Institute, Shahid Beheshti University, Tehran, Iran.

Behjat Javadi
Department of Traditional Pharmacy, School of Pharmacy, Mashhad University of Medical Sciences, Mashhad, Iran.

Maryam Kabiri
Arnold & Marie Schwartz College of Pharmacy and Health Sciences, Long Island University, New York, USA.

Seyedeh Mahnaz Karimi
Department of Traditional Pharmacy, School of Persian Medicine, Tehran University of Medical Sciences, Tehran, Iran.

Mehrdad Karimi
Department of Traditional Persian Medicine, School of Persian Medicine, Tehran University of Medical Sciences, Tehran, Iran.

Seyede Nargess Sadati Lamardi
Department of Traditional Pharmacy, School of Persian Medicine, Tehran University of Medical Sciences, Tehran, Iran.

Raefeh Mardi
Department of Traditional Persian Medicine, School of Persian Medicine, Tehran University of Medical Sciences, Tehran, Iran.

Mozhgan MehriArdestani
Department of Persian Medicine, Faculty of Medicine, AJA University of Medical Sciences, Tehran, Iran.

Zahra Memariani
Traditional Medicine and History of Medical Sciences Research Center, Health Research Institute, Babol University of Medical Sciences, Babol, Iran.

Reihaneh Moeini
Traditional Medicine and History of Medical Sciences Research Center, Health Research Institute, Babol University of Medical Sciences, Babol, Iran.

Abdolali Mohagheghzadeh
Department of Phytopharmaceuticals (Traditional Pharmacy), Faculty of Pharmacy, Shiraz University of Medical Sciences, Shiraz, Iran; and Pharmaceutical Sciences Research Center, Shiraz University of Medical Sciences, Shiraz, Iran.

Ghazaleh Mosleh
Department of Phytopharmaceuticals (Traditional Pharmacy), Faculty of Pharmacy, Shiraz University of Medical Sciences, Shiraz, Iran.

Ayeh Naghizadeh
Department of Traditional Persian Medicine, School of Persian Medicine, Tehran University of Medical Sciences, Tehran, Iran.

Parva Namiranian
Department of Traditional Persian Medicine, School of Persian Medicine, Tehran University of Medical Sciences, Tehran, Iran.

Samaneh Noroozi
Department of Traditional Persian Medicine, School of Persian Medicine, Tehran University of Medical Sciences, Tehran, Iran.

Mohadeseh Ostovar
Research Center for Traditional Medicine and History of Medicine, Department of Persian Medicine, School of Medicine, Shiraz University of Medical Sciences, Shiraz, Iran.

Roja Rahimi
Department of Traditional Pharmacy, School of Persian Medicine, Tehran University of Medical Sciences, Tehran, Iran.
PhytoPharmacology Interest Group (PPIG), Universal Scientific Education and Research Network (USERN), Tehran, Iran.

Hossein Rezaeizadeh
Department of Traditional Persian Medicine, School of Persian Medicine, Tehran University of Medical Sciences, Tehran, Iran.

Najmeh Sasani
Nutrition Research Center, School of Nutrition and Food Sciences, Shiraz University of Medical Sciences, Shiraz, Iran.

Asie Shojaii
Department of Traditional Pharmacy, School of Persian Medicine, Institute for Studies in Medical History, Persian and Complementary Medicine, Iran University of Medical Sciences, Tehran, Iran.

Zahra Sobhani
Department of Traditional Pharmacy, School of Pharmacy, Mashhad University of Medical Sciences, Mashhad, Iran.

Zahra Taghipour
Department of Traditional Pharmacy, School of Persian Medicine, Tehran University of Medical Sciences, Tehran, Iran.

Meysam Zaeri
Department of Phytopharmaceuticals (Traditional Pharmacy), Faculty of Pharmacy, Shiraz University of Medical Sciences, Shiraz, Iran.

Azadeh Zarei
Department of Traditional Persian Medicine, School of Persian Medicine, Tehran University of Medical Sciences, Tehran, Iran.

Arman Zargaran
Department of Traditional Pharmacy, School of Persian Medicine, Tehran University of Medical Sciences, Tehran, Iran.

Mohammad M. Zarshenas
Medicinal Plants Processing Research Center, Shiraz University of Medical Sciences, Shiraz, Iran; and Department of Phytopharmaceuticals (Traditional Pharmacy), School of Pharmacy, Shiraz University of Medical Sciences, Shiraz, Iran.

Abbreviations

6-OHDA	6-hydroxydopamine
8-OHdG	8-hydroxy-2′-deoxyguanosine
α-SMA	alpha smooth muscle actin
α-syn	alpha-synuclein
AchE	acetylcholinesterase
ACT	Asthma Control Test
ADAS	Alzheimer's Disease Assessment Scale
ADI	Acne Disability Index
AGEs	advanced glycation end products
AKT	protein kinase B
ALP	alkaline phosphatase
ALT	alanine transaminase
ALX	alloxan
APACHE	Acute Physiology and Chronic Health Evaluation
ApoB	apolipoprotein B
ARDS	acute respiratory distress syndrome
AST	aspartate transaminase
bFGF	basic fibroblast growth factor
BMI	body mass index
BP	blood pressure
BUN	blood urea nitrogen
BW	body weight
CAT	catalase
CBS	cystathionine-β-synthase
CCl_4	carbon tetrachloride
COPD	chronic obstructive pulmonary disease
COVID-19	coronavirus disease of 2019
CRP	C-reactive protein
CT	computed tomography
CTGF	connective tissue growth factor
CVD	cardiovascular diseases
DSS	dextran sodium sulfate
ECG	electrocardiogram
EPS	extrapyramidal symptoms
ERK	extracellular signal-regulated kinase
FBS	fasting blood sugar
FEV1	forced expiratory volume in 1 second
FPI	fasting plasma insulin
FSH	follicle stimulating hormone
GABA	gamma amino butyric acid
GAD	generalized anxiety disorder
GERD	gastroesophageal reflux disease
GFR	glomerular filtration rate
GGT	γ-glutamyl transpeptidase
GI	gastrointestinal
Gpx	glutathione peroxidase
GR	glutathione reductase

GSH	reduced glutathione
GSRS	Gastrointestinal Symptom Rating Scale
HDL-C	high-density lipoprotein cholesterol
HIF	hypoxia-inducible factor
HIV	human immunodeficiency virus
HMG-CoA	3-hydroxy-3-methylglutaryl coenzyme A
HO-1	heme-oxygenase-1
HOMA-IR	Homeostatic Model Assessment for Insulin Resistance
HPV	human papilloma virus
hs-CRP	high-sensitivity C-reactive protein
HSV	herpes simplex virus
HTN	hypertension
IBD	inflammatory bowel disease
IBS	irritable bowel syndrome
ICAM-1	intercellular adhesion molecule 1
ICU	intensive care unit
IFN	interferon
Ig	immunoglobulin
IGA	Investigator's Global Assessment
IL	interleukin
iNOS	inducible nitric oxide synthase
INR	international normalized ratio
LD	low dose
LDH	lactate dehydrogenase
LDL-C	low-density lipoprotein cholesterol
LH	luteinizing hormone
LPO	lipid peroxidation
LPS	lipopolysaccharide
MAO	monoamine oxidase
MAP	mean arterial pressure
MCP	monocyte chemoattractant protein
MDA	malondialdehyde
MIC	minimum inhibitory concentration
MMP	matrix metalloproteinase
MPO	myeloperoxidase
MS	multiple sclerosis
mTOR	mammalian target of rapamycin
NAFLD	nonalcoholic fatty liver disease
NASH	nonalcoholic steatohepatitis
NF-κB	nuclear factor-kappa-light-chain-enhancer of activated B cells
NLRP3	NBD leucine-rich family pyrin-containing 3
NO	nitric oxide
NSAID	nonsteroidal anti-inflammatory drug
OCD	obsessive compulsive disorder
OCP	oral contraceptive
OFT	open field test
PAI	plasminogen activator inhibitor
PASI	Psoriasis Area and Severity Index
PCOS	polycystic ovary syndrome
PEG	polyethylene glycol

PG	prostaglandin
PGP	P-glycoprotein
PI3K	phosphoinositide 3-kinase
PKC	protein kinase C
PMDD	premenstrual dysphoric disorder
PMS	premenstrual syndrome
PPARγ	peroxisome proliferator-activated receptor gamma
PT	prothrombin time
PTZ	pentylenetetrazole
QUICKI	Quantitative Insulin Sensitivity Check Index
RCT	randomized controlled trial
REM	rapid eye movement sleep
RT-PCR	reverse-transcription polymerase chain reaction
SCFA	short-chain fatty acids
SDH	succinate dehydrogenase
SOD	superoxide dismutase
SpO_2	oxygen saturation
SSRI	selective serotonin reuptake inhibitor
STZ	streptozotocin
T2DM	type 2 diabetes mellitus
TAC	total antioxidant capacity
TAG	triacyl glycerol
TC	total cholesterol
TEWL	transepidermal water loss
TGF-β	transforming growth factor beta
TNBS	2,4,6-trinitrobenzene sulfonic acid
TNF-α	tumor necrosis factor α
TSH	thyrotropin
UV	ultra violet
VAS	Visual Analogue Scale
VASI	Vitiligo Area Scoring Index
VCAM-1	vascular cell adhesion molecule 1
VEGF	vascular endothelial growth factor
VLDL-C	very low-density lipoprotein cholesterol
vWF	von Willebrand factor
WBC	white blood cell
WC	waist circumference

1 Medicinal Plants in Traditional Persian Medicine

Basics and Principles

Roja Rahimi

INTRODUCTION

Traditional Persian Medicine (TPM) is an old medical discipline that consists of knowledge, skill, and practices based on the theories, beliefs, and experiences of Persian civilization and is used in the maintenance of health as well as in the prevention, diagnosis, improvement, or treatment of physical and mental illnesses (WHO, 2013). The history of ancient Persia goes back to about 10,000 years ago, and the development of pharmaceutical science and practice was particularly notable. Zoroaster, a religious reformer and founder of Zoroastrianism in Persia (more than 25 centuries ago), divides physicians into three groups in his book *Avesta*: surgeons, physicians who worked with herbal medicines, and physicians who treated with holy words (Zargaran et al., 2012). Different treatment modalities have been recommended in TPM for the management of diseases, which can be divided into two categories: pharmacological interventions and non-pharmacological interventions.

Pharmacological interventions include natural pharmaceutical dosage forms that originated from plants, animals, and/or minerals. Medicinal plants are the most used components in natural pharmaceutical dosage forms in TPM. According to the Sassanid Pahlavic manuscript known as the *Bondahesh* (written more than 2,000 years ago), plants have been categorized into eleven groups, one of them being medicinal plants. The medicinal plants used in ancient Persia had been divided into a number of subgroups, including antiseptics, analgesics, sedatives, oils, poisons, antidotes, abortifacients, balms for ulcers, and cosmetics (Zargaran et al., 2012).

Different ancient pharmaceutical devices and tools have been discovered in Persian territory, such as various types of mortars (green stone mortar and admiralty metal mortar from the Achaemenid period [550–330 BC] and earthen mortar from the Parthian period [247 BC–224 AD]), distillation vessels (first millennium BC), earthen baby drinking cup (found in the Kurdistan province, first millennium BC), gun metal pediatric medicine dropper from the Sassanid period (224–637 AD), and drug storage vessel from the Parthian period (Zargaran et al., 2012).

BOOKS ON MEDICINAL PLANTS IN TPM

The knowledge of TPM has been transferred from generation to generation verbally. About medicinal plants used in TPM, more than the regional and folklore experiences about them, various handwritten manuscripts were left behind by Persian scholars that describe their pharmacological properties. One of the most famous handwritten manuscripts devoted to *Materia medica* is *al-Abnie an-al Haghayegh-al-Advia*, which was written by Abu Mansur Heravi in 10th century AD. In addition to its medicinal value, this book has a historical worthiness; it has been recorded as the oldest

DOI: 10.1201/b22971-1

Persian-written manuscript in the world (Khosrobeigi and Azadi, 2018). Volumes 20 and 21 of the book *al-Hawi* (*Liber continens*), written by Rhazes (9–10th century AD), specifies the natural components used as remedy in TPM (Richter-Bernburg, 2003). Moreover, Avicenna in his book *Al-Qanun fi al-Teb* (*The canon of medicine*), one of the main medical references in Europe until the 16th century AD, also describes the pharmacological activities of medicinal plants (Zargaran et al., 2012). Other books that focused on natural substances, especially medicinal plants, in TPM include *Ekhtiyarat Badiee* (by Ansari Shirazi, 15th century AD) and *Tohfe-al–Momenin* (by Momen Tonkaboni, 17th century AD). But the most famous and comprehensive encyclopedia of *Materia medica* in TPM is *Treasury of drugs* (*Makhzan al-Advia*), written by Mohammad Hosein Aghili Khorasani in 1771 AD (Aghili Khorasani 1771) (See Figure 1.1.). In *Makhzan al-Advia*, Aghili also mentions the viewpoints of other physicians and pharmacologists in cases where there is no consensus on a certain characteristic or when prominent scholars like Avicenna and Momen Tonkaboni have other opinions. *Makhzan al-Advia* contains a total of 1,629 natural substances, including 1,114 plants, 294 drugs of animal origin, and 221 minerals. The medicinal plants belong to 66 different families, the most common of them being Fabaceae, Asteraceae, Lamiaceae, and Apiaceae (Naghizadeh et al., 2020).

STRUCTURES OF BOOKS ON MEDICINAL PLANTS IN TPM

In all the books mentioned earlier, each medicinal plant has its own monograph, and drug monographs are composed of some sections including synonyms, identity, temperament (*Mizaj*), therapeutic use, dose, adverse reactions, use during pregnancy and lactation, and substitute.

SYNONYMS

The initial part of each monograph includes popular synonyms and translations of the name of a medicinal plant in other languages and dialects. About 70 languages and dialects have been applied in *Makhzan al-Advia*, the most common of which include Persian, Arabic, Hindi and Greek.

IDENTITY

In the section on identity, the origin of medicinal plants, types, and botanical characteristics are provided. For example, whether wild or cultivated, the morphological characteristics of leaves, bark, flower, or fruit, and countries and geographical habitat, as well as its medicinal part(s) are described in this section.

TEMPERAMENT

According to TPM, all that exists in the universe is composed of four elements, namely air, fire, water, and earth, and each of these elements has its specific quality: air is hot and wet, fire is hot and dry, water is cold and wet, and earth is cold and dry. The differences and diversities between objects are because of the different ratios of these four elements in their structures. Hence, every object in the world has a specific quality based on the dominant element(s) in its structure. This specific quality is known as temperament. For example, if elemental water is dominant, the object has a cold and wet temperament, and if elemental water and earth are dominant, the object has a cold temperament (Table 1.1). Belief in temperament existed not only in TPM but also in many other traditional medical theories, including Unani (Greek), Arabic, Roman, Indian, European, and Chinese traditional medicines.

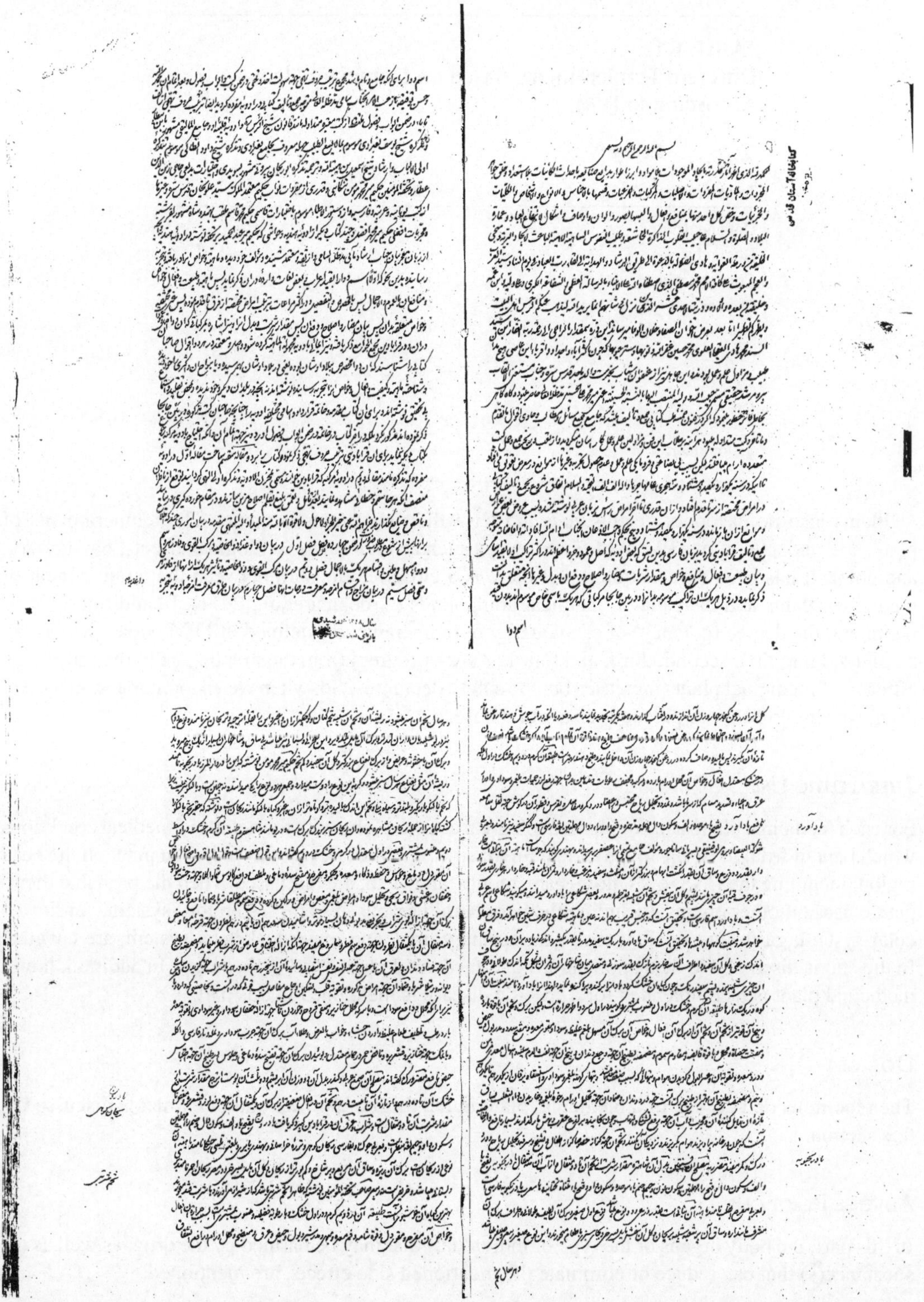

FIGURE 1.1 A handwritten manuscript from the book *Makhzan-al-Advia* compiled by Aghili in the 18th century (deposited in Astan Qods Razavi Library, Mashhad, Iran). (a) Introduction. (b) Monograph of lemon balm.

TABLE 1.1
Different Temperaments Based on Dominant Element(s) According to TPM

Temperament \ Element	Fire	Air	Water	Earth
Hot and dry	√			
Hot and wet		√		
Cold and wet			√	
Cold and dry				√
Hot	√	√		
Cold			√	√
Wet		√	√	
Dry	√			√

√: dominant

Plants also no exception to this rule and have their own temperaments. The temperaments of plants are understood in TPM by different ways such as their pharmacological effects, flavor, odor, and color. It has been demonstrated that there is a close relationship between the temperament of medicinal plants and their major chemical compounds (Ardekani et al., 2011). In addition to temperament, the degree (potency) of each quality of temperament is defined in TPM books, which can be divided into first, second, third, and fourth. As we progress from the first degree to the fourth, the efficacy of medicinal plants increases but the safety decreases. So, when we encounter a more potent drug, we should be more precautious about its use.

Therapeutic Use

For each medicinal plant, a list of pharmacological actions along with the details of medical conditions which benefit from the drug are provided. Firstly, the possible effects of a medicinal plant on the head region, including the CNS, eyes, nose, ears, mouth, and teeth, are discussed. Then the probable therapeutic uses on other organs, including the peripheral nervous system, respiratory system, cardiovascular system, gastrointestinal system, genitourinary tract, and musculoskeletal system, are covered. In the end is discussed topical applications of a medicinal plant for skin disorders. In addition, how a medicinal plant is recommended for a specific disease is mentioned in this part.

Dosage

The recommended dosage of a medicinal plant in the form of powder and/or extract is discussed in this section.

Adverse Reactions

In this part, the body organs or the type of individuals that may be harmed by the drug, as well as the substance(s) that can reduce or eliminate the mentioned side effects, are mentioned.

Use during Pregnancy and Lactation

A medicinal plant considered emmenagogue or abortifacient is contraindicated during pregnancy. Some medicinal plants like celery should not be used during pregnancy. Purgatives like senna leaves and aloe juice, as well as some laxative herbs like sweet violet flowers, mallow flowers, and marshmallow flowers are prohibited during pregnancy.

Concerning breastfeeding, some herbs are directly implied to not be used, like celery. Some herbs, like spearmint and chives, are concerned with changing the milk taste, making it unpleasant for babies. Furthermore, some medicinal components are described to be present in secreted milk; for example, when a lactating mother consumes aloe juice, known as a wormicide in TPM, its wormicidal effects can be transferred from the mother's milk to the infant.

Substitute

In TPM, a substitute drug has similar pharmacological activity to the original drug. For example, fennel seed is a good substitute for aniseed (Aghili Khorasani 1771).

CONCLUSION

While the manuscripts written about medicinal plants in TPM date back to more than 1,000 years ago, many tips from modern phytotherapy are considered in these books, including botanical characteristics, medicinal part(s), pharmacological activities and indications, dosage, adverse events, and use during pregnancy and lactation. However, there are some elements in modern phytotherapy books that do not exist in TPM. One of them is the scientific name of medicinal plants. Notably, *Makhzan al-Advia* (1771 AD), the most popular book on *Materia medica* in TPM, was written simultaneously or around the time of the formalization of binomial nomenclature by Carl Linnaeus (1740–1760s AD). Moreover, contraindications and drug interactions are not discussed in TPM manuscripts. On the other hand, there are some elements in *Materia medica* books that are not available in modern phytotherapy literature. One of them is the temperament of medicinal plants, which is so important in TPM. Another missing information is substances that can reduce or eliminate adverse side effects. For example, while aloe juice can be harmful to the gastrointestinal tract, rose petals and mastic can reduce its adverse events. The last thing that is special to TPM but does not exist in modern phytotherapy is substitute—a substance with similar pharmacological activity to the original drug.

Finally, it seems that TPM manuscripts are invaluable sources for identifying medicinal plants with novel pharmacological activities and for designing preclinical and clinical studies to confirm the claimed biological properties of medicinal plants in these manuscripts.

REFERENCES

Aghili Khorasani MH 1771. *Makhzan-al-Adviah* (*The treasury of drugs*) (rewritten by Shams Ardakani MR, Rahimi R, Farjadmand F, 1st ed). Tehran: Tehran University of Medical Sciences; 2009.

Ardekani MR, Rahimi R, Javadi B, Abdi L, Khanavi M. Relationship between temperaments of medicinal plants and their major chemical compounds. J Tradit Chin Med. 2011;31(1):27–31.

Khosrobeigi H, Azadi N. Structural analysis of pharmacology in the book of "Al-Abnieh An Haghayegh Al-Advieh" by Abu Mansour Heravi. J Islam Iran Trad Med. 2018;9(3):193–210.

Naghizadeh A, Hamzeheian D, Akbari S, et al. UNaProd: A universal natural product database for *Materia Medica* of Iranian traditional medicine. Evid Based Complement Alternat Med. 2020;2020:3690781.

Richter-Bernburg L. Ḥāwi, al-. In: Yarshater E (ed.), *Encyclopædia Iranica, vol. XII/1: Harem I–Hedāyat al-mota'allemin*. London: Routledge & Kegan Paul; 2003:64–67.

World Health Organization. *WHO traditional medicine strategy: 2014–2023*. Geneva: WHO; 2013.

Zargaran A, Ahmadi SA, Daneshamouz S, Mohagheghzadeh A. Ancient Persian pharmaceutical vessels and tools in Iranian archaeological museums. Pharm Hist (Lond). 2012;42(4):68–71.

Zargaran A, Mehdizadeh A, Yarmohammadi H, Mohagheghzadeh A. Zoroastrian priests: Ancient Persian psychiatrists. Am J Psychiatry. 2012;169:3.

Zargaran A, Mehdizadeh M, Zarshenas M, Mohagheghzadeh A. Avicenna (980–1037 AD). J Neurol. 2012;259(2):389–390.

2 The History of Medicinal Plants in Traditional Persian Medicine

Shahrzad Irannejad

INTRODUCTION

The Iranian plateau has for centuries been a crucial part of a corridor between Central Asia, Europe, and North Africa through which actors, goods, foodstuffs and drugs, concepts, ideas, technologies, and manuscripts have circulated. What has sedimented through these circulations has fermented into a landscape of knowledge distinct from its Greco-Arabic predecessor and such temperamental medical systems as Unani medicine, Ayurveda, and TCM. In contemporary Iran, researchers, teachers, and practitioners of Traditional Persian Medicine (TPM) have taken it upon themselves to transform this distinct body of knowledge into a field applicable in integrative medical healthcare, offering fresh solutions in terms of hygiene, prevention, diagnosis, therapeutics, and drug development. Based mainly on the heritage of Greco-Arabic humoral medicine, TPM is a recapitulation of centuries of codified experience, including with medicinal plants, in the Iranian plateau, calibrated for contemporary healthcare provision. While drawing on ethnic knowledge of medicinal plants, TPM as a knowledge system relies mainly on the theoretical framework of humoral paradigm. Within this paradigm, *Materia medica* (of three sources: mineral, plant, and animal, with medicinal plants having a central place) is regarded as possessing a binary of qualities (hot and cold, dry and wet) and degrees of powers, which can be used to retain health as a balance in an individual's temperament, or its restoration when a disease has occurred.

ROOTS AND ROUTES

Humoral medicine in the Persianate context, namely TPM as taught and practiced in contemporary Iran, looks back on centuries of Persian, Greek, and Indian heritage. While the Persian and Indian shares of the heritage are under-researched (for one of the few recent studies, see Kahl, 2015), the Greek heritage is the most well-researched as the theoretical framework into which centuries of trials and errors have been codified. The roots of humoral pathophysiology are conventionally sought in the Hippocratic corpus. Although the theoretical framework that emerges by looking into the entirety of this corpus is somewhat contradictory, it is customary to regard the treatise *On the Sacred Disease* as a turning point in ancient medicine, as the treatise calls for looking into the "natural" causes of diseases (Van der Eijk, 2005). In the Hippocratic text *On the Nature of Man*, the contemporaneous classic Greek cosmology was concocted into a medical system in which a balance of four humors (blood, phlegm, yellow bile, and black bile) and their corresponding binary qualities (cold/hot and wet/dry) was regarded as health, and their imbalance would bring about disease (Pormann, 2019).

DOI: 10.1201/b22971-2

In the fourth century BCE, Aristotle of Stagira undertook systematic examinations in, and delineated, many fields of knowledge that we recognize as such today. Aristotle established that the sublunar sphere is made up of the four elements of earth, water, air, and fire. Hence, Aristotelian physics consolidated the concepts of the four elements and their qualities, on which humoral ideas were further instituted. Following in his footsteps in the methods of inquiry into the natural world, his student Theophrastus (b. *c.*370 BC) attempted a collection of knowledge of plants and their functions among the drug vendors (*pharmakopolai*) and root cutters (*rhizotomoi*) in the Attic marketplace. Following Aristotle's *Historia Animalium* and *De Partibus Animalium*, Theophrastus authored *Historia Plantarum*, in the ninth book of which he analyzed the therapeutic properties of about 60 herbs and herbal preparations (Scarborough, 2006). While Theophrastus can be regarded as the earliest botanist in the Greek tradition, Dioscorides is regarded as the earliest *medical* botanist, and much of the knowledge in Theophrastus's work is traceable in the *Materia medica* of Dioscorides (Scarborough, 1978). *De materia medica* of Pedanius Dioscorides of Anazarbus, written in the second half of the first century AD, had two main features that were widely received in the Islamicate tradition: first, its underlying principle that each substance has specific properties (*dunameis*), such as cooling/warming, binding, softening, etc., and, second, organizing knowledge regarding each *Materia medica* in a certain order: "morphology, habitat(s), relative qualities, methods of preparation, general properties and specific therapeutic applications, adulteration, compounding, and directions for storage" (Beck, 2005). The work included about 600 plants (along with 35 from animal and 90 from mineral sources) and was extensively illustrated (Yildirim, 2013).

With the highly influential figure of Galen of Pergamon (*c.*129–216) came the full realization of Aristotelian doctrine in the field of medicine and pharmacognosy. Several key Galenic concepts also continued to play central roles in the theory of humoral medicine: for instance, the concepts of nature, innate heat and radical moisture, and *krasis* (temperament). Furthermore, Galen's system of describing *Materia medica* in terms of their primary and secondary qualities and degrees of powers created a frame into which later Indian and Persian *Materia medica* and drug lore was integrated (Pormann, 2019). Following in the footsteps of the Hippocratic corpus and Aristotle, for Galen, the *primary* qualities of a medicinal substance are identical with the elementary qualities of hot and cold, dry and wet. Each substance is a mixture (*krasis*) of one of the active qualities (hot and cold) with one of the passive qualities (dry and wet). The secondary qualities are those that can only be determined in terms of their effect on the body, for instance, heating, drying, purging, suppurating, etc. Galen also described drugs in terms of the degrees of their power and categorized them in four levels in accordance with the intensity of their effect on the body. In his relevant works, Galen discusses 440 plants, but notes the degrees of power for only about a third of this number (Vogt, 2008). Still, the systematic nature of Galen's observations and his writings established him as the main medical figure whose work was received in the Islamicate tradition.

In the seventh century CE, Islam emerged in a world where humoral medical paradigm had long been established in the Sassanid and Byzantine lands that it conquered. A significant role was played in the introduction of "new" drugs to the Islamicate lands by the cosmopolitan culture of the Sasanian empire (King, 2015). The emergence of Islam and its expansion reshuffled power structures and borders and allowed for a new circulation of actors, manuscripts, foodstuffs, and *Materia medica* that were to be instrumental in the further development of humoral medicine and its drug lore in the Islamicate lands. For instance, Nestorian Christian physicians from the renowned Bukhtishū' family from Gondēšāpur (in present-day Khūzestān) were invited to the Abbasid court in Baghdad; medical and philosophical manuscripts traveled along new routes; and there was an influx of new foodstuff and *Materia medica* from the Iranian plateau and the Indian subcontinent that needed to be added to the corpus of tools at the disposal of physicians.

The result of this reshuffled mobility was a multilingual, multicultural, multifaith world which was still a culturally distinguishable region with Islam acting as a cultural, unifying force. Perhaps most importantly for the history of knowledge, new linguistic dynamics also emerged in the early centuries of Islam. Arabic emerged as the lingua franca of the Islamicate world, facilitating intellectual encounters from the Iranian plateau to North Africa; only in later centuries substantial knowledge started being produced in such local languages as Persian. To address the pragmatic needs of a new state on the scene, knowledge in various fields needed to be translated into the language of the empire. Translations into Arabic that had already begun under the Umayyads gained momentum during the Abbasid reign (Gutas, 1998).

From mid-eighth century till roughly mid-tenth century, the Abbasid translation movement emerged and flourished through the patronage of intelligentsia of the Abbasid court, and to cater to a burgeoning knowledge scape. While translations were mainly made from Greek into Arabic (often mediated by Syriac), some texts were also translated from other languages, from Sanskrit, for instance, through the patronage of the Barmakid family (Dols, 2011). With these translation activities, Arabic developed a hegemony which "shaped the structure of pharmacological discourse" in Islamicate lands (King, 2015). The ensuing multilingual nature of this new knowledge landscape framed by Arabic as the lingua franca is best shown in the case of pharmocognosy in *Kitāb al-Ṣaydana fi al-ṭibb* (*Book of pharmacy in medicine*) by al-Bīrūnī (d. *c.*1048). In this monumental work written in Arabic, while quoting Galen and Dioscorides extensively, al-Bīrūnī provides the names of the plants he discusses in Arabic, Persian, Latin, Greek, and "Indian" (Chipman, 2019).

It is also important to note that the medieval Islamicate medical tradition was governed by two further forces: it was part of a broader manuscript culture and relied on an encyclopedic tradition. The textual dissemination of knowledge was bound by the mechanics and economy of manuscript production and trade, and the working of both professional scribes and those who copied texts by hand for their personal use (van Leeuwen, 2016). The manuscripts were stored in the libraries of scholars, rulers, caliphs, schools, and hospitals (Brentjes, 2018) and traveled along various routes: whether during knowledge-seeking quests, or even as gifts from one ruler to the other. Furthermore, the textual transfer of knowledge, whether synchronic or diachronic, was influenced by the convention, inherited from earlier traditions, of organizing knowledge in the form of encyclopedia, that is, structuring what knowledge was deemed relevant and crucial in medical compendia (Biesterfeldt, 2011). This convention affected the circulation of knowledge, as medical ideas presented in individual treatises were circulated differently from those ideas canonized in medical encyclopedias. Such compendia played a central role in the learning and practice of medicine and canonizing the knowledge of drug lore.

The Canon and *The Treasury*

Against a background governed by these mentioned forces, various fields of knowledge, including medicine and drug lore, flourished in the medieval Islamicate tradition. From within this context emerged the likes of Rhazes (Kahl, 2011) and Avicenna (Ullmann, 1970). Abū ʿAlī al-Ḥusayn ibn ʿAbd Allāh ibn al-Ḥasan ibn ʿAlī ibn Sīnā (980 Bukhara–1037 Hamedan), conveniently known to the Latin-speaking world as Avicenna, stands out in the history of medicine as a figure whose stature equals that of Hippocrates and Galen in influencing medical thought and knowledge for many centuries (Reisman, 2013). By virtue of the Abbasid translation movement, Avicenna had access to much of the Hellenic heritage, and his philosophical and medical works stand in a manifest dialectical relationship to the Aristotelian and Galenic heritage (Gutas, 2014). He was a great systematizer of knowledge and wrote prolifically within the encyclopedic tradition, often in Arabic, and at times in Persian, which was his mother tongue. His most influential medical work was an encyclopedia of medicine written in Arabic, named *Al-Qānūn fi-ṭ-Ṭibb* (*The canon of medicine*).

As an encyclopedia covering all that Avicenna deemed necessary in the teaching of medicine, *The canon of medicine* comprises five volumes. Volume 1 deals with the principles of medicine; volumes 2 and 5 deal with simple and compound drugs, respectively; volume 3, following the preceding medical encyclopedic tradition, discusses diseases *a capite ad calcem*; and volume 4 discusses diseases affecting the entire body (Veit, 2012). Book 2 of *The canon* comprises two sections: the first section provides a summary of the theoretical background of pharmacology; the second section offers, in 752 chapters in an alphabetical order, a collection of *Materia medica* (mainly plants), their qualities, and therapeutic properties, both in general and on various organs of the body. With regard to the theory of pharmacognosy, Avicenna's "major contribution could be identified in the clarification, the re-organisation, the systematisation, and the further expansion and development of the theoretical fundaments of the Galenic pharmacology." Although Dioscorides and Galen are the two most quoted sources in this volume of *The canon*, Galen's influence seems to be contained to the section on theory: Avicenna does not seem to be relying on Galen in the case of descriptive pharmacology of the second section of the second book of *The canon* (Ventura, 2019). Rather, this section is a culmination of inherited knowledge of *Materia medica*, knowledge produced within the Islamicate lands, and Avicenna's observations.

With this comprehensive and neatly organized compendia written in Arabic, the theoretical framework of humoral medicine was consolidated in the Islamicate tradition, along with the knowledge of medicinal plants (and other *Materia medica*). Around the same time, and in the succeeding generations, apart from engaging with the Avicennian heritage in the forms of commentary and abridgement, translations into and commentaries in Persian also emerged, along with texts originally written in Persian (Vesel and Brentjes, 2021). An early such example is Abū Manṣūr Heravī's *Ketāb al-abnīa ʿan ḥaqāʾeq al-adwīa*, the earliest extant text in Persian on *Materia medica*, in which he presents the names (in Persian, Greek, Syriac, and Indian) and properties of 584 items of *Materia medica* in order of the Arabic alphabet (Richter-Bernburg, 1983). A more recent example is Mohammad Hossein Aghili Khorasani's *Makhzan al-Adwiya* (*Treasury of drugs*) written at the beginning of the nineteenth century CE. This text is the epitome of knowledge of medicinal plants in the Persianate context, comprising 1629 monographs of *Materia medica*. Following in the footsteps of Galen and Avicenna and within the theoretical frame established by them, Aghili provides in each monograph names of the respective simple drug (in different languages and local dialects), its physical description, where it is endemic to, its temperament, secondary properties and indications, dosage, adverse effects and ameliorators (*muṣliḥāt*), and substitutes (*abdāl*) (Shams Ardakani et al., 2018).

Despite regional variations, especially with regard to *Materia medica* and therapeutic techniques, the overall theoretical framework of humoral medicine in the Perso-Islamicate tradition was somewhat of a constant. The central idea was that balance in the temperament of a body constitutes health, as in the Islamicate tradition the concept of temperament played a more prominent role than that of humors (Savage-Smith, 2013). Things integral to the body and its health were discussed under the title of seven naturals: element (*rukn*/*rokn*), temperament (*mizāj*/*mezāj*), humor (*khilṭ*/*khelṭ*), organ (*ʻuẓw*/*ozv*), pneuma (*rawḥ*/*rūḥ*), faculty (*quwwa*/*qovve*), and function (*fiʻl*/*fe'l*). And six necessary causes (non-naturals) were discussed as having effect on health: air, movement and rest, sleep and wakefulness, eating and drinking, retention and evacuation, and psychic accidents (mental and emotional states) (Pormann and Savage-Smith, 2007). As everything in the sublunar world was regarded to be made up of elements, and by extension having its own temperament, each of the necessary causes was at the disposal of the physician to restore the balance in a sick body. In a therapeutic spectrum having diet and surgery as its two extremes, and an array of foods and drugs in the middle, the prescription of medicinal plants had a central place.

EARLY MODERN TIMES TO CONTEMPORARY IRAN

The story of the integration of medicinal plants in the framework of temperamental medicine in Islamicate context is one of both continuation and innovation (Pormann, 2011). This framework of humoral/temperamental medicine held unrivalled sway in Iran until early modern times. Within this medical paradigm, as mentioned, it is the imbalance in the temperament of a certain body that causes diseases in that very same body. No canonized notion, then, existed in this framework of a body being capable of engendering diseases in another body. Among the six non-naturals, only one could have been used metaphorically to account for the etiology of contagious diseases: air. To borrow Vivian Nutton's words, "Given that none of the infective agents could be observed, let alone identified, until the nineteenth century, it is hardly surprising that the debate [around transmission of diseases], if such there was, centered on metaphors, or that the process of disease transmission was associated most often with the air, whose foulness could be perceived by smell and occasionally sight" (Nutton, 2017, 161). There were, of course, observations regarding contagious diseases, and the concept was heavily debated (Stearns, 2017); however, the concept was never canonized and integrated into the theoretical framework of the paradigm.

The nineteenth century CE in Iran witnessed the supposed paradigm shift in medicine during the Qajar era. The limitations of the humoral/temperamental paradigm in explaining *transmissibility* of contagious diseases were one of the reasons for its demise in early modern Iran, in a society going through rapid demographic changes. Apart from this theoretical reason, other forces were also at play: reception of "Western" medicine against a broader backdrop of modernization in times of the constitutional revolution; transformation of institutions such as hospitals and universities; the need for national measures against contagious diseases; and the emergence of systematic licensing of practitioners of medicine (Ebrahimnejad, 2014). With the founding of the Polytechnic University (Dār al-Fonūn) in 1825, and the presence of such actors as Jakob Eduard Polak as teacher of "modern" medicine (Gächter, 2019), humoral/temperamental medicine was gradually omitted from scholarly discourse.

Despite this omission from scholarly and official discourse, many key concepts, ideas, and categories of humoral/temperamental medicine continued living a parallel life, at times intermingled with folk medicine: much survived as intermingled with Persianate culture; for instance, its ideas regarding what constitutes food and medicament, the temperament of foodstuffs, and a meticulous quest for balance survived as sublimated in classic Persian cuisine (Alimi and Irannejad, 2019); the teaching of the principles of humoral/temperamental medicine continued in seminaries, and from one generation of healers to the next; its practice continued by sages or *hakīms*; and, last but not least, its drug lore survived in the institution of *attārī*: dispensaries of *Materia medica* still found around every corner on the streets of Iran. Therefore, despite this omission from scholarly and official discourse, Iran has, for well over a century, been a "medically pluralistic society" where patients have sought care from various medical paradigms and have consumed medicinal plants alongside allopathic medications (Loeffler, 2017).

In line with the global complementary and alternative medicine movement in recent decades, Iran has witnessed a local revival of humoral/temperamental medicine in the frame of TPM as complementary healthcare provision (Ghaffari et al., 2010). The revival is meeting fertile ground in the Iranian society; as mentioned earlier, humoral/temperamental ideas are embedded in Persian culture and are familiar to many, and the consumption of medicinal plants in various forms at the intersection of medicine and cuisine is a common practice. The revival is also partially grounded in readdressing a medieval textual corpus: more effort is now being dedicated to the study of its underlying manuscript culture and editing of historical texts; these resurfacing texts, such as *The canon of medicine* and *The treasury of drugs*, are not being dogmatically reread; rather, they are being creatively reinterpreted to benefit healthcare provision in the contemporary world. The schools of TPM are dedicated to research and education and oversee the practice of TPM in their clinics and provision of (mostly plant-based) medicaments in their pharmacies. In contemporary Iran, then, humoral/temperamental medicine is once again a fully living body of knowledge, with the prescription and consumption of medicinal plants having a central role.

REFERENCES

Alimi K, Irannejad S. Cuisine as a mirror for the state of medicine in Qajar Persia. Qajar Studies. 2019;16:265–271.

Beck LY. *De materia medica by Pedanius Dioscorides*. Hildesheim / Zürich / New York: Olms-Weidmann; 2005.
Biesterfeldt HH. Medieval Arabic encyclopedias of science and philosophy. In: Pormann PE (ed.), *Islamic medical and scientific tradition, vol. 1*. London / New York: Routledge; 2011:48–67.
Brentjes S. *Teaching and learning the sciences in Islamicate societies (800–1700)*. Turnhout: Brepols; 2018.
Chipman L. The reception of Galenic pharmacology in the Arabic tradition. In: Bouras-Vallianatos P, Zipser B (eds.), *Brill's companion to the reception of Galen*. Leiden / Boston: Brill; 2019:304–316. doi:10.1163/9789004394353_018.
Dols M. The origins of the Islamic hospital: Myth and reality. In: Pormann PE (ed.), *Islamic medical and scientific tradition, vol. 1*. London / New York: Routledge; 2011:109–135.
Ebrahimnejad H. *Medicine in Iran: Profession, practice and politics, 1800–1925*. New York: Palgrave Macmillan; 2014.
Gächter A. *Der Leibarzt Des Schah: Jacob E. Polak 1818–1891. Eine West-Östliche Lebensgeschichte*. Vienna: New Academic Press; 2019.
Ghaffari F, Naseri M, Khodadoost M. Traditional Iranian medicine and the need for its revival and development. Teb va Tazkieh. 2010;19(3):63–71.
Gutas D. *Avicenna and the Aristotelian tradition: Introduction to reading Avicenna's philosophical works. Including an inventory of Avicenna's authentic works*. 2nd ed. Leiden / Boston: Brill; 2014.
Gutas D. *Greek thought, Arabic culture: The Graeco-Arabic translation movement in Baghdad and early 'Abbasaid society (2nd–4th/5th–10th c.)*. London: Routledge; 1998.
Kahl O. The pharmacological tables of Rhazes. J Semit Stud. 2011;56(2):367–399.
Kahl O. *The Sanskrit, Syriac and Persian sources in the comprehensive book of Rhazes*. Leiden: Brill; 2015.
King A. The new materia medica of the Islamicate tradition: The pre-Islamic context. J Am Orient Soc. 2015;135(3):499–528.
Loeffler A. *Health and medical practice in Iran: Traditional culture and modern medicine*. London / New York: IB Tauris; 2017.
Nutton V. Did the Greeks have a word for it? Contagion and contagion theory in classical Antiquity. In: Wujastyk D, Conrad LI (eds.), *Contagion: Perspectives from pre-modern societies*. New York: Routledge; 2017:137–162.
Pormann PE. The formation of the Arabic pharmacology between tradition and innovation. Ann Sci. 2011;68(4):493–515. doi:10.1080/00033790.2011.594619.
Pormann PE. Medical conceptions of health from antiquity to the renaissance. In Adamson P (ed.), *Health*. Oxford: Oxford University Press; 2019:43–74.
Pormann PE, Savage-Smith E. *Medieval Islamic medicine*. Edinburgh: Edinburgh University Press; 2007.
Reisman DC. The life and times of Avicenna. In: Adamson P (ed.), *Interpreting Avicenna: Critical essays*. Cambridge: Cambridge University Press; 2013:21–41.
Richter-Bernburg L. Abū Manṣūr Heravī. In: *Encyclopædia Iranica, vol. 2*. 1983:336–337.
Savage-Smith E. Were the four humours fundamental to medieval Islamic medical practice? In: Horden P, Hsu E (eds.), *The body in balance: Humoral theory in practice*. Oxford: Berghahn Books; 2013:89–106.
Scarborough J. Drugs and drug lore in the time of theophrastus: Folklore, magic, botany, philosophy and the rootcutters: keynote address. In: *Acta classica: Proceedings of the Classical Association of South Africa, vol. 49*. Cape Town: Classical Association of South Africa; 2006:1–29.
Scarborough J. Theophrastus on herbals and herbal remedies. J Hist Biol. 1978;11(2):353–385.
Shams Ardakani MRS, Farjadmand F, Rahimi R. Makhzan al Adviyeh and pointing to the scientific names of medicinal plants for the first time in a Persian book. Trad Integr Med. 2018;3(4): 186–195.
Stearns JK. *Infectious ideas: Contagion in premodern Islamic and Christian thought in the western Mediterranean*. Baltimore: JHU Press; 2011.
Ullmann M. *Die Medizin Im Islam*. Leiden / Köln: E. J. Brill; 1970.
Van der Eijk PJ. *Medicine and philosophy in classical antiquity: Doctors and philosophers on nature, soul, health and disease*. Cambridge: Cambridge University Press; 2005.
van Leeuwen J. Manuscripts. In: Lightman BV (ed.), *A companion to the history of science*. Chichester, UK / Malden, MA: John Wiley & Sons; 2016:331–343.
Vedat Yildirim R. Studies on De Materia Medica of Dioscorides in the Islamic era. Asclepio. 2013;65(1):1–7. doi:10.3989/asclepio.2013.07.
Veit R. Greek roots, Arab authoring, Latin overlay: Reflections on the sources for Avicenna's canon. In: Fraenkel C, Fumo JC, Wallis F, Wisnovsky R (eds.), *Vehicles of transmission, translation, and transformation in medieval textual culture*. Turnhout: Brepols; 2012:353–370.

Ventura I. Galenic pharmacology in the Middle Ages: Galen's *On the capacities of simple drugs* and its reception between the sixth and fourteenth century. In: *Brill's companion to the reception of Galen*. Leiden / Boston: Brill; 2019:393–433.

Vesel Ž, Brentjes S. Science in Persian. In: Utas B (ed.), *Persian prose*. London / New York: I.B. Tauris; 2021:217–273.

Vogt S. Drugs and pharmacology. In: Hankinson RJ (ed.), *The Cambridge companion to Galen*. Cambridge: Cambridge University Press; 2008:304–322.

3 *Aloe vera* (L.) Burm.f.

Ghazaleh Mosleh and Abdolali Mohagheghzadeh

Scientific name: *Aloe vera* (L.) Burm.f., (syn. *Aloe barbadensis* Mill.)
Family: Asphodelaceae
Common names:

- **English:** Aloe, true aloe, medicine aloe, common aloe, yellow-flowered aloe
- **Persian:** *ṣabr, ṣabr-e zard, šabyār, ṣabr-e barbad*
- **Arabic:** *ṣabr, al-maqr, ṣabbārā, ṣabbārah, ṣabar*

Medicinal part(s): Dried mass of the extracted liquid (exudate) from the ground and squeezed whole aloe leaves (Figure 3.1)
Temperament (nature): Hot in the second degree and dry in the second degree
Major chemical constituents:

- **Anthraquinones:** Aloins A and B (barbaloin and iso-barbaloin), aloinosides A and B, aloe-emodin, emodin, and chrysophanol
- **Chromones:** Aloesin, aloeresin E, isoaloeresin D, and furoaloesone
- Volatile oil and a large quantity of a resinous mass
- Protein moiety (higher amounts in the leaf rind than in the inner gel)
- **Organic acids:** Citric acid, isocitric acid, malic acids, and isocitric acid lactone are the major organic acids of the rind. A considerable amount of isocitrate is found in aloe rind while lacking in the inner leaf. So, isocitric acid and its lactone are markers to distinguish whole aloe leaf from the gel (Williamson and Baxter, 2009; Reynolds, 2004; Capasso and Gaginella, 1997; Shimo et al., 2017, Zhang, 2018).

THERAPEUTIC USE

TPM Literature

Aloe exudate is considered to be a general laxative in TPM because of its deep cleansing effects on different parts of the body including brain, stomach, blood vessels, and joints by expelling the pathologic humors, especially black bile and different forms of pathologic phlegm humor. On the other hand, it is considered a hypnotic remedy and is suggested for the treatment of melancholia. Topical use of aloe exudate is an eye tonic and is suggested for the treatment of several ocular problems such as eye pain and itching. Inhalation and smoking of aloe exudate is helpful in asthma. It can tonify the stomach, reduce the false thirst (i.e., thirst caused by the accumulation of thick phlegm humor in gut), and bring back lost appetite. As a laxative, its administration to the infant or his/her mother can treat constipation because the therapeutic effect will be delivered to the infant via mother's milk. It can treat liver obstruction and has been used in the treatment of jaundice. Also, it can relieve several mental diseases associated with gut–brain axis due to beneficial effects on both brain and the GI tract. Enema is recommended for hemorrhoids, and the alcoholic extract is suggested for anal fissure.

DOI: 10.1201/b22971-3

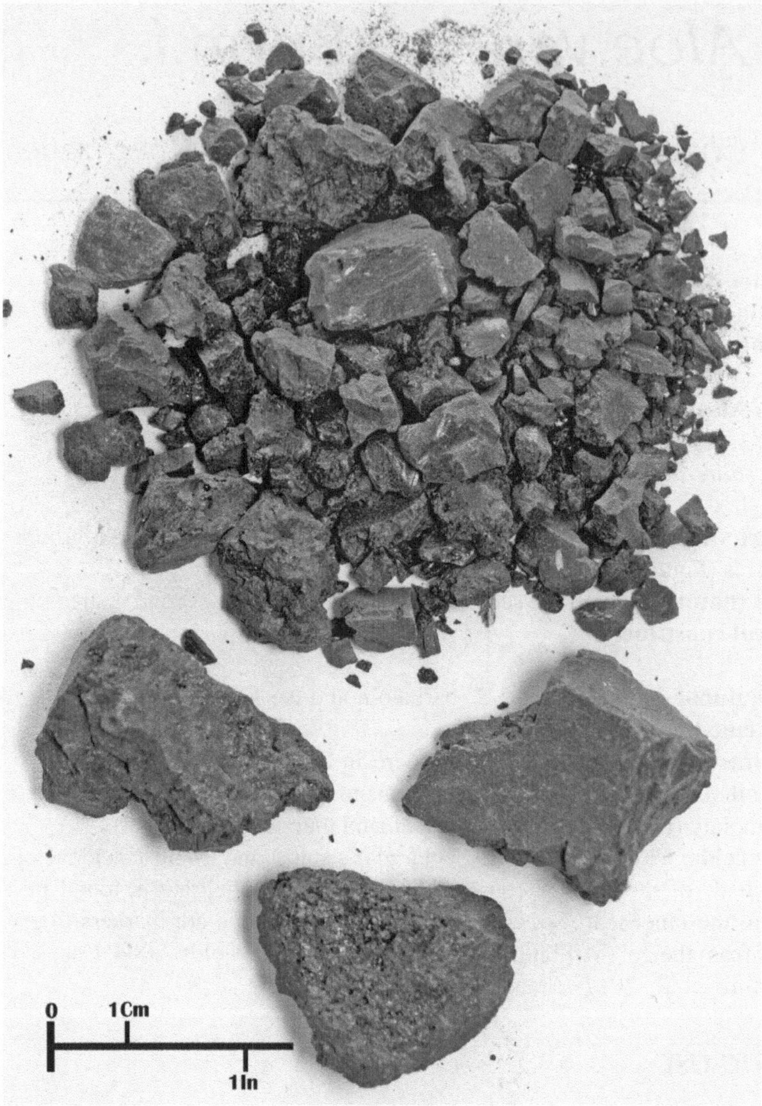

FIGURE 3.1 Dried aloe exudate.

In topical application, a lotion of the alcoholic extract is considered to be an anti-hair loss medicine. It is good for patients with genital, anal, nasal, and oral ulcers due to its intense wound-healing and antiseptic properties. Dried aloe exudate as a topical powder is recommended for wound-healing (Aghili Khorasani 1771; Avicenna 1025).

CURRENT EVIDENCE

Clinical Evidence

Diabetes: A meta-analysis and systematic review of aloe's effects in glycemic control conducted on eight clinical trials including 470 patients (235 prediabetes and 235 type 2 diabetes) showed significant improvement of FBS with no effect on HbA1c in prediabetes. However, the study indicated a probable marginal amelioration in FBS and a meaningful HbA1c improvement in type 2 diabetic patients. Most of the included RCTs used a dose range of 600–1400 mg of dried aloe extract; however, aloe juice or commercial products were also used in some studies, which may have contained only the inner leaf (gel) extract (Suksomboon et al., 2016).

Autoimmunity and thyroid function: Based on a clinical study on 30 women with consecutive Hashimoto's thyroiditis, high thyroperoxidase autoantibodies, and levothyroxine-untreated subclinical hypothyroidism, a commercial aloe juice could improve the autoimmunity and thyroid function. After 9 months of daily intake of 50 mL aloe juice, a significant improvement in serum TSH, free thyroxine (FT4), and thyroperoxidase autoantibodies was observed. However, free triiodothyronine (FT3) significantly decreased in the third month and had no further reduction in the ninth month. So, the FT4:FT3 ratio significantly increased. In addition, 9 months consumption of 100 mL aloe juice per day lowered the autoimmune thyroid inflammation. Aloe juice protects thyrocyte function via decreasing the conversion of T4 into T3 and inhibiting the deiodination of T4 (Metro et al., 2018).

Psoriasis: In a double-blind, placebo-controlled RCT, a hydrophilic cream containing 0.5% aloe exudate showed significant therapeutic effects on 60 patients with chronic plaque-type psoriasis whose PASI scores were 4.8–16.7. The cream was administered topically, trice daily on 5 consecutive days each week for 16 weeks with weekly examination and 12 months of monthly follow-up. A progressive reduction of wounds and desquamation, as well as a lowered PASI score and decreased infiltration and erythema were considered healing signs. According to the results, the aloe cream had a cure rate of 83.3% compared to 6.6% by the placebo, without any side effects (Syed et al., 1996).

Genital herpes: A double-blind, placebo-controlled RCT assessed the efficacy of 0.5% aloe exudate in a hydrophilic cream on 60 male patients with the first episodes of genital herpes. They applied the cream trice daily for 5 consecutive days and the active treatment period was 1 or 2 weeks. The patients were followed up after 16 weeks, continuing monthly up to 20 months. Reepithelialization of lesions with some residual erythema was proposed as healing signs. The results indicated that aloe exudate cream has a significantly faster healing time and higher healing rate for patients than the placebo group. After 15 months, the recurrence rate was determined at 13.6% (Syed et al., 1997).

Preclinical Evidence

Diabetes: The effect of aloe exudate was investigated on blood glucose levels in alloxan-induced diabetics in mice. A dose of 5 mg/kg intraperitoneal injection of aloe bitter or an oral dose of 500 mg/kg of aloe exudate were administered to animals as single dose or chronic treatment. The study showed no decrease in the FBS level in animals treated with a single dose of 500 mg/kg aloe exudate. In contrast, chronic oral administration of aloe exudate (500 mg/kg twice a day for 5 days) significantly lowered the FBS level (Ajabnoor, 1990).

Constipation: The ethanol extract of aloe leaf showed laxative effects in loperamide-induced constipation in rats. One week's consumption of 50, 100, and 200 mg/kg of the extract could improve intestinal motility, normalize body weight, and increase fecal volume in rat constipation models. This laxative effect was comparable with Gaviscon as a standard laxative medicine (Ashafa et al., 2011). The aloe's anthraquinone glycosides are chemically stable in the gastric acid and liver detoxification process. Thus, they act as a laxative prodrug in the large intestine. Furthermore, aloe resins are as active as the anthraquinones in the induction of laxative effects (Reynolds, 2004).

Ulcerative colitis: In an in vivo study conducted on 50 rats, oral administration of aloe aqueous extract (18 and 72 mg/kg) for 10 days ameliorated DSS-induced colitis in rats via preventing colon length shortening and mitigation of colonic pathological features. Proinflammatory mediators such as TNF-α, IL-1β, and IL-6 were downregulated, while IL-10 was upregulated. In addition, aloe enhanced colon mucus barrier functions by increasing mucin proteins and mucus layer thickness in the colon. It increased the expression of p-ERK and p-PKC, while reducing p-AKT and p-PI3K expression (Shi et al., 2021). According to another in vivo study conducted on 70 Wistar rats, rectal administration of 400 mg/kg aloe hydroalcoholic extract for 1 week could significantly reduce TNF-α, IL-6, NO, MDA, and MPO levels compared to the untreated colitis group. Furthermore, colonic weight:length ratio and body weight were improved. The results indicated that the rectal administration of aloe extract was more potent than the oral administration (Naini et al., 2021).

Peptic ulcer: Commercial aloe extract (150 mg/kg) was administered to rats with indomethacin-induced gastric ulcer. A protective effect was observed by improving cytokine-induced neutrophil chemoattractant-1, TNF-α, and gastric MDA, as well as decreasing gastric erosions, neutrophil infiltration, and IL-18-positive cells (Werawatganon et al., 2014). In HCl-induced mucosal injury in rats, intraperitoneal injection of aloe ethanolic extract prevented gastric acid secretion in a dose-dependent manner and exhibited a gastroprotective effect at a dose of 25 mg/kg (Yusuf et al., 2004).

Liver toxicity: Aloe leaves exhibited a hepatoprotective effect against pesticides (malathion and cartap)-induced toxicity in rats. The results indicated that 15-day administration of 420 mg/kg aloe aqueous leaf extract significantly reduced hepatic MDA, AST, ALT, ALP, and LDH while increasing the antioxidant factors including GSH, CAT, and SOD (Gupta et al., 2019).

Brain edema: According to a study on Wistar rats with a traumatic brain injury, 200 or 400 mg/kg aqueous extract of aloe leaf represented an antiedema effect. The elevated levels of IL-1β in serum and brain were reduced in the high-dose aloe group. Also, aloe lowered TNF-α and TGF-β levels in the brain after trauma (Shahryari et al., 2021).

Seizure: Oral administration of 100, 200, and 400 mg/kg aloe leaf aqueous extract showed a significant anticonvulsant activity in the mouse model. It reduced the duration of tonic hind limb extension response and clonic convulsion while increasing seizure threshold current and latency to onset in the acute model of epilepsy. Besides, it decreased MDA levels and increased GSH levels in the brain and inhibited the progression of kindling in a chronic study on PTZ-kindled mice (Rathor et al., 2014).

Neuropathy: Oral administration of 100 and 300 mg/kg aloe dried leaf ethanolic extract showed therapeutic effects on neuropathic pain in adult female albino rats. It increased the nociception threshold, decreased LPO, and improved antioxidant parameters. Also, it decreased serum calcium, protein, nitrite, and MPO levels, representing protection against injury derived from sciatic nerve ligation. The therapeutic effect on neuropathic pain may be associated with the reduced migration of neutrophils and antioxidant mechanisms of action (Kanyadhara et al., 2014).

ADVERSE REACTIONS

TPM Literature

Aloe exudate may harm weak stomach, liver, intestine, or anus, so that it can cause anal bleeding or intestinal ulcers. To prevent these side effects, it is recommended to be taken together with tragacanth in patients with intestinal weakness, damask rose petals and mastic gum in patients with liver or stomach weakness, and guggul gum to prevent side effects involving the anus. Also, rubbing rose oil or sweet violet oil on the anus can prevent its side effects. Generally, the intake of aloe exudate with one of the mentioned plants, as well as hot spice decoction, honey drink, or macerating the latex in rose water, can prevent its side effects (Aghili Khorasani 1771; Avicenna 1025).

Current Evidence

Individuals report cramp-like distresses in the GI tract and diarrhea after oral intake of aloe exudate. The dosage should be reduced in such cases (Blumenthal et al., 2000; Ulbricht, 2010). Also, high doses of aloe exudate can lead to abdominal discomfort, nausea, vomiting, gastritis, muscle weakness, bloody diarrhea, and violent purgation (Capasso and Gaginella, 1997; Aronson, 2009). Dependency may occur after taking aloe for more than 7 days. After that, worsening constipation may occur by aloe discontinuation (Ulbricht, 2010). Other probable adverse events associated with the ingestion of aloe exudate are nose bleeds, nausea, vomiting, hematuria, albuminuria, diarrhea, bloody stool, and colitis (Gardner and McGuffin, 2013). Pseudomelanosis coli, as a harmless adverse effect of aloe anthraquinones, usually reverses after drug discontinuation. Long-term use of stimulating laxatives can lead to an increase in sluggish bowel transit (Blumenthal et al., 2000). In addition, a case of small bowel obstruction due to *A. vera* bezoars is reported after excessive use of *A. vera* in a patient with diabetic gastroparesis (Hong et al., 2017). Prolonged use of aloe exudate is also correlated with vomiting, abdominal pain, and cathartic colon (Blumenthal et al., 2000). Besides, long-term consumption of anthraquinone laxatives might be associated with the development of colon cancer (Gorkom, 1999). The increased risk of colorectal cancer is reported after prolonged use of aloe extract for more than 1 year (Ulbricht, 2010). Overdose (1 g/day for several days) of aloe exudate products can produce bleeding diarrhea, colonic perforation, kidney damage, and even death (Gardner and McGuffin, 2013).

In long-term use, electrolyte balance disturbances, exclusively potassium deficiency, hematuria, and albuminuria may occur. Hypokalemia, especially by concurrent use of diuretics, cardiac glycosides, and corticosteroids, may result in heart disorders and muscle weakness (Blumenthal et al., 2000). Imbalances of blood electrolytes may be worse in people with kidney disease or diabetes. Also, ingestion of aloe may lower blood glucose levels (Ulbricht, 2010). Aloe in high doses can lead to peripheral edema, cardiac dysrhythmias, weight loss, and dehydration (Aronson, 2009). A 47-year-old man who had taken an oral formulation containing *Cape aloe* at least thrice a month before his visit was diagnosed with acute oliguric renal failure (Luyckx et al., 2002).

Overdosage of aloe can lead to harmless urine red coloration (Aronson, 2009). Acute hepatitis was reported after oral consumption of aloe capsules (500 mg aloe leaf powder) in a 73-year-old woman, whose liver markers were normalized after its discontinuation (Bottenberg et al., 2007). Also, acute hepatitis was observed in a 57-year-old woman after ingesting dried extract of aloe leaves (Rabe et al., 2005). Acute liver damage and toxic hepatitis were seen in a healthy young man after taking aloe capsules (500 mg of aloe exudate/day) for 3 weeks (Kanat et al., 2006; Gardner and McGuffin, 2013).

Extensive intraoperative bleeding is reported in a 35-year-old woman who had taken aloe tablets for 14 days before surgery. Aloe can decrease prostaglandin synthesis and inhibit secondary platelet aggregation. Because both aloe and Sevoflurane (a general anesthetic) have antiplatelet effects, the herb–drug interaction may lead to massive bleeding (Lee et al., 2004). Furthermore, using aloe on surgical ulcers slows wound healing (Ulbricht, 2010).

Allergic contact dermatitis was observed in a 72-year-old woman using homemade aloe juice on her legs for pain relief. The patch test revealed positive reactions to aloe leaf and its macerated jelly (Ferreira et al., 2007). Furthermore, a Henoch–Schonlein purpura case caused by aloe was reported in a 45-year-old man with a rash on his lower legs and generalized edema. The patient confessed that a month before admission, he had used aloe extracts for 1 week to improve his health (Kim et al.,

2007). Another case of Henoch-Schonlein purpura was reported in a 52-year-old man 10 days after aloe juice consumption. Nephritis and renal dysfunction were considered a result of consuming high doses of aloe (Cholongitas et al., 2005).

High doses of aloe exudate can lead to redness, rash, itching, and pruritus (Aronson, 2009). Rash has been reported in sun-exposed areas after aloe application. Topical use of aloe juice on the face after dermabrasion may cause burning and redness. On the other hand, injections of aloe should be avoided because it has been correlated with death in undetermined circumstances (Ulbricht, 2010).

Daily oral gavage of freeze-dried powder of aloe whole leaf (400, 1,200, 2,000 mg/kg) for 28 days to Sprague–Dawley rats, followed by a 14-day recovery phase, could lead to a significant decrease in white blood cell and lymphocyte counts. Also, soft changes in feces and increased mucosal thickness of the colon were noted. Furthermore, organ-to-brain weight and organ-to-body weight ratios of kidneys showed a significant increase in a dose of 2,000 mg/kg (Chen et al., 2017).

CONTRAINDICATIONS

TPM Literature

None.

Current Evidence

Patients with intestinal obstruction, a prolonged period without defecation, severe abdominal pain of unclear origin, IBD, ileus, or appendicitis should not take aloe exudate orally (Ulbricht, 2010; Blumenthal et al., 2000). Other contraindications include spastic constipation, chronic constipation, constipation derived from bowel alterations (proctitis, irritability, etc.), diarrhea, long-term therapy, obesity, and fluid retention (Reynolds, 2004). Also, it is contraindicated in people with hemorrhoids, melanosis coli, liver disease, kidney dysfunction, severe dehydration, or menstruation (Gardner and McGuffin, 2013). It should not be prescribed to children under 12 years of age (Blumenthal et al., 2000). On the other hand, individuals with heart disease, thyroid disorders, electrolyte abnormalities, kidney disease, or diabetes should take aloe only under medical supervision (Ulbricht, 2010).

PREGNANCY AND LACTATION

TPM Literature

Based on Persian medicine, aloe can pass into breastmilk and its therapeutic effects can be delivered to the infant via mother's milk.

Current Evidence

Aloe intake is discouraged for females during lactation, pregnancy, or menstruation. According to studies, rhein, one of aloe's active metabolites, can be present in breastmilk, but no laxative effect has been reported in nursing infants (Reynolds, 2004). In fact, topical administration of aloe is implausible to be dangerous during breastfeeding or pregnancy; however, its oral intake is not suggested because of the possibility of stimulated uterine contractions and increased risk of miscarriage or premature labor (Panel, 2007; Ulbricht, 2010). No experimental or clinical evidence is found for aloe abortifacient action in the literature (Reynolds, 2004). Thus, according to some references, the application of aloe exudate in scheduled doses is considered appropriate during second or third trimesters of pregnancy (Gardner and McGuffin, 2013).

DRUG INTERACTIONS

Corticosteroids: Concurrent use of aloe exudate with corticosteroids is cautioned (Gardner and McGuffin, 2013). Theoretically, increased risk of hypokalemia is predicted in patients using corticosteroids who ordinarily use or abuse aloe (taking more than recommended doses). According to a case report, excessive loss of water and potassium in chronic diarrhea (associated with prolonged use or abuse of aloe) has resulted in metabolic acidosis (Williamson and Baxter, 2009). Topical use of aloe with steroid creams such as hydrocortisone may improve its absorption (Ulbricht, 2010).

Digitalis glycosides: Coadministration of aloe exudate with antiarrhythmic and cardiac glycoside drugs is cautioned (Gardner and McGuffin, 2013). In theory, digitalis toxicity is probable if patients routinely use or abuse aloe. Hypokalemia induced by chronic diarrhea (associated with prolonged use or abuse of aloe) can develop digitalis toxicity and cardiac arrhythmias (Williamson and Baxter, 2009; Blumenthal et al., 2000).

Potassium-sparing diuretics: In theory, excessive potassium loss is probable in patients who routinely use or abuse aloe. Moreover, potassium-sparing diuretics such as loop diuretics or thiazides may lead to potassium depletion (Williamson and Baxter, 2009; Blumenthal et al., 2000).

Sevoflurane: Coadministration of aloe exudate and sevoflurane has led to massive bleeding during surgery in a 35-year-old female due to their synergistic inhibitory effects on platelet function (Aronson, 2009; Baxter and Preston, 2013).

Vitamins C and E: Aloe may increase the absorption of vitamin C or E (Ulbricht, 2010).

Others: Concurrent use of laxative drugs with aloe exudate may increase the risk of electrolyte imbalance, potassium depletion, dehydration, and pH changes in blood (Ulbricht, 2010). Moreover, because aloe exudate may decrease GI transit time, it reduces the absorption of orally consumed drugs (Gardner and McGuffin, 2013). Additionally, oral aloe can decrease blood glucose levels, and caution is warranted when taking supplements or herbs that may lower blood glucose. Moreover, caution is noted with concurrent use of aloe with phytoestrogens, cancer drugs, and antiviral agents. Preliminary reports indicate that ingestion of aloe may increase the levels of azidothymidine. Furthermore, coadministration of aloe exudate with licorice or quinidine is cautioned (Ulbricht, 2010; Gardner and McGuffin, 2013).

METHOD OF ADMINISTRATION

TPM Literature

Aloe exudate in the form of powder or electuary can be used for oral administration. Besides, the powder is indicated topically for some ocular diseases, wound healing, hemorrhoids, and swellings. Inhalation and smoke of aloe are recommended for respiratory problems. Furthermore, enema and lotion are indicated for local treatments (Aghili Khorasani 1771; Avicenna 1025).

Current Evidence

Powders, capsules, tablets, aqueous or hydroalcoholic extracts in liquid or powder form, or other similar products are recommended (Reynolds, 2004; Blumenthal et al., 2000).

DOSAGE

The recommended dose for constipation is the smallest amount to maintain a soft stool. Typically, oral intake of 40–170 mg dried juice (containing 10–30 mg hydroxyanthraquinones) is advised. Alternatively, a daily indication of 150 mg dried aloe juice in combination with psyllium (50 mg) and celandine (300 mg) has shown acceptable laxative effects (Ulbricht, 2010). According to other studies, taking 0.25 mg (Reynolds, 2004) or 250 mg (Capasso and Gaginella, 1997) aloe can produce laxative effects after 6–12 hours via loose bowel movements and abdominal pain (Reynolds, 2004). Also, a single dose of 50–300 mg aloe exudate at bedtime is recommended (Gardner and McGuffin, 2013). Long-term use (more than 1–2 weeks) of aloe exudate for self-treatment of constipation is not allowed (Reynolds, 2004; Gardner and McGuffin, 2013).

REFERENCES

Aghili Khorasani MH 1771. *Makhzan-al-Adviah* (*The treasury of drugs*) (rewritten by Shams Ardakani MR, Rahimi R, Farjadmand F, 1st ed). Tehran: Tehran University of Medical Sciences; 2009.

Ajabnoor MA. Effect of aloes on blood glucose levels in normal and alloxan diabetic mice. J Ethnopharmacol. 1990;28(2):215–220.

Aronson JK. *Meyler's side effects of herbal medicines*. Amsterdam: Elesevier Science; 2009.

Ashafa AOT, Sunmonu TO, Abass AA, et al. Laxative potential of the ethanolic leaf extract of *Aloe vera* (L.) Burm. f. in Wistar rats with loperamide-induced constipation. J Nat Pharmaceut. 2011;2(1):158–162.

Avicenna 1025. *Al-Qanoon fi al-Tibb* (*The canon of medicine*) (rewritten by Masoudi A, ed.). Tehran: Almaei; 2015.

Baxter K, Preston CL, eds. *Stockley's drug interactions*. London: Pharmaceutical Press; 2013.

Blumenthal M, Goldberg A, Brinckmann J. *Herbal medicine: Expanded Commission E monographs*. Newton, MA: Integrative Medicine Communications; 2000.

Bottenberg MM, Wall GC, Harvey RL, et al. Oral *Aloe vera*-induced hepatitis. Ann Pharmacother. 2007;41(10):1740–1743.

Capasso F, Gaginella TS. *Laxatives: A practical guide*. Milano: Springer; 1997.

Chen T, Wang L, Hu C. Treatment-related changes after short-term exposure of SD rats to *Aloe vera* whole-leaf freeze-dried powder. Int J Exp Pathol. 2017;98(5):248–259.

Cholongitas E, Katsoudas S, Dourakis S. Henoch-Schonlein purpura associated with *Aloe vera* administration. Eur J Intern Med. 2005;16(1):59–60.

Ferreira M, Teixeira M, Silva E, et al. Allergic contact dermatitis to *Aloe vera*. Contact Dermatitis. 2007;57(4):278–279.

Gardner Z, McGuffin M. *Botanical safety handbook*. Boca Raton, FL: Taylor & Francis Group; 2013.

Gorkom BV, de Vries EG, Karrenbeld A, et al. Review article: Anthranoid laxatives and their potential carcinogenic effects. Aliment Pharmacol Ther. 1999;13(4):443–452.

Gupta VK, Siddiqi NJ, Ojha AK, et al. Hepatoprotective effect of *Aloe vera* against cartap- and malathion-induced toxicity in Wistar rats. J Cell Physiol. 2019;234(10):18329–18343.

Hong IT, Cha JM, Ki HJ, et al. Small bowel obstruction caused by *Aloe vera* bezoars: A case report. Korean J Gastroenterol. 2017;69(5):312–315.

Kanat O, Ozet A, Ataergin S. *Aloe vera*-induced acute toxic hepatitis in a healthy young man. Eur J Intern Med. 2006;17(8):589.

Kanyadhara S, Dodoala S, Sampathi S, et al. Ethanolic extract of *Aloe vera* ameliorates sciatic nerve ligation induced neuropathic pain. Anc Sci Life. 2014;33(4):208–215.

Kim EJ, Kim HJ, Kim SG, et al. Aloe-induced Henoch-Schonlein purpura. Nephrology (Carlton). 2007;12(1):109.

Lee A, Chui PT, Aun CS, et al. Possible interaction between sevoflurane and *Aloe vera*. Ann Pharmacother. 2004;38(10):1651–1654.

Luyckx VA, Ballantine R, Claeys M, et al. Herbal remedy-associated acute renal failure secondary to Cape aloes. Am J Kidney Dis. 2002;39(3):E13.

Metro D, Cernaro V, Papa M, et al. Marked improvement of thyroid function and autoimmunity by *Aloe barbadensis* Miller juice in patients with subclinical hypothyroidism. J Clin Transl Endocrinol. 2018;11:18–25.

Naini MA, Zargari-Samadnejad A, Mehrvarz S, et al. Anti-inflammatory, antioxidant, and healing-promoting effects of *Aloe vera* extract in the experimental colitis in rats. Evid Based Complement Alternat Med. 2021;2021:9945244.

Panel CE. Final report on the safety assessment of *Aloe andongensis* extract, *Aloe andongensis* leaf juice, *Aloe arborescens* leaf extract, *Aloe arborescens* leaf juice, *Aloe arborescens* leaf protoplasts, *Aloe barbadensis* flower extract, *Aloe barbadensis* leaf, *Aloe barbadensis* leaf extract, *Aloe barbadensis* leaf juice, *Aloe barbadensis* leaf polysaccharides, *Aloe barbadensis* leaf water, *Aloe ferox* leaf extract, *Aloe ferox* leaf juice, and *Aloe ferox* leaf juice extract. Int J Toxicol. 2007;26 suppl 2:1–50.

Rabe C, Musch A, Schirmacher P, et al. Acute hepatitis induced by an *Aloe vera* preparation: A case report. World J Gastroenterol. 2005;11(2):303–304.

Rathor N, Arora T, Manocha S, et al. Anticonvulsant activity of *Aloe vera* leaf extract in acute and chronic models of epilepsy in mice. J Pharm Pharmacol. 2014;66(3):477–485.

Reynolds T. *Aloes: The genus aloe*. Boca Raton, FL: CRC Press; 2004.

Shahryari M, Bibak B, Khaksari M, et al. Anti-edema effect of *Aloe vera* leaf extract following traumatic brain injury: Role of pro-inflammatory cytokines. Avicenna J Phytomed. 2021;11(4):380–393.

Shi G, Jiang H, Feng J, et al. *Aloe vera* mitigates dextran sulfate sodium-induced rat ulcerative colitis by potentiating colon mucus barrier. J Ethnopharmacol. 2021;279:114108.

Shimo K, Zhao X, Yue Lu, et al. Main anthraquinone components in *Aloe vera* and their inhibitory effects on the formation of advanced glycation end-products. J Food Process Pres. 2017;41(5):e13160.

Suksomboon N, Poolsup N, Punthanitisarn S. Effect of *Aloe vera* on glycaemic control in prediabetes and type 2 diabetes: A systematic review and meta-analysis. J Clin Pharm Ther. 2016;41(2):180–188.

Syed TA, Afzal M, Ashfaq Ahmad S, et al. Management of genital herpes in men with 0.5% *Aloe vera* extract in a hydrophilic cream: A placebo-controlled double-blind study, J Derm Treat.1997;8(2):99–102.

Syed TA, Ahmad SA, Holt AH, et al. Management of psoriasis with *Aloe vera* extract in a hydrophilic cream: A placebo-controlled, double-blind study. Trop Med Int Health. 1996;1(4):505–509.

Ulbricht CE. *Mosby's natural standard herb & supplement guide*. St. Louis, MO: Elsevier; 2010.

Werawatganon D, Rakananurak N, Sallapant S, et al. *Aloe vera* attenuated gastric injury on indomethacin-induced gastropathy in rats. World J Gastroenterol. 2014;20(48):18330–18337.

Williamson E, Baxter K. *Stockley's herbal medicines interactions*. London: Pharmaceutical Press; 2009.

Yusuf S, Agunu A, Diana M. The effect of *Aloe vera* A. Berger (Liliaceae) on gastric acid secretion and acute gastric mucosal injury in rats. J Ethnopharmacol. 2004;93(1):33–37.

Zhang Y, Bao Z, Ye X, et al. Chemical investigation of major constituents in *Aloe vera* leaves and several commercial aloe juice powders. J AOAC Int. 2018;101(6):1741–1751.

4 *Althaea officinalis* L.

Roodabeh Bahramsoltani and Mehdi Sabet Jahromi

Scientific name: *Althaea officinalis* L.
Family: Malvaceae
Common names:

- **English**: Marshmallow, moorish mallow, cheeses, mallards, white mallow
- **Persian**: *ḫatmī, ḫetmī, ḫeyrū*
- **Arabic**: *ḫatmī*

Medicinal part(s): Flowers, leaves, fruits, roots (Figure 4.1)
Temperament (nature): Moderate in hotness and coldness, wet in the first degree
Major chemical constituents:

- **Mucilage (10–20%):** arabans, neutral glucans, neural arabinogalactans, galacturonic rhamnans
- **Pectins and starch**
- **Flavonoids:** quercetin, kaempferol, scopoletin
- **Phenolic acids:** caffeic acid, syringic acid, ferulic acid, chlorgenic acid (WHO, 2002; Mahboubi 2020)

THERAPEUTIC USE

TPM Literature

Generally, the roots, leaves, and seeds of marshmallow are considered more potent than its flowers; however, the flowers are commonly available in herbal market. Topical application of marshmallow leaves is useful to reduce inflammation and pain due to swelling in different organs (such as brain, ears, breasts), anusitis, and blepharitis. Warm boiled or raw fruit mucilage sweetened with sugar shows soothing effect on cough and hemoptysis. Also, chewing the fruit can suppress thirst. Both marshmallow root and seeds are well-known emollients and used for the management of colitis, gastrointestinal ulcers and obstructions, burning diarrhea, and subsequent intestinal inflammation. Marshmallow flowers are useful for dysuria, kidney and bladder stones, and urinary hesitancy. They also improve wound healing, bone fracture repair, sciatica, and joint pain due to hotness. Topical application of leaves in combination with oils or fats relieves fire burn, bee/insect bites, tremor, joint pain, and sciatica. Cooked plant with oil can provide a fast relief for hot swellings. Sitz bath with leaves decoction is helpful for anusitis and some types of female infertility and, interestingly, is also recommended for joint stiffness. Additionally, washing hair with marshmallow decoction prevents trichoptilosis and trichorrhexis nodosa (Aghili Khorasani 1771; Avicenna 1025).

 DOI: 10.1201/b22971-4

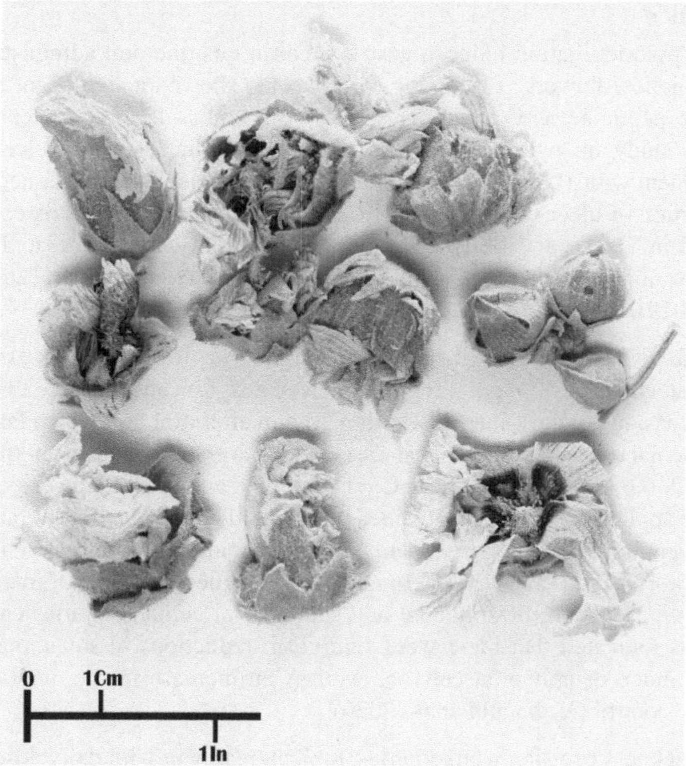

FIGURE 4.1 Marshmallow flower.

Current Evidence

Clinical Evidence

Atopic dermatitis: In a double-blind RCT, a topical liposomal formulation of marshmallow flower hydroethanolic extract (10%) was administered to 40 patients with moderate to severe allergic atopic eczema for 4 weeks. Patients received topical corticosteroid on the left hand and placebo (eucerin) or marshmallow cream on the right hand. As a result, all marshmallow-treated group had better decreasing effects in severity scoring of atopic dermatitis (SCORAD) than the placebo group. Also, the efficacy of marshmallow was similar to topical hydrocortisone or triamcinolone as active control (Khalighi et al., 2021). Another double-blind, active-controlled, pilot RCT investigated the effects of marshmallow flower ethanolic extract in the treatment of atopic dermatitis. For this, 22 children aged between 3 months and 12 years with mild to moderate atopic dermatitis were treated with 1.5 mL marshmallow ointment (1%) twice a day in the first week and three times per week in the next 3 weeks, which resulted in significant improvement of symptoms in comparison to 1% hydrocortisone as the control (Naseri et al., 2021).

Breast engorgement: In an RCT on 40 lactating women with breast engorgement, the alleviating effect of marshmallow in combination with warm and cold compresses was assessed. Patients were treated with warm compress before nursing and a cold compress after nursing six times for 2 days, while the intervention group received a topical marshmallow compress prepared by maceration of marshmallow leaf powder in cooled boiling water. The overall breast engorgement severity was noticeably decreased in the marshmallow group vs. control (Khosravan et al., 2017).

Preclinical Evidence

Gastric ulcer: In pyloric ligation-induced gastric ulcer in rats, the oral administration of aqueous extracts of marshmallow flowers (100 mg/kg for 2 weeks) showed a significant reduction in ulcer index and number, peptic activity, histamine, and gastric mucosal MDA content (Zaghlool et al., 2015). In another study on pyloric ligation/indomethacin-induced gastric ulcer in rats, 2-week prophylactic treatment with 100 mg/kg marshmallow flower aqueous extract, once daily, resulted in a significant reduction of ulcer number and ulcer index vs. negative control. A considerable reduction was observed in TNF-α and IL-1β contents, peptic activity, histamine, and gastrin contents, as well as the elevation of gastric mucosal PG-E2 and PG-I2 contents, CBS and HO-1 activities (Zaghlool et al., 2019).

Cough: The acidic polysaccharide extract from marshmallow flowers was assessed orally in non-anesthetized cats at a dose of 50 mg/kg. Results showed a significant decrease in cough efforts and frequency, as well as cough attack intensity within 30 min after oral use, which lasted for 5 hours in either tracheobronchial or laryngopharyngeal area (Sutovska et al., 2007). In another study, different concentrations (0.2, 0.6, 2.6, 6.6, 14.6 μg/mL) of both methanolic and aqueous extracts of marshmallow roots were applied on isolated rat trachea segments. The contractions of rat tracheobronchial smooth muscles were inhibited upon treatment with marshmallow extract, while it had no effect on β-adrenergic receptors (Alani et al., 2015). In a rat model, aqueous extract of marshmallow flowers was assessed for the treatment of epithelial and submucosal cellular injuries caused by cigarette smoke. The results indicated that there were significant reductions in squamous metaplasia, cell injuries, and reid index of epithelial cells, as well as an increase in the number of goblet cells compared with the control (Mahboubi et al., 2020).

Wound: In full-thickness excision wound in rats, topical treatment with daily doses of 5% and 10% marshmallow whole-plant hydroethanolic extract incorporated in hydrogel base for 2 weeks showed a significant improvement in hair follicles, mean diameter of vessels, and fibroblast population in the dermis in both groups. Significantly higher volume densities of collagen bundles were also observed in 10% marshmallow-treated group (Mohsenikia et al., 2020). In another study using excision wound model rats, hydroethanolic extract of marshmallow leaves was topically administered at a daily dose of 0.5 g (based on the wound area) and wound margins were measured up to 21 days. In comparison with the control group, considerable improvements were observed in wound epithelization and wound healing after 3 weeks of intervention, along with a low cellular density, brief inflammation, and matured granulation of fibrosis tissues (Rezaei et al., 2015).

ADVERSE REACTIONS

TPM Literature

Since the plant is wet-tempered, it can cause indigestion in long-term use and in people with cold and wet temperament. In such cases, it is better to be taken with barberry, fennel, or honey. It may also cause irritation in lungs and thus is recommended to be taken with honey (Aghili Khorasani 1771).

Current Evidence

Marshmallow is generally regarded as safe on healthy subjects. According to preclinical studies, marshmallow may decrease blood sugar level, and thus diabetic patients are advised to monitor their blood glucose when taking marshmallow preparations. Allergic reactions may also occur (Ulbricht, 2010).

CONTRAINDICATIONS

TPM Literature

None.

Current Evidence

None.

PREGNANCY AND LACTATION

TPM Literature

It is contraindicated during pregnancy.

Current Evidence

No specific warnings or adverse events during pregnancy and lactation is reported for marshmallow; however, some reference suggest to stay on the safe side as the safety cannot be guaranteed (Tobyn et al., 2011; Gardner and MacGaffin, 2013).

DRUG INTERACTIONS

Due to its high mucilage content, the absorption of other drugs may be delayed in simultaneous intake with marshmallow; thus, other medicines should be taken an hour before or several hours after marshmallow consumption (Gardner and MacGaffin, 2013).

METHOD OF ADMINISTRATION

TPM Literature

The decoction or infusion can be orally taken (may be sweetened with sugar or honey) or topically used as a compress for skin complications or as a hair mask. All plant parts can also be used topically in the form of poultice. Also, the decoction can be used as sitz bath for vaginal, uterine, and bladder problems (Aghili Khorasani 1771; Avicenna 1025).

Current Evidence

The aqueous extracts of cut leaves or ground root are administrated for internal use. In addition, marshmallow syrup is only permitted for dry cough treatment (Gruenwald et al., 2007).

DOSAGE

Leaves: 5 g daily.
Root: 6 g daily.
Whole plant: 2 g (Skidmore-Roth, 2010).

REFERENCES

Aghili Khorasani MH 1771. *Makhzan-al-Adviah* (*The treasury of drugs*) (rewritten by Shams Ardakani MR, Rahimi R, Farjadmand F, 1st ed.). Tehran: Tehran University of Medical Sciences; 2009.

Alani B, Zare M, Noureddini M. Bronchodilatory and B-adrenergic effects of methanolic and aqueous extracts of Althaea root on isolated tracheobronchial smooth rat muscle. Adv Biomed Res. 2015;4:78.

Avicenna 1025. *Al-Qanoon fi al-Tibb* (*The canon of medicine*) (rewritten by Masoudi A, ed.). Tehran: Almaei; 2015.

Gardner Z, McGuffin M, eds. *American Herbal Products Association's botanical safety handbook*. Boca Raton: CRC Press; 2013.

Gruenwald J, Brendler T, Jaenicke C. *PDR for herbal medicines*. Montvale: Thomson Reuters; 2007.

Khalighi N, Jabbari-Azad F, Barzegar-Amini M, et al. Impact of *Althaea Officinalis* extract in patients with atopic eczema: A double-blind randomized controlled trial. Clin Phytoscience. 2021;7(1):1–6.

Khosravan S, Mohammadzadeh-Moghadam H, Mohammadzadeh F, et al. The effect of Hollyhock (*Althaea officinalis* L) leaf compresses combined with warm and cold compress on breast engorgement in lactating women: A randomized clinical trial. J Evid Based Complementary Altern Med. 2017;22(1):25–30.

Mahboubi M. Marshmallow (*Althaea officinalis* L.) and its potency in the treatment of cough. Complement Med Res. 2020;27(3):174–183.

Mohsenikia M, Rafiee S, Rozei LS, et al. *Althaea officinalis* improves wound healing in rats: A stereological study. Drug Discov Ther. 2020;14(5):239–242.

Naseri V, Chavoshzadeh Z, Mizani A, et al. Effect of topical marshmallow (*Althaea officinalis*) on atopic dermatitis in children: A pilot double-blind active-controlled clinical trial of an in-silico-analyzed phytomedicine. Phytother Res. 2021;35(3):1389–1398.

Rezaei M, Alirezaei M. Protective effects of *Althaea officinalis* L. extract in 6-hydroxydopamine-induced hemi-Parkinsonism model: Behavioral, biochemical and histochemical evidence. J Physiol Sci. 2014;64(3):171–176.

Rezaei M, Dadgar Z, Noori-Zadeh A, et al. Evaluation of the antibacterial activity of the *Althaea officinalis* L. leaf extract and its wound healing potency in the rat model of excision wound creation. Avicenna J Phytomed. 2015;5(2):105–112.

Skidmore-Roth L. *Mosby's handbook of herbs & natural supplements*. St. Louis: Elsevier Health Sciences; 2010.

Sutovska M, Nosalova G, Franova S, Kardosova A. The antitussive activity of polysaccharides from Althaea officinalis l., var. Robusta, Arctium lappa L., var. Herkules, and Prunus persica L., Batsch. Bratislavske lekarske listy. 2007;108(2):93–9.

Tobyn G, Denham A, Whitelegg M. Althaea officinalis, marshmallow; Malva sylvestris, common mallow; Alcea rosea, hollyhock. Medical Herbs. The Western Herbal Tradition. Chapter 8: 67–78. 2011.

Ulbricht CE. *Mosby's natural standard herb & supplement guide*. St. Louis, MO: Elsevier; 2010.

WHO. *WHO monographs on selected medicinal plants*, volume 2. Malta: World Health Organization; 2002.

Zaghlool SS, Abo-Seif AA, Rabeh MA, et al. Gastro-protective and anti-oxidant potential of *Althaea officinalis* and *Solanum nigrum* on pyloric ligation/indomethacin-induced ulceration in rats. Antioxidants. 2019;8(11):512.

Zaghlool SS, Shehata BA, Abo-Seif AA, Abd El-Latif HA. Assessment of protective effects of extracts of *Zingiber officinale* and *Althaea officinalis* on pyloric ligation-induced gastric ulcer in experimental animals. J Pharm Biosci. 2015;3(4):48–57.

5 *Boswellia serrata* Roxb., *Boswellia carteri* Birdw.

Parmis Badr and Fatemeh Etemadpour

Scientific name: *Boswellia serrata* Roxb., *Boswellia carteri* Birdw.
Family: Burseraceae
Common names:

- **English:** Frankincense, salai, salai guggul, shallaki, Indian olibanum
- **Persian:** *kondor*
- **Arabic:** *lubān, lubān ḏakar*

Medicinal part(s): Oleo-gum resin (Figure 5.1)
Temperament (nature): Hot and dry in the second degree
Major chemical constituents:

- **Resins (60%):** Pentacyclic triterpene acids such as α-boswellic acid, β-boswellic acid, 11-keto-β-boswellic acid, and acetyl-11-keto-β-boswellic acid
- **Volatile oil (5–9%):** Chief components are 1-octyl acetate (60%), 1-octanol (12.7%), α-pinene (3.5%), and incensol (2.7%).
- Mucilages (12–20%) (Gruenwald et al., 2007; Williamson et al., 2009)

THERAPEUTIC USE

TPM Literature

Frankincense is used as a memory enhancer, especially daily intake of macerate in the morning on empty stomach. In TPM, frankincense is highly recommended as one of the main ingredients in ophthalmic formulations for the improvement of eyesight, eye injuries and itching, excessive tearing, and eye infections. Frankincense can be used against respiratory infections and is effective in the treatment of productive coughs. Its oral intake with sugar acts as a carminative, digestive, antiemetic, and antidiarrheal tonic. Topical application of frankincense acts as a promising wound-healing agent and can prevent bleeding from different parts such as meninges, uterus, rectum, and hemorrhoids. Moreover, it is topically helpful for the relief of joint and bone pain (Aghili Khorasani 1771; Avicenna 1025).

Current Evidence

Clinical Evidence

Osteoarthritis: In a meta-analysis, seven randomized controlled trials assessing the effects of frankincense or its extracts in 545 patients with osteoarthritis were included. Compared with the control group, frankincense and its extracts (at doses of 100–250 mg of the extract, or 7.2–15 mg of boswellic acid taken for at least 4 weeks) were reported to relieve pain and stiffness and improved

DOI: 10.1201/b22971-5

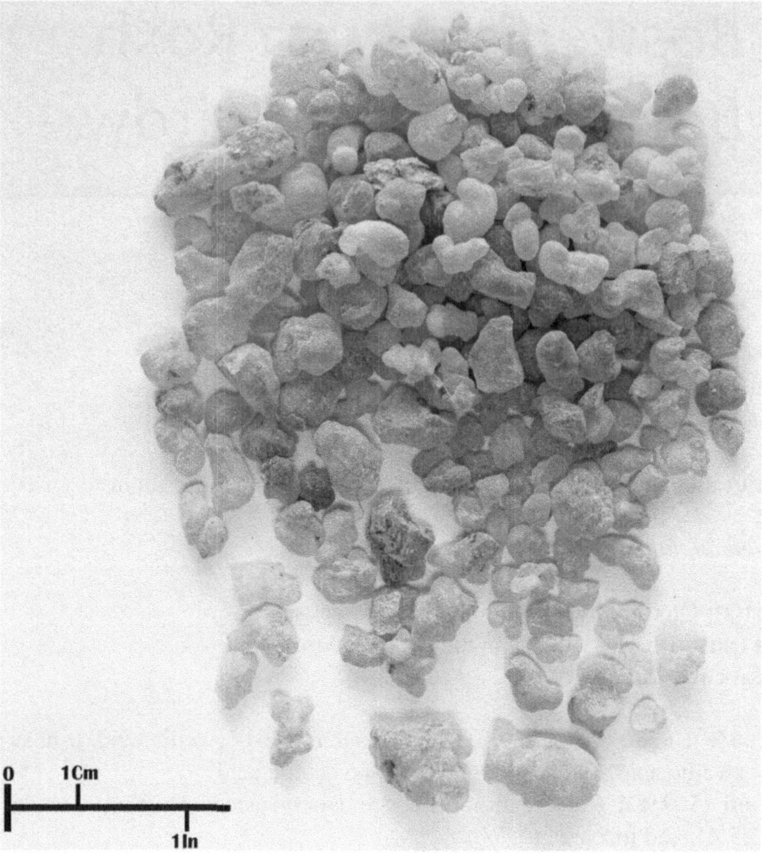

FIGURE 5.1 Frankincense oleo-gum-resin.

joint function (Yu et al., 2020). Based on another meta-analysis including four studies on 216 patients with knee osteoarthritis, frankincense was more effective than placebo in relieving pain and improving functions while having fewer side effects (Bannuru et al., 2018).

Dermatological problems: A placebo-controlled RCT was carried out on 114 women with breast carcinoma. Fifty-five patients used 2% frankincense cream two times a day (after radiation therapy and at bedtime on radiotherapy days; and other days in the morning and at night). The other 59 patients applied a placebo cream. The frankincense cream prevented erythema and decreased the intensity of skin reactions, thus reducing the need for topical cortisteroid (Togni et al., 2015). In a single-blind, pilot study, physical skin damage was created by stripping test and mechanical skin damage was induced by UV on 30 healthy volunteers. Then, an emulsion containing 1% *B. serrata* extract was topically applied twice a day for 1 week. *B. serrata* extract proved to be effective on stripping damage as well as for treating mechanical skin damage (Rigano et al., 2015).

Wounds: In a controlled RCT on primiparous women with singleton pregnancies after normal vaginal delivery, women received either 10 min sitz bath of *B. carteri* extract or betadine twice a day for 1 week. The results indicated that *B. carteri* was almost as effective as betadine sitz bath in improving episiotomy wound healing since the total REEDA (Redness, Edema, Ecchymosis, Discharge, Approximation) score was not statistically different between these two groups on second and seventh postpartum days (Faraji et al., 2021).

In a double-blind RCT, the healing effect of a 40% *B. carteri* formulation was compared with 1% silver sulfadiazine cream in the management of second-degree burn wounds. Seventeen patients from the silver sulfadiazine group and 15 patients from the frankincense group finished the trial. Both groups had a progressive healing trend during study time. Topical formulation of frankincense had a wound-healing effect similar to the standard 1% silver sulfadiazine treatment. Both healing time and healing indices were statistically similar between the groups on each day of study (Badr et al., 2023).

Heavy menstrual bleeding: In a placebo-controlled RCT, patients with menorrhagia received capsules containing either 300 mg *B. serrata* or lactose as placebo for 7 days of the menstrual cycle. Also, all patients received ibuprofen as a conventional painkiller. The results indicated that *B. serrata* as a complementary adjuvant to NSAIDs could be effective in reducing the duration and amount of bleeding, leading to increased quality of life (Eshaghian et al., 2019).

Pain: To assess the analgesic activity of *B. serrata*, a randomized, double-blind, placebo-controlled, cross-over study was performed on 12 healthy volunteers using a mechanical pain model (Randall selitto test). Two capsules each containing 125 mg *B. serrata* were administered as a single dose to one group, while the other group received a placebo. As a result, the pain threshold force and time increased significantly in 2 and 3 hours after drug administration. The most remarkable increase in pain tolerance force was observed after 2 and 3 hours, and for pain tolerance time, it was after 2 hours (Prabhavathi et al., 2014). The effect of topical application of *B. carteri* was examined in a triple-blind, placebo-controlled RCT with 28 patients suffering from carpal tunnel syndrome. A topical formulation was prepared according to TPM methods by dissolving frankincense in sesame oil as an oleogel. Intervention and placebo products were administered as 1.5 fingertip unit twice daily for 6 weeks. *B. carteri* was effective in alleviating pain and improving functions in comparison to the placebo (Karimi et al., 2021).

Cognitive impairment: Mild to moderate cognitive impairment happens in about 50% of patients with MS, affecting white and gray matters in the brain, which is accompanied by a rise in proinflammatory mediators. Sixty patients with relapsing-remitting MS without major depression participated in a double-blind, placebo-controlled RCT. Thirty patients received capsules containing 450 mg *B. serrata* two times a day for 2 months. As a result, the California Verbal Learning Test-Total Learning (CVLTII-TL) and Brief Visuospatial Memory Test-Total Learning (BVMTR-TL) were significantly improved in comparison to the placebo (Majdinasab et al., 2016). A double-blind, placebo-controlled RCT was carried out on 118 patients with mild cognitive impairment. The test group received capsules containing 300 mg *B. serrata* twice a day. Three and six months later, Montreal Cognitive Assessment (MoCA) showed a significant improvement in patients with memory impairment compared to the placebo (Rezakhani et al., 2020).

Dyslipidemia: In an RCT, 900 mg/day frankincense was given to 30 diabetic patients for 6 weeks and the results were compared to 30 other patients in the control group who received no intervention. The study indicated increased levels of HDL-C, reduced LDL-C, TC, and fructosamine levels, and improved activities of serum AST and ALT (Ahangarpour et al., 2014).

Ulcerative colitis: In a study, *B. serrata* gum resin (900 mg/day in three doses) was given to 20 patients with chronic active ulcerative colitis (15 with grade 2 and 5 with grade 3). Other 10 patients (six with grade 2 and four with grade 3) received Sulfasalazine (3 g daily in three doses). After 6 weeks, 18 out of 20 faced disease remission. After 1 year of observation, relapse occurred in 6 out of 18 patients who had initially responded to frankincense. Of the six patients who were successfully treated with sulfasalazine, relapse was observed in two after a year. Biochemical and hematological assaying confirmed this gum to be effective for IBD and the relapse is believed to be due to low doses of frankincense and short duration of treatment (Gupta et al., 2001). A 6-week randomized, double-blind, placebo-controlled study was performed on patients with collagenous colitis and chronic diarrhea. Patients in the test group were given 400 mg *B. serrata* extract orally three times a day. The results showed that compared with placebo, a higher number of patients remained on remission in the *B. serrata* arm; however, no difference was observed in histology and quality of life, which might be due to small sample size (Madisch et al., 2008).

Preclinical Evidence

Wound: The wound-healing potential of *B. serrata* was examined in STZ-induced diabetic rats. Foot ulcers were created on the dorsal surface of rat paw. *B. serrata* was administered orally in doses of 100, 200, and 400 mg/kg for 16 days. As a result of 200 and 400 mg/kg of *B. serrata* administration, the rate of wound contraction enhanced significantly due to different mechanisms such as increasing collagen synthesis, angiogenesis, and reduction in cellular necrosis. Different oxido-inflammatory markers such as TNF-α, interleukins, oxido-nitrosative stress, and NF-κB were inhibited. Furthermore, the inhibition of apoptosis was observed due to the modulation in Bcl-2-associated X protein expression. On the other hand, TGFβ-1 and VEGF were promoted (Pengzong et al., 2019).

Inflammation: In an LPS-induced model of oxidative damage and inflammation in rats, ethyl acetate extract of *B. serrata* was administered intraperitoneally 30 min before LPS. Rats were divided into four groups, including control, LPS, LPS plus 100 mg/kg of extract, and LPS plus 200 mg/kg of extract. During 3 weeks of the study, observations of renal and hepatic functions showed a decrease in ALT, AST, ALP, creatinine, IL-6, BUN, and MDA levels, while endogenous antioxidant defense mechanisms, including total thiol and protein, CAT, and SOD levels, increased in the treatment group (Marefati et al., 2022).

ADVERSE REACTIONS

TPM Literature

Frankincense might cause headache in people with hot temperament and may also cause irritation and agitation. Black patches and spots on skin may occur (Aghili Khorasani 1771).

Current Evidence

In a clinical trial, 18% of patients with ulcerative colitis who received 1.5 g daily frankincense for 6 weeks experienced epigastric pain, abdominal fullness, gastroesophageal reflux, and nausea, but long-term use did not cause any ulceration. The results of a systematic review of clinical trials showed that the adverse effects reported for frankincense, including diarrhea, abdominal pain, and nausea, were not serious and also not different from those of control or placebo groups (Gardner and McGuffin, 2013; Ulbricht, 2010). One case of allergic contact dermatitis from frankincense extract was reported in a young woman with atopic background after using a topical *B. serrata* formulation for a second-degree burn wound on her thigh. After 5 days, an intense eczematous local cutaneous reaction with bullae developed, needing systemic and topical corticosteroids (Acebo et al., 2004).

CONTRAINDICATIONS

TPM Literature

None.

Current Evidence

Individuals with known allergy to *Boswellia* or members of Burseraceae family should not use related preparations (Ulbricht, 2010).

PREGNANCY AND LACTATION

TPM Literature

No precautions during pregnancy and lactation have been recorded in TPM manuscripts. But in folkloric medicine of some regions of Iran, it is believed that taking frankincense during pregnancy will enhance the memory of born child. However, TPM practitioners believe that it can cause some neurological disturbances in the fetus, which might lead to attention-deficit hyperactivity disorder in born child. Thus, it is not safe to use during pregnancy.

Current Evidence

Frankincense is likely unsafe during pregnancy. It can be emmenagogue and induce abortion (Ulbricht, 2010). There is lack of data about the safety of frankincense during lactation (Gardner and McGuffin, 2013).

DRUG INTERACTIONS

Lipid-lowering drugs: Frankincense may lower cholesterol and increase the effects of lipid-lowering agents.
Drugs for osteoarthritis: It may act additively with agents used in the treatment of osteoarthritis, such as glucosamine and chondroitin (Ulbricht, 2010).

METHOD OF ADMINISTRATION

TPM Literature

For memory enhancement, frankincense may be chewed or macerated in water and taken daily on empty stomach in the morning. It may also be taken with sugar as a carminative and digestive.

For topical administration, frankincense may be mixed with oil or fat and applied as a poultice (Aghili Khorasani 1771).

Fine powder of frankincense may be used for ocular indications.

Current Evidence

Capsules containing frankincense in powder form are used (Ulbricht, 2010).

DOSAGE

300–1,200 mg frankincense is taken orally three times daily (Ulbricht, 2010).

REFERENCES

Acebo E, Ratón JA, Sautúa S, et al. Allergic contact dermatitis from *Boswellia serrata* extract in a naturopathic cream. Contact Derm. 2004;51(2):91–92.

Aghili Khorasani MH 1771. *Makhzan-al-Adviah* (*The treasury of drugs*) (rewritten by Shams Ardakani MR, Rahimi R, Farjadmand F, 1st ed.). Tehran: Tehran University of Medical Sciences; 2009.

Ahangarpour A, Heidari H, Fatemeh RA, et al. Effect of *Boswellia serrata* supplementation on blood lipid, hepatic enzymes and fructosamine levels in type2 diabetic patients. J Diabetes and Metab Disord. 2014;13:1–5.

Avicenna 1025. *Al-Qanoon fi al-Tibb* (*The canon of medicine*) (rewritten by Masoudi A, ed.). Tehran: Almaei; 2015.

Badr P, Afsharypuor S, Tohidinik HR, et al. Burn wound healing effect of a sterilized traditional formulation of *Boswellia carteri* vs. silver sulfadiazine cream 1% in patients presenting second-degree burn wounds: A randomized, double-blind clinical trial. Iran J Med Sci. 2023;48(2):137–145.

Bannuru RR, Osani MC, Al-Eid F, Wang C. Efficacy of curcumin and Boswellia for knee osteoarthritis: Systematic review and meta-analysis. Semin Arthritis Rheum. 2018;48(3):416–429.

Eshaghian R, Mazaheri M, Ghanadian M, et al. The effect of frankincense (*Boswellia serrata*, oleoresin) and ginger (*Zingiber officinale*, rhizoma) on heavy menstrual bleeding: A randomized, placebo-controlled, clinical trial. Complement Ther Med. 2019;42:42–47.

Faraji A, Aghdaki M, Hessami K, et al. Episiotomy wound healing by *Commiphora myrrha* (Nees) Engl. and *Boswellia carteri* Birdw. in primiparous women: A randomized controlled trial. J Ethnopharmacol. 2021;264:113396.

Gardner Z, McGuffin M. *Botanical safety handbook*. London: CRC Press; 2013.

Gruenwald J, Brendler T, Jaenicke C. *PDR for herbal medicines*. Montvale: Thomson Reuters; 2007.

Gupta I, Parihar A, Malhotra P, et al. Effects of gum resin of *Boswellia serrata* in patients with chronic colitis. Planta Med. 2001;67(5):391–395.

Karimi M, Rohani S, Akbari MG, et al. The efficacy of *Boswellia carterii* oleogel in pain relief and functional improvement among patients with carpal tunnel syndrome: A triple-blind randomized, controlled trial. Shiraz E Med J. 2021;22(9):e107952.

Madisch A, Miehlke S, Eichele O, et al. *Boswellia serrata* extract for the treatment of collagenous colitis: A double-blind, randomized, placebo-controlled, multicenter trial. Int J Colorectal Dis. 2008;22:1445–1451.

Majdinasab N, Siahpush A, Mousavinejad SK, et al. Effect of *Boswellia serrata* on cognitive impairment in multiple sclerosis patients. J Herb Med. 2016;6(3):119–127.

Marefati N, Beheshti F, Etemadizadeh P, et al. Gum resin extract of *Boswellia serrata* attenuates lipopolysaccharide-induced inflammation and oxidative damage in hepatic and renal tissues of rats. Asian Pac J Trop Biomed. 2022;12(1):20–25.

Pengzong Z, Yuanmin L, Xiaoming X, et al. Wound healing potential of the standardized extract of *Boswellia serrata* on experimental diabetic foot ulcer via inhibition of inflammatory, angiogenetic and apoptotic markers. Planta Med. 2019;85(8):657–669.

Prabhavathi K, Chandra US, Soanker R, Rani PU. A randomized, double blind, placebo controlled, cross over study to evaluate the analgesic activity of *Boswellia serrata* in healthy volunteers using mechanical pain model. Indian J Pharmacol. 2014;46(5):475.

Rezakhani S, Sedighi B, Pardakhty A, Shafiee K. Effects of *Boswellia serrata* on improvement of memory impairment in patients with mild cognitive impairment: A double-blind, randomized, placebo-controlled study. J Kerman Universit Med Sci. 2020;27(4):348–355.

Rigano L, Maramaldi G, Bonfigli A, et al. Skin-damage protective and recovery properties of an activated olibanum extract (from *Boswellia serrata*) on mechanical and physical skin damage: A single-blind evaluation on healthy volunteers. Esper Dermatol. 2015;17(4):139–142.

Togni S, Maramaldi G, Bonetta A, et al. Clinical evaluation of safety and efficacy of Boswellia-based cream for prevention of adjuvant radiotherapy skin damage in mammary carcinoma: A randomized placebo controlled trial. Eur Rev Med Pharmacol Sci. 2015;19(8):1338–1344.

Ulbricht CE. *Natural standard herb & supplement guide: An evidence-based reference*. St. Luis: Elsevier; 2010.

Williamson E, Driver S , Baxter K. *Stockley's herbal medicines interactions*. London: Pharmaceutical Press; 2009.

Yu G, Xiang W, Zhang T, Zeng L, Yang K, Li J. Effectiveness of Boswellia and Boswellia extract for osteoarthritis patients: A systematic review and meta-analysis. BMC Complement Med Ther. 2020;20(1):225.

6 *Cassia fistula* L.

Babak Daneshfard

Scientific name: *Cassia fistula* L.
Family: Fabaceae
Common names:

- **English:** Golden shower tree, golden rain, purging cassia, pudding-pipe tree
- **Persian:** *folūs, ḫiyār čanbar*
- **Arabic:** *ḫiyār šanbar*

Medicinal part(s): Flowers, fruit pulp and seeds (Figure 6.1)
Temperament (nature): Hot and wet in the first degree
Major chemical constituents:

- **Monosaccharides/oligosaccharides (50%):** Particularly saccharose
- **Anthracene derivatives (1% in the mesocarp):** Sennosides
- Fixed oil (in seeds)
- **Steroids:** Sterols (in the seeds) including β-sitosterol
- **Alpha-hydroxy acids:** Citric acid (Gruenwald et al., 2007)

THERAPEUTIC USE

TPM Literature

Purging cassia is used in the treatment of hot-tempered swellings and ulcers in the mouth and pharynx. It is a safe laxative for children and pregnant women; however, it has a slow onset of action. In combination with other substances, it is used for expelling pathologic humors and in the treatment of jaundice, hepatic and intestinal obstructions, and acute fever. Its topical ointment is useful in treating joint pain, gout, and hot swellings (Aghili Khorasani 1771; Avicenna 1025).

Current Evidence

Clinical Evidence

Constipation: In an RCT on 70 old-aged patients with constipation, 30 mL/day of purging cassia fruit pulp syrup for 2 weeks resulted in a significantly higher frequency of weekly defecation compared to lactulose. In addition, quality of life, hard stool, straining, pain during defecation, and stool consistency were significantly better in the intervention group (Sepehr et al., 2022). An RCT on 81 children with functional constipation revealed that an oral emulsion of purging cassia fruit could be more effective than mineral oil in providing relief. In this study, 0.1 g/kg/day of emulsion was compared with 1 mL/kg/day of mineral oil in a 3-week intervention. A significant improvement was observed in the emulsion group regarding frequency of defecation, severity of pain during defecation, and stool consistency (Mozaffarpur et al., 2012). Another open-labeled RCT on 109 pediatric patients with functional constipation compared the effect of 4-week administration of oral

DOI: 10.1201/b22971-6

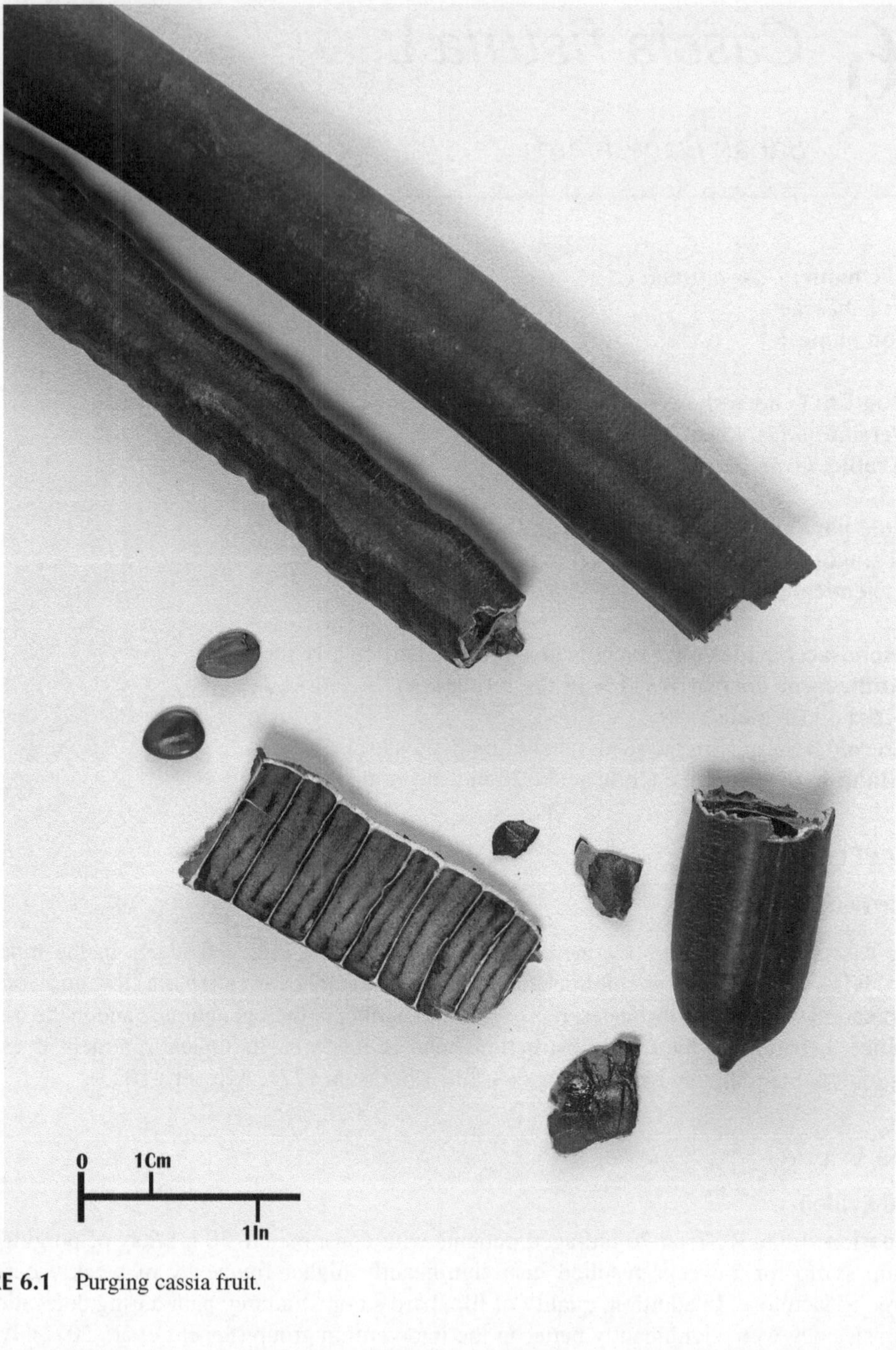

FIGURE 6.1 Purging cassia fruit.

emulsion of purging cassia fruit vs. PEG. The herbal intervention showed similar efficacy to PEG in all assessed outcomes, including pain severity, stool consistency, fecal incontinence, and retentive posturing; however, it significantly improved the frequency of defecation, without any considerable side effects, compared to PEG (Esmaeilidooki et al., 2016).

Pemphigus vulgaris: The efficacy of purging cassia fruit gel on cutaneous lesions of 82 patients with pemphigus vulgaris has been investigated as an adjuvant therapy in a double-blind RCT. The topical formulation was prepared by extracting the fruit palp in sesame oil, followed by the addition of oil (33%) to a gel base, which was equivalent to 8.3% concentrated pulp extract. Epithelialization index in the intervention group was significantly higher compared to the placebo on day 10 and 20 of study (Atarzadeh et al., 2018).

Skin aging: In a pilot placebo-controlled study on 13 healthy adult males, a patch containing 5% oil-in-water emulsion of purging cassia pod hydromethanolic extract was prepared. Individuals were instructed to apply the herbal patch on one of their forearms and the placebo patch on the other forearm for a period of 12 weeks. Purging cassia patch showed significant improvement in stratum corneum hydration, skin barrier function, and water-holding function, along with less wrinkles, dryness, and roughness, suggesting the plant to be a promising anti-aging candidate for topical application (Khan et al., 2015).

Preclinical Evidence

Liver toxicity: In a rat model of thioacetamide-induced hepatotoxicity, ethyl acetate fraction from purging cassia has shown significant hepatoprotective potentials. It reduced oxidative stress via downregulating p-PI3K, p-Akt, and p-mTOR expression and modulating antioxidant enzymes (Kaur et al., 2019). In another animal study, CCl_4-induced liver damage in albino rats was treated with 200 mg/kg/day purging cassia fruit pulp aqueous extract. Five days of intervention significantly reduced the levels of AST, ALT, ALP, and total bilirubin, along with an increase in total protein. It also prevented fatty changes, necrosis, and fibrosis in the liver (Das et al., 2008).

Diabetes: The protective effect of an hydroethanolic extract of purging cassia pods on STZ-induced diabetic rats was investigated. Three different doses (100, 250, and 500 mg/kg/day) of purging cassia extract for 60 days resulted in significant improvement in total protein concentration, serum insulin level, relative weight, and antioxidant markers in the pancreas. In addition, histomorphological evaluations revealed marked restoration of Langerhans islet morphology (Jangir and Jain, 2018). In another study, 20 mg/kg of novel triterpenoid compounds were orally administered to STZ-induced diabetic rats for 60 days. This intervention significantly decreased FBS, increased the glycogen content of liver and skeletal muscles, and normalized the levels of glucokinase and glucose 6-phosphatase (Indu et al., 2021).

Hyperlipidemia: The efficacy of purging cassia leaves aqueous extract was studied in a mouse model of diet-induced hyperlipidemia. A dosage of 500 mg/kg of this extract more effectively increased HDL-C and decreased TAG, TC, and LDL-C compared to simvastatin (Nawaz et al., 2019). Another study investigated the antihyperlipidemic effects of an hexane extract of purging cassia barks in STZ-induced diabetic rats. Treatment with 0.45 g/kg of the extract for 30 days improved TAG, TC, LDL-C, VLDL-C, and HDL-C compared to control animals (Nirmala et al., 2008).

Infected wound: The efficacy of an ointment formulated from the ethanolic extract of purging cassia leaves (10% in ointment base) was studied in infected wound model of rats. Compared to the control group, a significantly better tissue regeneration and wound closure, in addition to a lower bacterial count in the granulation tissue, was observed in purging cassia group. This ointment also improved histopathological parameters of wound healing such as collagen and protein content in the granulation tissue of infected rats (Kumar et al., 2006).

Pain: An animal study on Wister rats and Swiss Albino mice revealed that intraperitoneal administration of methanolic extract of purging cassia (500 mg/kg) could significantly inhibit the pain response induced by mechanical, thermal, and writhing stimuli (Sheikh et al., 2010). In another experiment on rats, 200 mg/kg of purging cassia bark extract showed a significant analgesic activity according to the reflex time in tail immersion, hot plate, and inhibition of writhing tests (Sharma et al., 2022).

ADVERSE REACTIONS

TPM Literature

It is nauseating and harmful for stomach; however, these side effects are decreased if taken with aniseed or mastic gum. It may cause intestinal cramps and ulceration; in order to prevent these adverse effects, the plant material should be mixed with sweet almond oil (Aghili Khorasani 1771).

Current Evidence

Upon a proper administration of standard therapeutic dosages of the herb, no adverse reaction has been observed (Gruenwald et al., 2007). However, in case of overdose, it may cause cramp-like GI complaints. Long-term use may also cause potassium loss, which in turn could lead to aldosteronism, hematuria, albuminuria, muscle weakness, and inhibition of intestinal motility. Rarely, it may lead to nephropathy, cardiac arrhythmia, edema, and accelerated osteoclasis (Gruenwald et al., 2007).

CONTRAINDICATIONS

TPM Literature

Purging cassia fruit should not be used unless after 1 year of harvest; otherwise it may cause hematuria (Aghili Khorasani 1771).

Current Evidence

Purging cassia is contraindicated in acute inflammatory diseases of intestine such as acute appendicitis and ileus. In addition, although it is considered a safe laxative in children according to TPM, modern evidence suggests that it should not be used by children under 12 years (Gruenwald et al., 2007). So, it is better to stay on the safe side and avoid use on children under 12.

PREGNANCY AND LACTATION

TPM Literature

It is considered safe.

Current Evidence

Purging cassia is contraindicated during pregnancy and lactation (Gruenwald et al., 2007). Although it is considered safe in pregnancy based on TPM, it is better to stay on the safe side and avoid use.

DRUG INTERACTIONS

Antiarrhythmics: Due to the possibility of electrolyte imbalance (particularly potassium loss) in case of toxicity, interaction with antiarrhythmics especially digoxin may occur (Gruenwald et al., 2007).

METHOD OF ADMINISTRATION

TPM Literature

The black pungent-smelling sweet pulp which sticks to the seeds is the most used part. It should be separated from other parts by heating. Then, it should be used orally with almond oil (Aghili Khorasani 1771).

Current Evidence

By maceration extraction, the pulps of purging cassia are used to prepare a soft extract for internal use (Gruenwald et al., 2007).

DOSAGE

Daily dosage is 4–8 g of the fruit pulp (Gruenwald et al., 2007).

REFERENCES

Aghili Khorasani MH 1771. *Makhzan-al-Adviah* (*The treasury of drugs*) (rewritten by Shams Ardakani MR, Rahimi R, Farjadmand F, 1st ed). Tehran: Tehran University of Medical Sciences; 2009.

Atarzadeh F, Kamalinejad M, Amin G, et al. Topical application of *Cassia fistula* L. fruit gel in management of cutaneous lesions of pemphigus vulgaris: A double-blind, placebo-controlled clinical trial. Avicenna J Phytomed. 2018;8(6):543–551.

Avicenna 1025. *Al-Qanoon fi al-Tibb* (*The canon of medicine*) (rewritten by Masoudi A, ed). Tehran: Almaei; 2015.

Das S, Sarma G, Barman S. Hepatoprotective activity of aqueous extract of fruit pulp of *Cassia fistula* (AFCF) against carbon tetrachloride (CCL4) induced liver damage in albino rats. J Clin Diagn Res. 2008;2(5):1133–1138.

Esmaeilidooki MR, Mozaffarpur SA, Mirzapour M, et al. Comparison between the *Cassia fistulas* emulsion with polyethylene glycol (peg4000) in the pediatric functional constipation: A randomized clinical trial. Iran Red Crescent Med J. 2016;18(7):e33998.

Gruenwald J, Brendler T, Jaenicke C. *PDR for herbal medicines*. Montvale: Thomson Reuters; 2007.

Indu S, Vijayalakshmi P, Selvaraj J, Rajalakshmi M. Novel triterpenoids from *Cassia fistula* stem bark depreciates STZ-induced detrimental changes in IRS-1/Akt-mediated insulin signaling mechanisms in type-1 diabetic rats. Molecules. 2021;26(22):6812.

Jangir RN, Jain GC. Evaluation of protective effects of hydroalcoholic extract of *Cassia fistula* Linn. pod on pancreas in streptozotocin-induced diabetic rats. Pharmacognosy Res. 2018;10(2):205–212.

Kaur S, Sharma D, Singh AP, Kaur S. Amelioration of hepatic function, oxidative stress, and histopathologic damages by *Cassia fistula* L. fraction in thioacetamide-induced liver toxicity. Environ Sci Pollut Res. 2019;26(29):29930–29945.

Khan BA, Akhtar N, Menaa A, Menaa F. A novel *Cassia fistula* (L.)-based emulsion elicits skin anti-aging benefits in humans. Cosmetics. 2015;2(4):368–383.

Kumar MS, Sripriya R, Raghavan HV, Sehgal PK. Wound healing potential of *Cassia fistula* on infected albino rat model. J Surg Res. 2006;131(2):283–298.

Mozaffarpur SA, Naseri M, Esmaeilidooki MR, et al. The effect of *Cassia fistula* emulsion on pediatric functional constipation in comparison with mineral oil: A randomized, clinical trial. DARU J Pharm Sci. 2012;20(83):1–9.

Nawaz U, Ilyas N, Ali H. Exploring lipid lowering activity of *Cassia fistula* and simvastatin, in hyperlipedimic mice. J Univ Med Dent Coll. 2019;10(2):1–6.

Nirmala A, Eliza J, Rajalakshmi M, et al. Effect of hexane extract of *Cassia fistula* barks on blood glucose and lipid profile in streptozotocin diabetic rats. Int J Pharmacol. 2008;4(4):292–296.

Sepehr F, Shirafkan H, Behzad C, et al. The effect of *Cassia fistula* L. syrup in geriatrics constipation in comparison with the lactulose: A randomized clinical trial. J Ethnopharmacol. 2022;297:115466.

Sharma DK, Sharma SK, Lonare MK, et al. Pharmacological evaluation of antipyretic, analgesic and anti-inflammatory activities of ethanolic extract of *Cassia fistula*. Indian J Anim Res. 2022;56(4):483–488.

Sheikh NW, Patel RD, Upwar NI, et al. Analgesic study of methyl alcohol extract of *Cassia fistula* Pod. J Pharmacy Res. 2010;3(9):2218–2219.

7 *Cichorium intybus* L.

Seyedeh Mahnaz Karimi

Scientific name: *Cichorium intybus* L.
Family: Asteraceae
Common names:

- **English:** Chicory, succory, coffeeweed
- **Persian:** *kāsnī*
- **Arabic:** *hindibā'*

Medicinal parts: Leaves, seeds, and roots (Figure 7.1)
Temperament (nature):

- **Fresh leaves:** Cold and wet in the first degree
- **Dried leaves:** Cold and dry in the third degree
- **Seeds:** Cold and dry in the second degree
- **Roots:** Hot in the first degree and dry in the second degree

Major chemical constituents:

- **Polysaccharide:** Inulin (up to 40%)
- **Sesquiterpenes:** Sesquiterpene lactones, especially lactucin, lactucopicrin, 8-deoxylactucin, Jacquilenin, 11β,13-dihydrolactucin, 11,13-dihydrolactucopicrin
- **Guaianolid glycosides:** Chicoroisides B and C, sonchuside C
- **Caffeic acid derivatives:** Chicoric acid, chlorogenic acid, isochlorogenic acid, dicaffeoyl tartaric acid
- **Hydroxycoumarins:** Umbelliferone
- **Flavonoids:** Hyperoside
- **Volatile oil:** Octane, octen-3-ol, 2-pentyl furan, (2*E*, 4*E*)-heptadienal, 1,8-cineole, benzene acetaldehyde, *n*-nonanal, camphor, (2*E*, 6Z)-nonadienal, (2*E*)-nonen-1-al, *n*-decanal (Street et al., 2013; Gruenwald et al., 2007)

THERAPEUTIC USE

TPM Literature

Topical application of chicory leaves on the head is helpful to relieve hot-tempered headaches. Compression with a poultice of leaves can alleviate conjunctivitis. Use of the root or seeds decoction as a mouthwash is helpful for toothache. Chicory is also a stomach tonic, especially for hot-tempered stomach, and can alleviate GI problems due to excessive accumulation of yellow bile humor, such as vomiting and diarrhea. Chicory is highly recommended for the treatment of a wide range of liver problems in TPM. The plant is a liver tonic and is useful in both hot-tempered and cold-tempered disorders of the liver. It acts as a potent liver cleanser and detoxifier so that it removes waste materials from hepatic tissues and opens obstructions. Due to improving the function of liver,

DOI: 10.1201/b22971-7

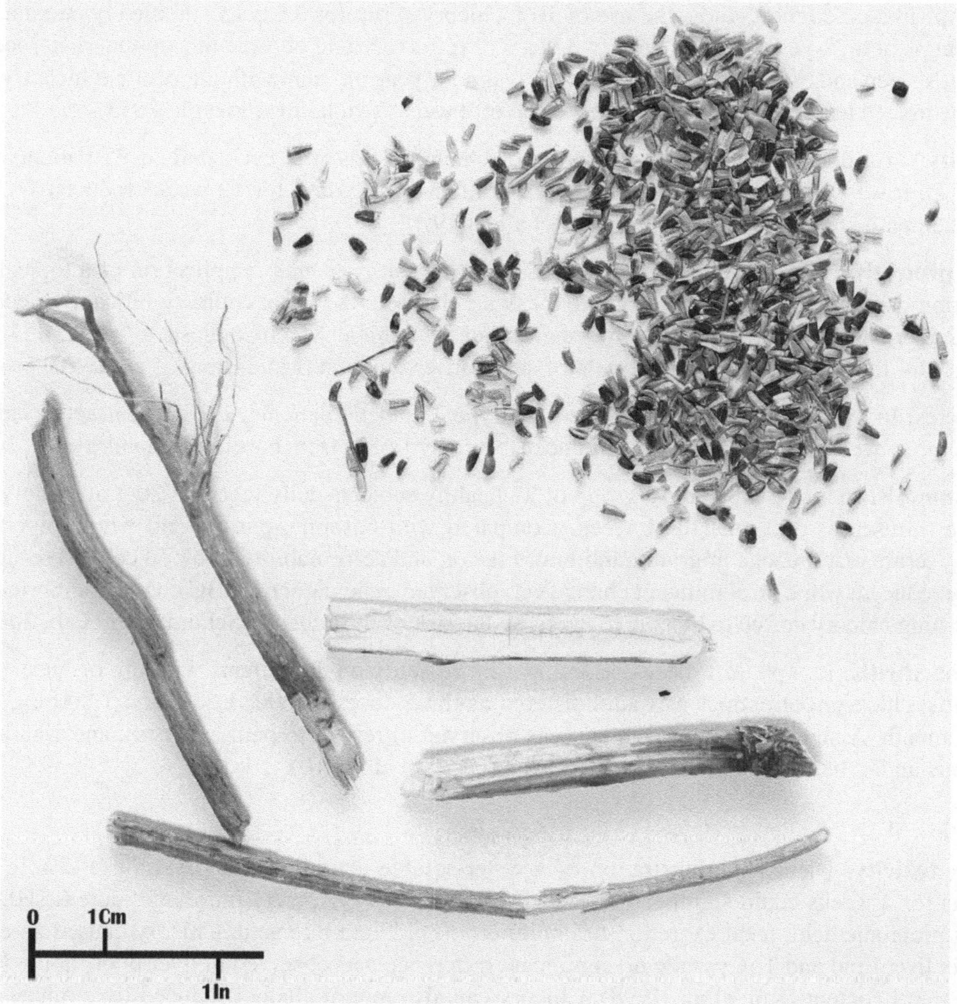

FIGURE 7.1 Chicory seeds (top) and roots (bottom).

chicory is highly recommended in jaundice, NAFLD, ascites, and peripheral edema. In addition to liver, it is also a cleanser of spleen and urinary tract. The more bitter the taste of chicory is, the better it acts as a cleanser of visceral organs. Moreover, it is useful for skin conditions caused by dysfunction of liver, e.g., urticaria and pruritus. Local use of extract and decoction is useful for healing insect bites such as bees and scorpions. Its leaf poultice regulates heart rate. Chicory seed is an appetizer and antipyretic. It can be used instead of chicory leaves for the abovementioned purposes. Chicory root is also useful for liver disorders. Furthermore, it is diuretic and blood purifier and is beneficial for visceral inflammation, ascites, and arthritis (Aghili Khorasani 1771; Avicenna 1025).

Current Evidence

Clinical Evidence

Jaundice: In an RCT on 64 term infants with neonatal jaundice, bath with 500 mL chicory root hydroethanolic extract before phototherapy, as well as 24 h and 48 after phototherapy caused a significant reduction of mean bilirubin level compared with infants who only received phototherapy (Mohammadi Pirkashani et al., 2017).

Hiccup: In a case report study, the use of 10% chicory syrup for 3 weeks completely cured a case of hiccups of a 78-year-old man with two years of refractory and chronic hiccup that disturbed the patient's sleep and eating. A second case who was a 54-year-old man with intermittent hiccup could also be treated using chicory syrup for a period of 2 weeks (Mohammadi et al., 2013).

Obesity: In a double-blind RCT, the effect of chicory seeds was evaluated in 92 patients with NAFLD. It was shown that taking chicory seed infusion (9 g/day) for 12 weeks reduced WC and BMI compared to placebo group (Ghaffari et al., 2019).

Skin protective: In a placebo-controlled RCT on 60 healthy women, application of a topical formulation containing the chicory root extract twice daily for 4 weeks could significantly decrease transepidermal water loss and improve microrelief vs. vehicle which suggests a "vitamin D-like" activity for the plant due to improvement of skin barrier function (Maia Campos et al., 2017).

Diabetes: In a placebo-controlled RCT on 150 type 2 diabetic patients, aqueous extract of chicory seeds for 12 weeks could significantly reduce HbA1c by 1.18% from baseline (Chandra et al., 2020).

Thrombosis: In a clinical study, a group of 27 healthy subjects daily received 20 g of chicory root coffee (infused as 300 mL) for 1 week. Compared with baseline, plasma and whole blood viscosity, serum macrophage migration inhibitory factor, and deformability of blood cells were significantly reduced; while no significant change was observed in hematocrit, RBC count, and fibrinogen, suggesting chicory coffee to be able to decrease the risk of thrombosis (Schumacher et al., 2011).

Osteoarthritis: In a phase I, dose-escalating clinical study on 40 patients with hip or knee osteoarthritis, chicory root extract was administered as three doses of 600, 1,200, and 1,800 mg daily for 1 month. A significant improvement was observed in regard to pain, stiffness, and walking in patients under therapy with chicory vs. placebo (Olsen et al., 2010).

Preclinical

Liver toxicity: Dietary administration of a water-soluble extract of chicory root (1–5% in diet) to rats for 4 weeks could significantly reduce LDL-C, Apo B/Apo A1 ratio, and increase HDL-C, cecal propionic acid, fecal excretion of cholesterol, lipid, and bile acid. Chicory caused an elevation in liver lipid and TAG; while no significant difference was observed in liver phospholipids and cholesterol content (Kim et al., 1998). Chicory can also inhibit alcohol-induced liver injury (Kim et al., 2021). The intraperitoneal administration of hydroalcoholic extract of chicory leaves (100, 200 and 400 mg/kg/day) showed hepatoprotective effects in a rat model of obstructive cholestasis. Chicory extract significantly decreased PT and the serum levels of AST, ALT, TNF-α, and NO, whereas increased albumin levels compared with the control group (Moloudi et al., 2021). The hepatoprotective activity of ethanolic extract of chicory root and leaves, as well as hydromethanolic extract of chicory seeds was confirmed in acetaminophen and CCl_4-induced hepatic damage at the dose of 500 mg/kg (Gilani and Janbaz, 1994; Elgengaihi et al., 2016). Also, different fractions of the seeds ethanolic extract were evaluated in CCl_4-induced hepatotoxicity in rats which showed the methanolic fraction to be the most potent one at the dose of 500 mg/kg due to the complete repair of hepatic tissue damage (Ahmed et al., 2003). The effect of aerial parts of chicory, administered as 10% in diet, was investigated in nitrosamine-induced oxidative stress and hepatotoxicity in rats. Chicory could successfully show a significant decrease in serum and hepatic LPO, AST, ALT, ALP, GGT, bilirubin, and TC, as well as an elevation of albumin, total protein, CAT, SOD, GSH, and GR (Hassan and Yousef, 2010).

Cardiac damage: Cardioprotective effects of hydroalcoholic extract of chicory leaves were investigated in a rat model of ischemia/reperfusion in three daily doses of 50, 100 or 200 mg/kg for 14 days. Infarct size, episodes of the ventricular ectopic beat, ventricular tachycardia, and QTc shortening were all improved by chicory. It stabilized the ST segment changes and increased heart rate during ischemia (Sedighi et al., 2021).

Brain damage: In an animal model of ethanol-induced brain damage, the aqueous extract of chicory root (200 mg/kg) could significantly reduce brain cyclin B1; while improved total antioxidant capacity vs. control group (Erkec et al., 2018).

Diabetes: Aqueous chicory seed extract (125 mg/kg) could improve renal damage upon 21 days of administration in STZ and STZ/niacinamide-induced type 2 diabetes in rats, evident by reduction of urinary α1-microgobulin, serum uric acid, and glomerular diameter vs. control. Metformin was more effective in case of uric acid, BUN, and urea (Pourfarjam et al., 2017). In another animal study using STZ-induced model of diabetes, chicory root extract (125 mg/kg/day) could significantly decrease FBS, TAG, TC, and LDL-C, along with a significant elevation of HDL-C, GSH, and SOD (Samarghandian et al., 2013). In another similar animal study, chicory whole plant ethanolic extract (125 mg/kg/day) in STZ-induced diabetic rats showed hypoglycemic and hypolipidemic effects by decreasing FBS, TAG, and TC, without any change in FPI (Pushparaj et al., 2007).

Gout: In a monosodium urate crystal-induced model of gout in rats, animals were orally administered with extract of chicory aerial parts (15 or 7.5 g/kg) or colchicine. The results confirmed that chicory extract can decrease ankle swelling and inflammation by inhibiting the NF-κB and NLRP3 signaling pathways (Wang et al., 2019).

Peptic ulcer: Chicory root extract (25 and 50 mg/kg daily), administered as a prophylaxis for 7 days, showed gastroprotective effect on pylorus ligation-induced peptic ulcer in rats due to the modulatory and cytoprotective properties on the secretory activity of the stomach (Krylova et al., 2015).

Poor appetite: Treatment of mice with a chicory decoction (equivalent to 7 mg of roasted root per animal), daily for 30 days, demonstrated significant prebiotic properties of chicory root via modulation of gut microbiota such as *Alloprevotella*, *Oscillibacter*, *Alistipes*, and *Blautia* (Foure et al., 2018).

ADVERSE REACTIONS

TPM Literature

Chicory leaf may worsen cough and should be used with sugar or sweet violet syrup. Chicory seed has a bad taste and induces nausea. Moreover, it is harmful to the spleen. Its management is by oxymel and fragrant herbs/spices (Aghili Khorasani 1771).

Current Evidence

Chicory in food amounts is likely safe. Occupational asthma and allergic skin reactions (rash and contact dermatitis) are reported due to the presence of sesquiterpene lactone compounds in the fresh, unroasted plant material. Cross sensitivity may occur with other plants of the Asteraceae family (Ulbricht, 2010; Gardner and McGuffin, 2013).

Due to induction of hypoglycemia in animal studies, diabetic patients are recommended to monitor their blood sugar (Gardner and McGuffin, 2013). Also, patients with gallbladder stone should be cautious due to bile-stimulating properties of chicory (Ulbricht, 2010).

Loss of appetite, weight loss, and myalgic encephalomyelitis are also reported. Mild GI complications (bloating, flatulence) may occur (Ulbricht, 2010). An inulin-rich soluble chicory extract was well tolerated using 8.1 g/day dose (containing 5 g inulin) in healthy individuals, but a 14 g daily dose (containing 7.8 g inulin) caused mild GI discomfort. GI discomfort by inulin is usually tolerable up to 20 g daily dose (Ripoll et al., 2010).

CONTRAINDICATIONS

TPM Literature

None.

Current Evidence

None.

PREGNANCY AND LACTATION

TPM Literature

None.

Current Evidence

Chicory should not be taken during pregnancy due to the possibility of abortion (Ulbricht, 2010).

DRUG INTERACTION

None.

METHOD OF ADMINISTRATION

TPM Literature

Its decoction (leaves) is administered orally for liver and digestive system disorders. Mouthwash with leaves decoction is recommended for mouth and throat problems. For topical administration, the dried or fresh plant material can be used as a poultice or the decoction may be used as a compress (Aghili Khorasani 1771).

Current Evidence

It is recommended to prepare an infusion by adding 2–4 g drug to the hot water and boiling for 10 minutes, then straining. A tea is prepared by brewing 2–4 g of the whole herb with 150–250 mL boiling water and then straining it after 10 minutes (Gruenwald et al., 2007).

DOSAGE

A common daily dosage is 3–6 g of the root. 2–4 g whole herb is recommended as an infusion (Gruenwald et al., 2007). While there is no advice about daily dose of chicory seed in modern phytotherapy, the recommended dose in TPM has been 6 g (Aghili Khorasani 1771).

REFERENCES

Aghili Khorasani MH 1771. *Makhzan-al-Adviah* (*The treasury of drugs*) (rewritten by Shams Ardakani MR, Rahimi R, Farjadmand F, 1st ed.). Tehran: Tehran University of Medical Sciences; 2009.

Ahmed B, Al-Howiriny TA, Siddiqui AB. Antihepatotoxic activity of seeds of *Cichorium intybus*. J Ethnopharmacol. 2003;87(2–3):237–240.

Avicenna 1025. *Al-Qanoon fi al-Tibb* (*The canon of medicine*) (rewritten by Masoudi A, ed.). Tehran: Almaei; 2015.

Chandra K, Jain V, Jabin A, et al. Effect of *Cichorium intybus* seeds supplementation on the markers of glycemic control, oxidative stress, inflammation, and lipid profile in type 2 diabetes mellitus: A randomized, double-blind placebo study. Phytother Res. 2020;34(7):1609–1618.

Elgengaihi S, Mossa AT, Refaie AA, Aboubaker D. Hepatoprotective efficacy of *Cichorium intybus* L. extract against carbon tetrachloride-induced liver damage in rats. J Diet Suppl. 2016;13(5):570–584.

Erkec OE, Arihan O, Colcimen N, et al. Effects of *Cichorium intybus* on serum oxidative stress, liver and kidney volume, and cyclin B1 and Bcl-2 levels in the brains of rats with ethanol induced damage. Mol Cell Biol. 2018;64(7):30–35.

Foure M, Dugardin C, Foligne B, et al. Chicory roots for prebiotics and appetite regulation: A pilot study in mice. J Agric Food Chem. 2018;66(25):6439–6449.

Gardner Z, McGuffin M, eds. *American Herbal Products Association's botanical safety handbook*. Boca Raton: CRC Press; 2013.

Ghaffari A, Rafraf M, Navekar R, et al. Turmeric and chicory seed have beneficial effects on obesity markers and lipid profile in non-alcoholic fatty liver disease (NAFLD). Int J Vitam Nutr Res. 2019;89(5–6):293–302.

Gilani AH, Janbaz KH. Evaluation of the liver protective potential of *Cichorium intybus* seed extract on Acetaminophen and CCl4-induced damage. Phytomedicine. 1994;1(3):193–197.

Gruenwald J, Brendler T, Jaenicke C. *PDR for herbal medicines*. Montvale: Thomson Reuters; 2007.

Hassan HA, Yousef MI. Ameliorating effect of chicory (*Cichorium intybus* L.)-supplemented diet against nitrosamine precursors-induced liver injury and oxidative stress in male rats. Food Chem Toxicol. 2010;48(8–9):2163–2169.

Kim J, Kim MJ, Lee JH, et al. Hepatoprotective effects of the *Cichorium intybus* root extract against alcohol-induced liver injury in experimental rats. Evid-Based Complement Altern Med. 2021;2021:6643345.

Kim M, Shin HK. The water-soluble extract of chicory influences serum and liver lipid concentrations, cecal short-chain fatty acid concentrations and fecal lipid excretion in rats. J Nutr. 1998;128(10):1731–1736.

Krylova SG, Vymyatnina ZK, Zueva EP, et al. Effects of *Cichorium intybus* L. root extract on secretory activity of the stomach in health and ulcer disease. Bull Exp Biol Med. 2015;159(5):638–642.

Maia Campos PM, Mercurio GD, Melo OM, Closs-Gonthier B. *Cichorium intybus* root extract: A "vitamin D-like" active ingredient to improve skin barrier function. J Dermatolog Treat. 2017;28(1):78–81.

Mohammadi PL, Asghari G, Marofi M, Barekatain B. Effect of chicory extract bath on neonatal bilirubin levels: A randomized clinical trial study. Int J Pediatr. 2017;5(12):6679–6688.

Mohammadi Q, Minae MB, Somi MH, et al. Novel use of chicory for the treatment of hiccups in liver obstruction in Iranian traditional medicine. Iran Red Crescent Med J. 2013;15(11):e6647.

Moloudi MR, Hassanzadeh K, Abdi M, et al. Hepatoprotective effect of the hydroalcoholic extract of *Cichorium intybus* in a rat model of obstructive cholestasis. Arab J Gastroenterol. 2021;22(1):34–39.

Olsen NJ, Branch VK, Jonnala G, et al. Phase 1, placebo-controlled, dose escalation trial of chicory root extract in patients with osteoarthritis of the hip or knee. BMC Musculoskelet Disord. 2010;11(1):156.

Pourfarjam Y, Rezagholizadeh L, Nowrouzi A, et al. Effect of *Cichorium intybus* L. seed extract on renal parameters in experimentally induced early and late diabetes type 2 in rats. Renal Failure. 2017;39(1):211–221.

Pushparaj PN, Low HK, Manikandan J, et al. Anti-diabetic effects of *Cichorium intybus* in streptozotocin-induced diabetic rats. J Ethnopharmacol. 2007;111(2):430–434.

Ripoll C, Flourié B, Megnien S, et al. Gastrointestinal tolerance to an insulin-rich soluble roasted chicory extract after consumption in healthy subjects. Nutrition. 2010;26(7–8):799–803.

Samarghandian S, Borji A, Hidar Tabasi S. Effects of *Cichorium intybus* linn on blood glucose, lipid constituents and selected oxidative stress parameters in streptozotocin-induced diabetic rats. Cardiovasc Hematol Disord Drug Targets. 2013;13(3):231–236.

Schumacher E, Vigh É, Molnár V, et al. Thrombosis preventive potential of chicory coffee consumption: A clinical study. Phytother Res. 2011;25(5):744–748.

Sedighi M, Ghorbanzadeh V, Abaszadeh S, et al. Up-regulation of chemokine receptor type 4 expression in the ischemic reperfused heart by alcoholic extract of *Cichorium intybus* rescue the heart from ischemia injury in male rat. J Pharm Pharmacol. 2021;73(10):1351–1360.

Street RA, Sidana J, Prinsloo G. *Cichorium intybus*: Traditional uses, phytochemistry, pharmacology, and toxicology. Evid-Based Complement Altern Med. 2013;2013:579319.

Ulbricht CE. *Natural standard herb & supplement guide: An evidence-based reference*. St. Louis: Elsevier; 2010.

Wang Y, Lin Z, Zhang B, et al. *Cichorium intybus* L. extract suppresses experimental gout by inhibiting the NF-κB and NLRP3 signaling pathways. Int J Mol Sci. 2019;20(19):4921.

8 *Cinnamomum verum* J.Presl

Mohadeseh Ostovar and Mohammad Hashem Hashempur

Scientific name: *Cinnamomum verum* J.Presl, syn. *Cinnamomum zeylanicum* Blume
Family: Lauraceae
Common names:

- **English**: Cinnamon
- **Persian**: *dārčīnī, dārčīn*
- **Arabic**: *dārṣīnī*

Medicinal part(s): Inner bark (Figure 8.1)
Temperament (nature): Hot and dry in the second to third degree
Major chemical constituents:

- **Volatile oil:** Chief components including cinnamaldehyde, eugenol, cinnamyl acetate, cinnamyl alcohol, *o*-methoxycinnamaldehyde
- **Organic acids:** Cinnamic acid
- **Diterpenes:** Cinncassiols
- **Oligomeric proanthocyanidins:** Cinnamtannins (Gruenwald et al., 2007; Williamson et al., 2013)

THERAPEUTIC USE

TPM Literature

Cinnamon acts as a general tonic for cold-tempered people. It has positive effects on mind and brain and is recommended for feeling heaviness in head, obsession, panic, and dementia. Also, the topical use of cinnamon oil can reduce tremor. For relieving cold headaches, it is recommended to use cinnamon oil topically on forehead and temples or as aromatherapy. Respiratory symptoms including cough, catarrh, coryza, and asthma can be treated by cinnamon. Cinnamon improves vision if applied across the eyelid and can relieve eyelid twitching as a topical compress on eye. Moreover, it relieves earache and improves hearing by applying drops of cinnamon oil in the ear. It is a hepatoprotective and gastroprotective herb, enhances the digestion, and can be effective in treatment of jaundice, ascites, bloating, bad breath, and hemorrhoid. The diuretic, emmenagogue, its effectiveness on relieving uterine/pelvic pain, as well as improvement of sexual desire, makes cinnamon a good choice for genitourinary system disorders (Aghili Khorasani 1771).

Eczema, freckles, and swellings have been mentioned to be treated using cinnamon oil (Avicenna 1025). Cinnamon was prescribed in cases of infections and it was used for wound healing, especially in infected wounds. Avicenna mentioned the effectiveness of cinnamon, especially when used topically on the body surface, to reduce chills and fever (Avicenna 1025). In addition, cinnamon is known as a powerful antidote against toxins of herbal, mineral, and animal origin and was widely used as scorpion sting antidote.

DOI: 10.1201/b22971-8

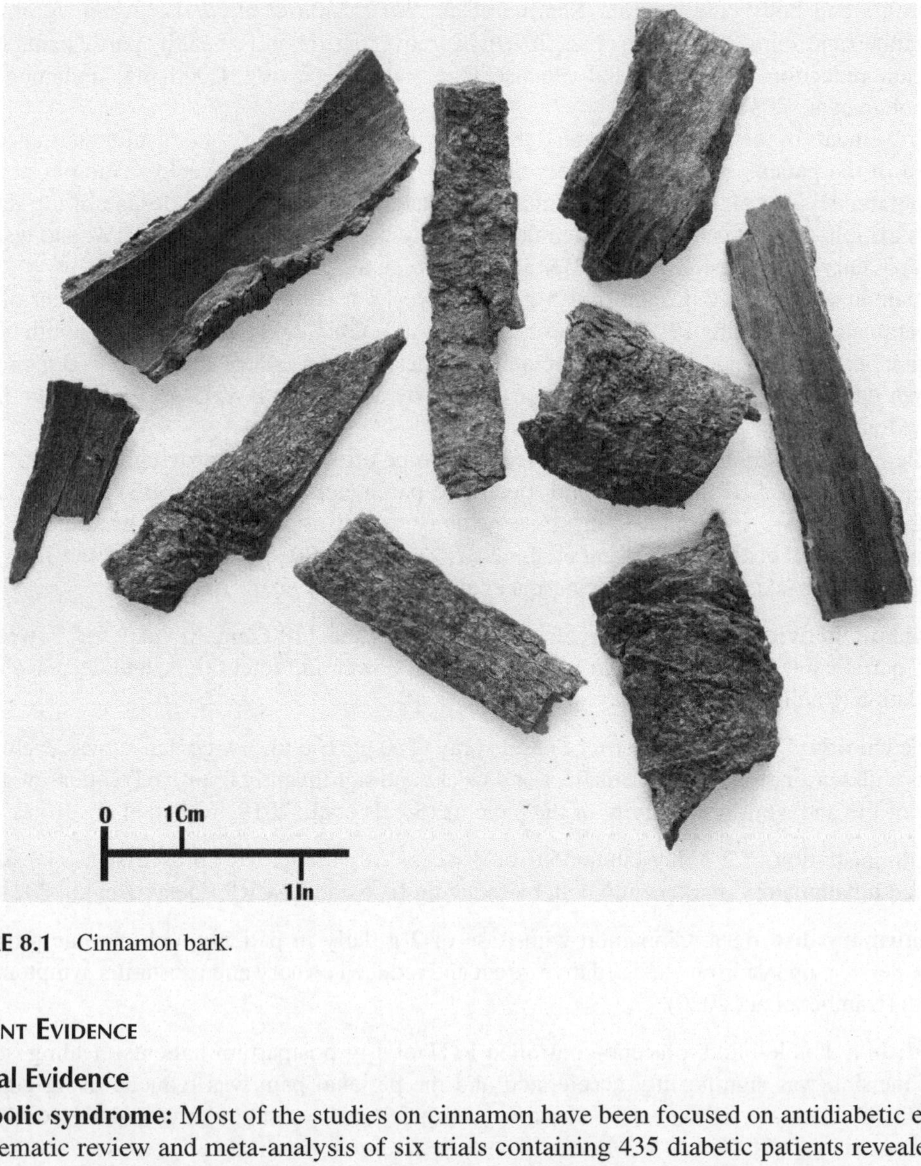

FIGURE 8.1 Cinnamon bark.

Current Evidence

Clinical Evidence

Metabolic syndrome: Most of the studies on cinnamon have been focused on antidiabetic effects. A systematic review and meta-analysis of six trials containing 435 diabetic patients revealed that using 1–6 g of cinnamon per day can significantly reduce HbA1c and FBS (Akilen et al., 2012). Also, another systematic review and meta-analysis of 10 RCTs containing 543 diabetic patients showed that cinnamon doses of 120 mg/day to 6 g/day for 4–18 weeks reduced FBS, TC, LDL-C, and TAG levels, and increased HDL-C levels (Allen et al., 2013). Several reviews have evaluated the studies on the hypoglycemic effect of cinnamon on diabetic patients and healthy volunteers (Qin et al., 2010; Deng, 2012; Anand et al., 2016; Ulbricht et al., 2011; Pathak and Sharma, 2021). The most important mechanisms of cinnamon in reducing metabolic syndrome complications include insulin-mimetic properties, inhibition of HMG-CoA reductase, reduction of ghrelin and insulin resistance, decrease in VCAM-1 expression, and antioxidant effects (Mollazadeh and Hosseinzadeh, 2016).

Clinical trials on patients with type 2 diabetes mellitus have shown that using cinnamon powder 50 mg to 6 g per day orally for 2–3 months has a positive effect on glycemic control, blood pressure, lipid profile and body composition (Sharma et al., 2012; Vafa et al., 2012; Azimi et al., 2016; Thiyagarajan and John, 2020; Zare et al., 2020). Moreover, a trial on 18 healthy participants showed significant reduction in postprandial glucose levels after receiving 1,000 mg cinnamon orally (Beejmohun et al., 2014).

Improvements of metabolic parameters, especially insulin sensitivity and insulin resistance, were reported in the patients with PCOS used cinnamon 1–1.5 g for 8–12 weeks (Wang et al., 2007; Hajimonfarednejad et al., 2018). In addition, oral intake of cinnamon with dosage of 6 g daily for 60 days exhibited significant hypolipidemic activity by improving lipid profile, BW, and waist–hip ratio in patients with primary hyperlipidemia (Agrawal et al., 2013).

Cinnamon with a daily dosage of 1.5 g for 12 weeks was effective in improvement of metabolic parameters, including FBS, lipid profile, ALT, AST, GGT, and CRP, in patients with NAFLD (Askari et al., 2014). Also, a systematic review and meta-analysis stated that using 1–3 g cinnamon orally per day for 8–16 weeks is effective on obesity by decreasing BW, BMI, WC, and fat mass in adults (Mousavi et al., 2020).

In the mentioned trials, cinnamon was reported to be effective in improving the cardiovascular parameters, such as SBP and DBP, and metabolic parameters, including FBS, HbA1c, LDL-C, HDL-C, VLDL, TAG, insulin level, insulin sensitivity, and insulin resistance (Agrawal et al., 2013; Hajimonfarednejad et al., 2018; Wang et al., 2007; Zare et al., 2020; Thiyagarajan and John, 2020; Vafa et al., 2012; Askari et al., 2014; Sharma et al., 2012; Azimi et al., 2016).

Antioxidant activity: Consumption of cinnamon with tea (100 mg/30 mL) for 2 weeks by healthy participants led to increase in total antioxidant power and total thiols, and decrease in lipid peroxidation (Ranjbar et al., 2006).

Allergic rhinitis: Cinnamon, in form of nasal spray (100 µg/100 µL, twice daily), was evaluated in patients with seasonal allergic rhinitis for 1 or 4 weeks and significantly improved clinical symptoms, quality of life and work productivity of the patients (Steels et al., 2019; Walanj et al., 2014).

MS: Administration of 2 g/day cinnamon for 8 weeks to patients with progressive-relapsing MS improved inflammatory markers and pain by reducing IL-6 and hs-CRP (Delaviz et al., 2021).

Genitourinary disorders: Cinnamon with dose of 2 g daily in patients with chronic prostatitis/chronic pelvic pain syndrome had sedative effect and reduced urinary and prostatitis symptoms after 1 month (Kamber et al., 2020).

Wound: In a double-blind, placebo-controlled RCT of 144 postpartum patients, healing of episiotomy incision was significantly accelerated and the perianal pain was reduced using cinnamon ointment (hydroethanolic extract of cinnamon with 2% concentration) twice daily for 10 days (Mohammadi et al., 2014).

Antimicrobial effect: A clinical trial on 105 dental and medical students demonstrated that using cinnamon mouthwash twice daily for 30 days can reduce plaque formation and gingivitis (Gupta and Jain, 2015). One pilot study of five patients with HIV showed that daily use of a cinnamon candy improved their oral candidiasis (Quale et al., 1996). Also, using ground cinnamon in some homogenized fruit three to four times a day by a 16-month infant with chronic salmonellosis resulted in negative stool cultures after 1 month (Rosti and Gastaldi, 2005). Additionally, 14 days consumption of cinnamon extract by 98 *H. pylori*-infected patients reduced clinical symptoms such as nausea, vomiting, diarrhea, constipation, blurred vision, headache, metallic flavor, epigastric pain, burp, and appetite (Imani et al., 2019).

Primary dysmenorrhea: In an RCT, administration of 1,260 mg/day cinnamon to 114 patients with primary dysmenorrhea in the first 24–72 h of the menstruation cycle reduced the severity and duration of pain, nausea, and vomiting. The effect was significantly higher than placebo, but lower than ibuprofen (1,200 mg/day) (Jaafarpour et al., 2015b; Jaafarpour et al., 2015a). In another study, administration of 1,000 mg of cinnamon powder to 60 subjects with primary dysmenorrhea three times per day for two menstrual cycles, significantly decreased the pain in comparison with placebo (Jahangirifar et al., 2018).

PCOS: An RCT of women with PCOS revealed that using 1,500 mg/day cinnamon for 6 months improves menstrual cyclicity. Cinnamon significantly changed the ovulatory progesterone and induced ovulatory menstruation cycles in these patients (Kort and Lobo, 2014).

Headache: In a placebo-controlled RCT, 50 patients with migraine headache received cinnamon powder with a dose of 600 mg, three times a day for 2 months. The results demonstrated a reduction in the frequency, severity, and duration of migraine headache. Also, the serum levels of inflammatory markers, such as IL-6 and NO were significantly decreased (Zareie et al., 2020).

Functional dyspepsia: In a double-blind, placebo-controlled RCT in 60 patients with functional dyspepsia, cinnamon oil (prepared by soaking cinnamon bark in sesame oil for 40 days based on the instructions of TPM) was prepared as soft capsules and administered three times a day for 6 weeks. No significant difference was observed between placebo and cinnamon oil group which may be due to high placebo effect in subjective diseases, including dyspepsia. Thus, cinnamon, at least in the form of oral oil, is not effective for the relief of dyspepsia (Zobeiri et al., 2021).

Preclinical Evidence

Liver damage: Multiple animal studies reported the hepatoprotective effect of cinnamon at oral doses of 10, 50, 100, and 200 mg/kg daily for 7–28 days (Moselhy and Ali, 2009; Quamuddin et al., 2021; Eidi et al., 2012). Cinnamon ethanolic extract could reduce the elevated levels of AST, ALT, ALP, total bilirubin, and TC. The decreased level of albumin and total protein was also significantly restored. It reversed histological alteration of hepatic damage and preserved the histoarchitecture of the liver tissue to near normal. The possible mechanism is reported to be due to radical scavenging by polyphenol compounds. Cinnamon significantly reduced liver MDA and increased the activity of endogenous enzymatic antioxidants such as SOD and CAT.

Alzheimer's disease: Aqueous extract of cinnamon with dosage of 50, 100 and 200 mg/kg for 20 days orally and 10 mL/kg injection was studied on rats with induced Alzheimer's disease and diabetic mice with impaired memory performance (Malik et al., 2015; Mesripour et al., 2016). Cinnamon decreased the transfer latency and improved cognitive deficit, memory performance, and discrimination between a familiar object and a novel object, representing the reversal of memory impairment.

Studies reported the probable cinnamon neuroprotective mechanism as interfering multiple oxidative stress and proinflammatory pathways, inducing Alzheimer's disease epigenetic modifications, reducing the filament formation and tau aggregation, inhibiting the formation of β-amyloid polypeptide and preventing the toxic effect of them on neuronal cells which are the main features of Alzheimer's disease (Anand et al., 2016; Momtaz et al., 2018; Frydman-Marom et al., 2011; Qin et al., 2010).

Parkinson's disease: Oral administration of 100 mg/kg cinnamon and 50 or 100 mg/kg sodium benzoate for 7 days in mouse models of Parkinson's disease revealed that it can prevent dopaminergic cell death, neurotransmitter dysregulation, and motor deficits disease. The probable mechanisms of its action include affecting the oligomerization process, inhibition of the excessive proinflammatory responses, autophagy regulation and its antioxidant effect (Angelopoulou et al., 2021).

Antidote effect: Dorri et al., reviewed the studies on antidote effect of cinnamon against natural and chemical toxins and reported that cinnamon and its main constituents have antidote activity against toxins in heart, liver, brain, kidney, spleen, reproductive system, embryo, and blood. It might be due to its anti-inflammatory, radical scavenging, and antioxidant, antimicrobial, and fungicidal activities, as well as modulation of enzymes and cytokines related to detoxification (Dorri et al., 2018).

Allergic rhinitis: Positive effects of intranasal treatment with 10 and 30 μg/kg or 40 μL of constituents of the cinnamon extract for 7 days on allergic rhinitis induced in rats and mice were reported in two studies (Aswar et al., 2015; Hancı et al., 2016). After receiving treatment with cinnamon, histopathological alterations such as decreased vascular congestion and inflammatory cell infiltration of nasal mucosa were observed and serum IgE, histamine, number of nasal rubbings, and sneezing were significantly decreased.

Asthma: Evaluation of the effect of cinnamon on airway hyper-responsiveness in laboratory animals exhibited significant improvement of lung function tests and the latency time to react to an antigen. In this study, type-A procyanidine polyphenol isolated from cinnamon with dosage of 100 mg/kg was administered orally to the rats. Moreover, cinnamon showed an anti-inflammatory activity as it reduced the cough frequency, infiltration of eosinophilic and inflammatory cells and goblet cell hyperplasia in lung tissue in asthmatic animals (Kandhare et al., 2013; Gupta et al., 2014).

Diuretic effect: An *in vivo* study on the rats demonstrated the marked diuretic action of 1,500, 2,250, and 3,000 mg/kg cinnamon extract compared to furosemide via loop diuretic mechanism and moderately by carbonic anhydrase inhibitory action (Jayaweera et al., 2018).

Depression: Intraperitoneal injection of 50, 100, 200, and 400 mg/kg of cinnamon hydroalcoholic extract revealed an antidepressant effect equal to fluoxetine in a mouse model of depression (Ghaderi et al., 2018).

Wound: Topical administration of cinnamon ointment with 2% and 4% cinnamon essential oil remarkably accelerated wound healing by upregulating the IGF-1, FGF-2, and VEGF expression and increasing cell proliferation, collagen synthesis, and re-epithelialization ratio in experimentally excisional infected wound model in mice (Seyed Ahmadi et al., 2019).

Peptic ulcer: Cinnamon with dosage of 300 and 400 mg/kg orally for 7 days revealed gastroprotective effect in rats with ethanol-induced gastric ulcer. The effect of oral use of cinnamon extract was more potent than ranitidine with the probable mechanism of decrease in acid-pepsin secretion and volume of gastric juice, reduction in the length of gastric ulcer and improvement of histopathological alterations of gastric mucosa (Amr and Maysa, 2010).

Infertility and testicular damage: Testosterone, as a hormone responsible of sexual desire, was increased upon treatment with cinnamon 75 mg/kg orally for 28 weeks or 10, 20 and 200 mg/kg intraperitoneally for 14 days, according to several animal studies reports (Fathiazad et al., 2013; Ahmed et al., 2013; Hemayatkhah Jahromi et al., 2011; Arisha et al., 2020; Modaresi et al., 2009; Khaki, 2015; Alahmadi, 2020). Results revealed improvement in testicular damage and significant increase in testicle length, width, and weight, the thickness of germinal epithelium, and the sperm number, motility, and viability in treated animals (Soleimani et al., 2019).

ADVERSE REACTIONS

TPM Literature

It is harmful for individuals with hot temperament. In addition, it may trigger headaches. It is also harmful for urinary bladder. Tragacanth and Asarum can decrease these side effects (Aghili Khorasani 1771).

Current Evidence

Food and Drug Administration listed cinnamon as a "Generally Recognized as Safe" herb (Muhammad and Dewettinck, 2017). Review articles suggest cinnamon to be a safe spice as a routine flavoring agent in diet; however, when taken in large doses or long durations, it may cause some minor adverse events, mainly minor gastrointestinal symptoms and allergic reactions with self-limiting nature (Hajimonfarednejad et al., 2019). Also, a systematic review including clinical studies on cinnamon suggest that there was no significant toxic or side effects between cinnamon group and placebo group regardless of dose and duration (Gu et al., 2022). Moreover, another study suggests that cinnamon toxicity is related to some of its phytochemicals that may exert their adverse effect at a dose of more than 3 g/kg (Singh et al., 2021).

There are many case reports about topical contact dermatitis (especially on the mouth or face) from cinnamon, its essential oil, and its active ingredients (Gardner and McGuffin, 2013).

CONTRAINDICATIONS

TPM Literature

None.

Current Evidence

Cinnamon should be avoided in those who have allergy or hypersensitivity to it or any members of the Lauraceae family, its ingredients, and/or Balsam of Peru (Ulbricht, 2010).

PREGNANCY AND LACTATION

TPM Literature

Cinnamon is an emmenagogue and mechanistically, it may induce abortion. It is mentioned as an abortifacient agent and is contraindicated in pregnancy.

Current Evidence

Its use during pregnancy is contraindicated. However, no concern has been identified for use during lactation (Gruenwald et al., 2007; Gardner and McGuffin, 2013).

DRUG INTERACTIONS

Antidiabetics: Cinnamon may interfere with the control of diabetes by conventional antidiabetic drugs, but controlled studies do not appear to support this suggestion (Williamson et al., 2013).

METHOD OF ADMINISTRATION

TPM Literature

It is commonly used orally as powder or decoction. A solution made from its powder and vinegar can be used for skin diseases. Also, topical use of its oil (made by adding cinnamon to olive oil and exposing it to sunlight for 40 days and then filtering) can be prescribed for tremor, fever and chills, and cold headaches. Its poultice may be used for hemorrhoid treatment. Aromatic water (distillate) may also be used orally and is said to have a faster effect than the plant powder (Aghili Khorasani 1771; Avicenna 1025).

Current Evidence

It is recommended as powder or infusion. Usually, hot water should be poured on its bark and strained after 10 minutes. Its drops and compound preparations can be used as bath additives (Gruenwald et al., 2007).

DOSAGE

1.5–4 g/day of its bark powder or one cup of its tea/infusion at mealtimes (2–3 times per day) can be used orally. Its essential oil may be used from 0.05 to 0.2 g (Gruenwald et al., 2007).

REFERENCES

Aghili Khorasani MH 1771. *Makhzan-al-Adviah* (*The treasury of drugs*) (rewritten by Shams Ardakani MR, Rahimi R, Farjadmand F, 1st ed.). Tehran: Tehran University of Medical Sciences; 2009.

Agrawal YB, Akhtar J, Shoaib M, Haque A. Clinical evaluation of Safoof-e-Darchini (*Cinnamomum zeylanicum* Blum.) in primary hyperlipidaemia. Hamdard Med. 2013;56(3):50–60.

Ahmed SA, Mohammad AA, Saadoon AH. Role of cinnamon extract on blood glucose and testosterone levels. Eng Technol J. 2013;31(1):8–13.

Akilen R, Tsiami A, Devendra D, Robinson N. Cinnamon in glycaemic control: Systematic review and meta-analysis. Clin Nutr. 2012;31(5):609–615.

Alahmadi BA. Effect of herbal medicine on fertility potential in experimental animals: An update review. Mater Socio Med. 2020;32(2):140–147.

Allen RW, Schwartzman E, Baker WL, et al. Cinnamon use in type 2 diabetes: An updated systematic review and meta-analysis. Ann Fam Med. 2013;11(5):452–459.

Amr AR, Maysa ME. Anti-ulcer effect of cinnamon and chamomile aqueous extracts in rat models. J Am Sci. 2010;6(12):209–216.

Anand V, Kumar S, Hedina A. *Cinnamomum zeylanicum* Linn: The spice with multi potential. Sys Rev Pharm. 2016;7(1):14–29.

Angelopoulou E, Paudel YN, Piperi C, Mishra A. Neuroprotective potential of cinnamon and its metabolites in Parkinson's disease: Mechanistic insights, limitations, and novel therapeutic opportunities. J Biochem Mol Toxicol. 2021;35(4):e22720.

Arisha SM, Sakr SA, Abd-Elhaseeb FR. *Cinnamomum zeylanicum* alleviate testicular damage induced by high fat diet in albino rats: Histological and ultrastructural studies. Heliyon. 2020;6(11):e05584.

Askari F, Rashidkhani B, Hekmatdoost A. Cinnamon may have therapeutic benefits on lipid profile, liver enzymes, insulin resistance, and high-sensitivity C-reactive protein in nonalcoholic fatty liver disease patients. Nutr Res. 2014;34(2):143–148.

Aswar UM, Kandhare AD, Mohan V, Thakurdesai PA. Anti-allergic effect of intranasal administration of type-A procyanidin polyphenols based standardized extract of cinnamon bark in ovalbumin sensitized BALB/c mice. Phytother Res. 2015;29(3):423–433.

Avicenna 1025. *Al-Qanoon fi al-Tibb* (*The canon of medicine*) (rewritten by Masoudi A, ed.). Tehran: Almaei; 2015.

Azimi P, Ghiasvand R, Feizi A, et al. Effect of cinnamon, cardamom, saffron and ginger consumption on blood pressure and a marker of endothelial function in patients with type 2 diabetes mellitus: A randomized controlled clinical trial. Blood Press. 2016;25(3):133–140.

Beejmohun V, Peytavy-Izard M, Mignon C, Muscente-Paque D, Deplanque X, Ripoll C, Chapal N. Acute effect of Ceylon cinnamon extract on postprandial glycemia: Alpha-amylase inhibition, starch tolerance test in rats, and randomized crossover clinical trial in healthy volunteers. BMC Complement Altern Med. 2014;14(1):351–362.

Delaviz E, Salehi M, Ahmadi A, et al. Effect of cinnamon on inflammatory factors, pain and anthropometric indices in progressive-relapsing multiple sclerosis patients: A randomized controlled trial. Jundishapur J Nat Pharm Prod. 2021;16(1):e14505.

Deng R. A review of the hypoglycemic effects of five commonly used herbal food supplements. Recent Pat Food Nutr Agric. 2012;4(1):50–60.

Dorri M, Hashemitabar S, Hosseinzadeh H. Cinnamon (*Cinnamomum zeylanicum*) as an antidote or a protective agent against natural or chemical toxicities: A review. Drug Chem Toxicol. 2018;41(3):338–351.

Eidi A, Mortazavi P, Bazargan M, Zaringhalam J. Hepatoprotective activity of cinnamon ethanolic extract against CCI4-induced liver injury in rats. EXCLI J. 2012;11:495–507.

Fathiazad F, Khaki A, Nouri M, Afshin KA. Effect of *Cinnamon zeylanicum* on serum testosterone and antioxidants levels in rats. Int J Women's Health Reprod Sci. 2013;1(1):495–507.

Frydman-Marom A, Levin A, Farfara D, et al. Orally administrated cinnamon extract reduces β-amyloid oligomerization and corrects cognitive impairment in Alzheimer's disease animal models. PloS One. 2011;6(1):e16564.

Gardner Z, McGuffin M (eds.). *American Herbal Products Association's botanical safety handbook.* Boca Raton: CRC Press; 2013.

Ghaderi H, Rafieian M, Nezhad H. Effect of hydroalcoholic *Cinnamomum zeylanicum* extract on reserpine-induced depression symptoms in mice. Pharmacophore. 2018;9(2):35–44.

Gruenwald J, Brendler T, Jaenicke C. *PDR for herbal medicines*. Montvale: Thomson Reuters; 2007.

Gu DT, Tung TH, Jiesisibieke ZL, et al. Safety of cinnamon: an umbrella review of meta-analyses and systematic reviews of randomized clinical trials. Front Pharmacol. 2022;12:790901.

Gupta A, Sharma PK, Sharma R, et al. Preparation and assessment of antiasthmatic activity of different extract of *Ipomoea aquatica*, *Cinnamomum zeylanicum*, and *Piper longum* containing polyherbal formuation. World J Pharm Res. 2014;4(1):801–808.

Gupta D, Jain A. Effect of cinnamon extract and chlorhexidine gluconate (0.2%) on the clinical level of dental plaque and gingival health: A 4-week, triple-blind randomized controlled trial. J Int Acad Periodontol. 2015;17(3):91–98.

Hajimonfarednejad M, Nimrouzi M, Heydari M, et al. Insulin resistance improvement by cinnamon powder in polycystic ovary syndrome: A randomized double-blind placebo controlled clinical trial. Phytother Res. 2018;32(2):276–283.

Hajimonfarednejad M, Ostovar M, Raee MJ, et al. Cinnamon: A systematic review of adverse events. Clin Nutr. 2019;38(2):594–602.

Hancı D, Altun H, Cetinkaya EA, et al. Cinnamaldehyde is an effective anti-inflammatory agent for treatment of allergic rhinitis in a rat model. Int J Pediatr Otorhinolaryngol. 2016; 84:81–87.

Hemayatkhah Jahromi V, Parivar K, Forozanfar M. The effect of cinnamon extract on spermatogenesis hormonal axis of pituitary gonad in mice. Iran J Appl Anim Sci. 2011;1(2):99–103.

Imani G, Dastan D, Imani B, Mehrpooya M. Effects of cinnamon extract on complications of treatment and eradication of *Helicobacter pylori* in infected people. J HerbMed Pharmacol. 2019;9(1):55–60.

Jaafarpour M, Hatefi M, Khani AL, Khajavikhan J. Comparative effect of cinnamon and ibuprofen for treatment of primary dysmenorrhea: A randomized double-blind clinical trial. J Clin Diagn Res. 2015a;9(4):QC04–07.

Jaafarpour M, Hatefi M, Najafi F, et al. The effect of cinnamon on menstrual bleeding and systemic symptoms with primary dysmenorrhea. Iran Red Crescent Med J. 2015b;17(4):e27032.

Jahangirifar M, Taebi M, Dolatian M. The effect of cinnamon on primary dysmenorrhea: A randomized, double-blind clinical trial. Complement Ther Clin Pract. 2018; 33:56–60.

Jayaweera G, Makuloluwa T, Perera K, et al. Oral diuretic activity of hot water extract of H-grade quills of *Cinnamomum zeylanicum* Blume in rats. Int J Pharm Pharm Sci. 2018;10(10):114–118.

Kamber HM, Al-Marzooq TJ, Hussein MA, et al. The use of cinnamon (Cinnamomum bark) for patients with chronic prostatitis/chronic pelvic pain syndrome: A randomized controlled trial. Open Access Maced J Med Sci. 2020;8(B):439–445.

Kandhare AD, Bodhankar SL, Singh V, et al. Anti-asthmatic effects of type-A procyanidine polyphenols from cinnamon bark in ovalbumin-induced airway hyperresponsiveness in laboratory animals. Biomed Aging Pathol. 2013;3(1):23–30.

Khaki A. Effect of *Cinnamomum zeylanicumon* on spermatogenesis. Iran Red Crescent Med J. 2015;17(2):e18668.

Kort DH, Lobo RA. Preliminary evidence that cinnamon improves menstrual cyclicity in women with polycystic ovary syndrome: A randomized controlled trial. Am J Obstet Gynecol. 2014;211(5):487–e1.

Malik J, Munjal K, Deshmukh R. Attenuating effect of standardized lyophilized *Cinnamomum zeylanicum* bark extract against streptozotocin-induced experimental dementia of Alzheimer's type. J Basic Clin Physiol Pharmacol. 2015;26(3):275–285.

Mesripour A, Moghimi F, Rafieian-Kopaie M. The effect of *Cinnamomum zeylanicum* bark water extract on memory performance in alloxan-induced diabetic mice. Res Pharm Sci. 2016;11(4):318–323.

Modaresi M, Messripour M, Rajaei R. The effect of cinnamon (bark) extract on male reproductive physiology in mice. Armaghane Danesh. 2009;14(1):67–77.

Mohammadi A, Mohammad-Alizadeh-Charandabi S, Mirghafourvand M, et al. Effects of cinnamon on perineal pain and healing of episiotomy: A randomized placebo-controlled trial. J Integr Med. 2014;12(4):359–366.

Mollazadeh H, Hosseinzadeh H. Cinnamon effects on metabolic syndrome: A review based on its mechanisms. Iran J Basic Med Sci. 2016;19(12):1258–1270.

Momtaz S, Hassani S, Khan F, et al. Cinnamon, a promising prospect towards Alzheimer's disease. Pharmacol Res. 2018;130:241–258.

Moselhy SS, Ali HK. Hepatoprotective effect of cinnamon extracts against carbon tetrachloride induced oxidative stress and liver injury in rats. Biol Res. 2009;42(1):93–98.

Mousavi SM, Rahmani J, Kord-Varkaneh H, et al. Cinnamon supplementation positively affects obesity: A systematic review and dose-response meta-analysis of randomized controlled trials. Clin Nutr. 2020;39(1):123–133.

Muhammad DR, Dewettinck K. Cinnamon and its derivatives as potential ingredient in functional food: A review. Int J Food Prop. 2017;20(supl. 2):2237–2263.

Pathak R, Sharma H. A review on medicinal uses of *Cinnamomum verum* (cinnamon). J Drug Deliv Ther. 2021;11(6S):161–166.

Qin B, Panickar KS, Anderson RA. Cinnamon: Potential role in the prevention of insulin resistance, metabolic syndrome, and type 2 diabetes. J Diabetes Sci Technol. 2010;4(3):685–693.

Quale JM, Landman D, Zaman MM, et al. In vitro activity of *Cinnamomum zeylanicum* against azole resistant and sensitive *Candida* species and a pilot study of cinnamon for oral candidiasis. Am J Chin Med. 1996;24(2):103–109.

Quamuddin M, Kumar S, Kumar P, Haque MR. Protective effect of cinnamomum zeylanicum bark against aceta-minophen induced hepatotoxicity in albino rats. Int J Pharm Sci Res. 2021;12(2):1074–1081.

Ranjbar A, Ghasmeinezhad S, Zamani H, et al. Antioxidative stress potential of *Cinnamomum zeylanicum* in humans: A comparative cross-sectional clinical study. Clin Pract. 2006;3(1):113–117.

Rosti L, Gastaldi G. Chronic salmonellosis and cinnamon. Pediatrics. 2005;116(4):1057.

Seyed Ahmadi SG, Farahpour MR, Hamishehkar H. Topical application of *Cinnamon verum* essential oil accelerates infected wound healing process by increasing tissue antioxidant capacity and keratin biosynthesis. Kaohsiung J Med Sci. 2019;35(11):686–694.

Sharma P, Sharma S, Agrawal RP, et al. A randomized double blind placebo control trial of cinnamon supplementation on glycemic control and lipid profile in type 2 diabetes mellitus. Aust J Herb Med. 2012;24(1):4–9.

Singh N, Rao AS, Nandal A, et al. Phytochemical and pharmacological review of *Cinnamomum verum* J. Presl-a versatile spice used in food and nutrition. Food Chem. 2021;338:127773.

Soleimani P, Chegini R, Sadeghi M, et al. Evaluation of hydroalcoholic extract of cinnamon effect on testicular tissue and fertility of busulfan-induced oligo-spermic model rats. J Babol Univ Med Sci. 2019;21(1):196–201.

Steels E, Steels E, Deshpande P, et al. A randomized, double-blind placebo-controlled study of intranasal standardized cinnamon bark extract for seasonal allergic rhinitis. Complement Ther Med. 2019;47:102198.

Thiyagarajan S, John S. Comparative study on the efficacy of *Cinnamomum zeylanicum* capsule and infusion on serum cholesterol level of subjects with type 2 diabetes. Hmlyn Jr Health Sci. 2020:32–36.

Ulbricht C, Seamon E, Windsor RC, et al. An evidence-based systematic review of cinnamon (*Cinnamomum* spp.) by the natural standard research collaboration. J Diet Suppl. 2011;8(4):378–454.

Vafa M, Mohammadi F, Shidfar F, et al. Effects of cinnamon consumption on glycemic status, lipid profile and body composition in type 2 diabetic patients. Int J Prev Med. 2012;3(8):531–536.

Valdivieso-Ugarte M, Gomez-Llorente C, Plaza-Díaz J, Gil Á. Antimicrobial, antioxidant, and immunomodulatory properties of essential oils: A systematic review. Nutrients. 2019;11(11):2786.

Walanj S, Walanj A, Mohan V, Thakurdesai PA. Efficacy and safety of the topical use of intranasal cinnamon bark extract in seasonal allergic rhinitis patients: A double-blind placebo-controlled pilot study. J Herb Med. 2014;4(1):37–47.

Wang JG, Anderson RA, Graham III GM, et al. The effect of cinnamon extract on insulin resistance parameters in polycystic ovary syndrome: A pilot study. Fertil Steril. 2007;88(1):240–243.

Williamson E, Driver S, Baxter K (eds.). *Stockley's herbal medicines interactions*. London: Pharmaceutical Press; 2013.

Zare R, Shams M, Heydari M, et al. Analysis of the efficacy of cinnamon for patients with diabetes mellitus type II based on traditional Persian medicine syndrome differentiation: A randomized controlled trial. Shiraz E-Med J. 2020;21(7):e95609.

Zareie A, Sahebkar A, Khorvash F, et al. Effect of cinnamon on migraine attacks and inflammatory markers: A randomized double-blind placebo-controlled trial. Phytother Res. 2020;34(11):2945–2952.

Zobeiri M, Parvizi F, Shahpiri Z, et al. Evaluation of the effectiveness of cinnamon oil soft capsule in patients with functional dyspepsia: A randomized double-blind placebo-controlled clinical trial. Evid-Based Complement Altern Med. 2021;2021:1–7.

9 *Commiphora mukul* (Hook. ex-Stocks) Engl.

Samaneh Noroozi and Hossein Rezaeizadeh

Scientific name: *Commiphora Mukul* (Hook. ex-Stocks) Engl..
Family: Burseraceae
Common names:

- **English:** Guggul, guggal, gum guggal, gum guggulu
- **Persian:** *moql*
- **Arabic:** *muql*

Medicinal part(s): Oleo gum resin (Figure 9.1)
Temperament (nature): Hot in the third degree and dry in the second degree
Major chemical constituents:

- Insoluble gum carbohydrates (55%)
- **Soluble guggulipid (45%):** Bases (0.3%), acids (4%), nonaromatic acids (e.g., ferulic acid), aromatic acids (phenolic and nonphenolic), neutral (80%), ketonic fraction (12%) including C21 and C27 steroids such as E-guggulsterone, nonketonic diterpenes, lignans, fatty acid alcohols (Pizzorno and Murray, 2013)

THERAPEUTIC USE

TPM Literature

Guggul has laxative properties which specifically expel excess phlegm humor, especially when ground and taken orally with warm water; thus, is highly useful in phlegmatic dystemperament. It is recommended for treatment of asthma, sore throat, productive coughs, and cleansing lung sputum. It is also used as a liver tonic. Guggul is a galactagogue and emmenagogue and is useful for amenorrhea, difficult birth, uterine discharges, and uterine adhesions in the form of enema and vaginal insert. Also, it can be topically used as a poultice for hemorrhoids, nerve stiffness, muscle injuries, swelling, ecchymosis, and hematoma. Oral intake of guggul relieves low back pain, sciatic pain, and gout. It is useful in urolithiasis. Guggul is also a libido booster, both topically and orally, especially when taken with fresh milk (Aghili Khorasani 1771; Avicenna 1025).

Current Evidence

Clinical Evidence

Hyperlipidemia: Data are controversial regarding the lipid-lowering properties of guggul which may be due to small sample sizes, variation in the baseline characteristics of patients in different studies such as race, and different guggul dosages. While some clinical trials have shown a significant effect of guggul administration on the reduction of LDL-C, TAG, and TC (Singh et al., 1994),

DOI: 10.1201/b22971-9

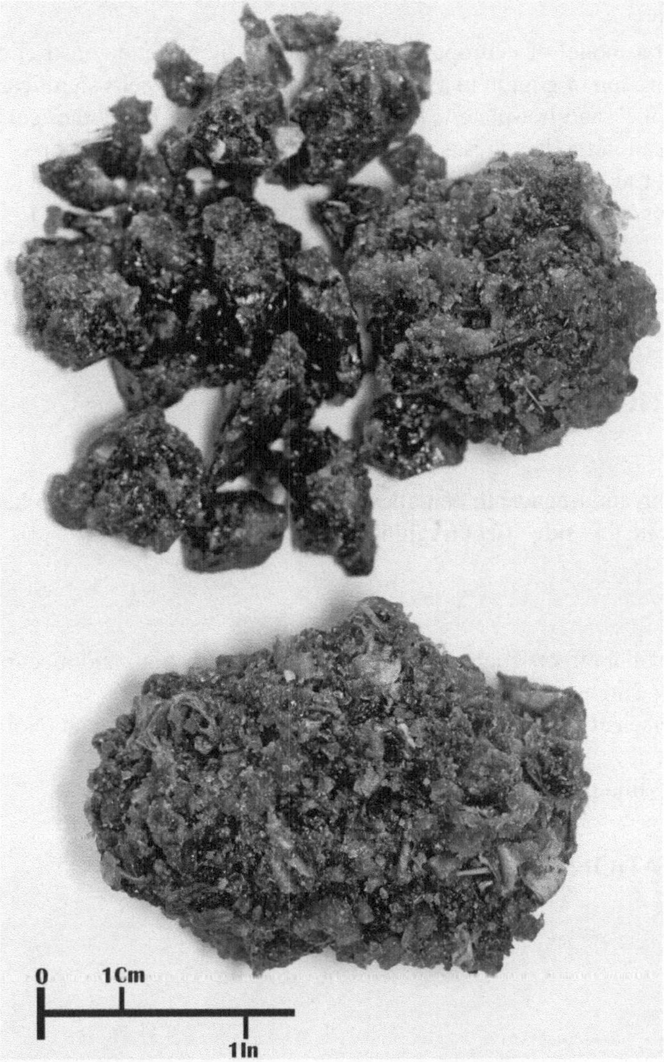

FIGURE 9.1 Guggul gum resin.

some other studies reported no significant change or even elevating effects of guggul on blood lipid levels (Szapary et al., 2003). A meta-analysis of seven RCTs involving 380 people demonstrated that guggul reduced TC and LDL-C levels in an average duration of 12 weeks (Gyawali et al., 2021); however, since the included clinical trials are rather old, future studies with larger sample size are still needed to clarify the role of guggul in hyperlipidemia.

Hemorrhoids: According to an RCT, 99 patients with grade 1 and 2 uncomplicated hemorrhoids randomly received oral guggul with a dose of 3 g/day for 1 month or a combination of lactulose and anti-hemorrhoid (lactulose syrup in laxative dose for 1 month and anti-hemorrhoid suppository daily for 10 days) as control group. Guggul was more effective than combination of lactulose syrup and anti-hemorrhoid suppository. Constipation and proctorrhagia in control group recurred significantly in 4-week follow-up after the treatment, whereas this recurrence in study group was not observed (Yousefi et al., 2013).

Preclinical Evidence

Sciatic pain: In a rat model of neuropathic pain induced by chronic constriction injury of sciatic nerve, oral administration of guggul in a dose of 200 mg/kg for 2 weeks significantly decreased pain as assessed by tail-flick and hot-plate tests (Mehta et al., 2015). In another study on sciatic nerve and spinal nerve ligation models in rats, 6-day intraperitoneal administration of 100 and 50 mg/kg of guggulipid, a neutral fraction of ethyl acetate extract of guggul, produced antinociceptive effects on the peripheral nerve injury models of neuropathic pain (Goyal et al., 2013).

Male infertility: A study in diabetic rats with sperm abnormalities showed daily gavage of 300 mg/kg guggul for 60 days increases total sperm count, sperm motility, and testosterone serum level, as well as reduction of sperms with abnormal morphology (Rezaei et al., 2020).

ADVERSE REACTIONS

TPM Literature

It is harmful for lung and tragacanth can alleviate its damage. It may be also harmful for liver and saffron can ameliorate this side effect (Aghili Khorasani 1771).

Current Evidence

Adverse gastrointestinal effects such as diarrhea, nausea, eructation, and hiccup (DerMarderosian, 2002; Spiteri, 2011; Singh et al., 1994).
Dermatologic hypersensitivity reaction (Szapary et al., 2003) and skin rash (Nohr et al., 2009).
Headache (Singh et al., 1994).
Rhabdomyolysis (Williamson et al., 2013).

CONTRAINDICATIONS

TPM Literature

None.

Current Evidence

It should be avoided in a known allergy and pregnancy (Spiteri 2011).

PREGNANCY AND LACTATION

TPM Literature

Due to emmenagogue properties, it should not be taken during pregnancy.

Current Evidence

It is contraindicated in pregnancy. There are no reports in the literature of guggul being either safe or contraindicated during lactation (Mills et al., 2006).

DRUG INTERACTIONS

Cardiovascular drugs: Absorption of propranolol and diltiazem was significantly reduced by guggul. Guggul can also potentially add to bleeding risk in patients taking anticoagulants/antiplatelet medication (DerMarderosian, 2002).

METHOD OF ADMINISTRATION

TPM Literature

It can be taken orally with water, or used topically as a poultice. It may also be used as fumigation and vaginal insert (Aghili Khorasani 1771).

Current Evidence

- **Oral:** crude oleoresin (gum guggul), alcohol extract, and petroleum ether
- **External use (gargle, rinse):** undiluted tincture (Spiteri, 2011; Pizzorno and Murray, 2013)

DOSAGE

Crude gum guggul: 10 g daily.
Alcoholic extract: 4.5 g daily.
Petroleum ether extract: 1.5 g daily (Pizzorno and Murray, 2013).
Guggulsterones: 25 mg three times daily, 50 mg twice daily (Ulbricht, 2010).

REFERENCES

Aghili Khorasani MH 1771. *Makhzan-al-Adviah* (*The treasury of drugs*) (rewritten by Shams Ardakani MR, Rahimi R, Farjadmand F, 1st ed.). Tehran: Tehran University of Medical Sciences; 2009.

Avicenna 1025. *Al-Qanoon fi al-Tibb* (*The canon of medicine*) (rewritten by Masoudi A, ed.). Tehran: Almaei; 2015.

DerMarderosian A, Beutler JA. *The review of natural products: The most complete source of natural product information*. 4th ed. St. Louis, MO: Facts and Comparisons; 2002.

Goyal S, Khilnani G, Singhvi I, et al. Guggulipid of *Commiphora mukul*, with antiallodynic and antihyperalgesic activities in both sciatic nerve and spinal nerve ligation models of neuropathic pain. Pharm Biol. 2013;51(12):1487–1498.

Gyawali D, Vohra R, Ormeh-Johnson D, et al. A systematic review and meta-analysis of ayurvedic herbal preparations for hypercholesterolemia. Medicina. 2021;57:1–24.

Mehta A, Tripathi C. *Commiphora mukul* attenuates peripheral neuropathic pain induced by chronic constriction injury of sciatic. Nutr Neur Sci. 2015;18(3):97–102.

Mills E, Dugoua JJ, Perri D, Koren G. *Herbal medicines in pregnancy and lactation: An evidence-based approach*. London: Taylor & Francis; 2006; 176–177.

Nohr L, Rasmussen L, Straand J. Resin from the mukul myrrh tree, guggul, can it be used for treating hypercholesterolemia? A randomized, controlled study. Complement Ther Med. 2009;17(1):16–22.

Pizzorno LU, Murray MT. *Natural medicine instructions for patients*. St. Louis: Elsevier; 2013; 690–693.

Rezaei AA, Salehi I, Karimi SA, et al. The effects of *Commiphora mukul* extract on spermatogenesis and testosterone levels in male diabetic rats. Clin Exp Reprod Med. 2020;47(1):34–41.

Singh R, Niaz M, Ghosh S. Hypolipidemic and antioxidant effects of *Commiphora mukul* as an adjunct to dietary therapy in patients with hypercholesterolemia. Cardiovasc Drugs Ther. 1994;8(4):659–664.

Spiteri M. *Herbal monographs including herbal medicinal products and food supplements*. Malta: Qormi; 2011; 116.

Szapary PO, Wolfe ML, Bloedon LT, et al. Guggulipid for the treatment of hypercholesterolemia: A randomized controlled trial. JAMA. 2003;290(6):765–772.

Ulbricht CE. *Natural standard herb & supplement guide: An evidence-based reference*. Elsevier Mosby; 2010.

Williamson E, Driver S, Baxter K (eds.). *Stockley's herbal medicines interactions*. London: Pharmaceutical Press; 2013.

Yousefi M, Vaez Mahdavi MR, Hosseini SM, et al. Clinical evaluation of *Commiphora mukul*, a botanical resin, in the management of hemorrhoids: A randomized controlled trial. Pharmacogn Mag. 2013;8(31):350–356.

10 *Coriandrum sativum* L.

Zahra Taghipour

Scientific name: *Coriandrum sativum* L.
Family: Apiaceae
Common names:

- **English:** Coriander
- **Persian:** *gešnīz*
- **Arabic:** *kuzbarah*

Medicinal part(s): Fruit and leaf (Figure 10.1)
Temperament (nature): Cold and dry in the third degree
Major chemical constituents:
Leaf:

- **Volatile oil (0.1%):** Decanal (19.09%), trans-2-decenal (17.54%), 2-decen-1-ol (12.33%) and cyclodecane (12.15%), cis-2-dodecenal (10.72%), dodecanal (4.1%), dodecan-1-ol (3.13%)
- **Flavonoids (0.13–10.71%):** Quercetin, kaempferol, among others.
- Phenolic acids (7.24–13.51%)
- Coumarins (1.4–6.83%) (Mahleyuddin et al., 2021)

Fruit:

- **Volatile oil (0.2–1.5%):** Linalool (58.0–80.3%), γ-terpinene (0.3–11.2%), α-pinene (0.2–10.9%), p-cymene (0.1–8.1%), camphor (3.0–5.1%), and geranyl acetate (0.2–5.4%)
- **Fatty oil (13–20%):** Petroselinic acid (68.8%), linoleic acid (16.6%), oleic acid (7.5%), and palmitic acid (3.8%) (Salem et al., 2022)

THERAPEUTIC USE

TPM Literature

Drinking coriander leaves extract is hypnotic. Dropping and covering eyes with leaves prevents eyes complication induced by diseases such as smallpox and measles and also improves its yellowing. Moreover, applying it topically with milk improves eye twitch and with dried bread improves eyelid thickening and conjunctivitis. Gargling the leaves improves mouth burn and relieves toothache. Chewing the leaves eliminates the smell of wine and drunkenness. Applying powder of dried leaves strengthens the gums and stops their bleeding. Dried leaves and fruits of coriander are useful for migraine headache and palpitation. Their extract sweetened with sugar is appetizer and prevents dyspepsia and sour burps. It also relieves gastritis and thirst, improves vomiting, and suppresses libido and erection. The extract of fresh leaves can be used topically for hot-tempered tumors and

DOI: 10.1201/b22971-10

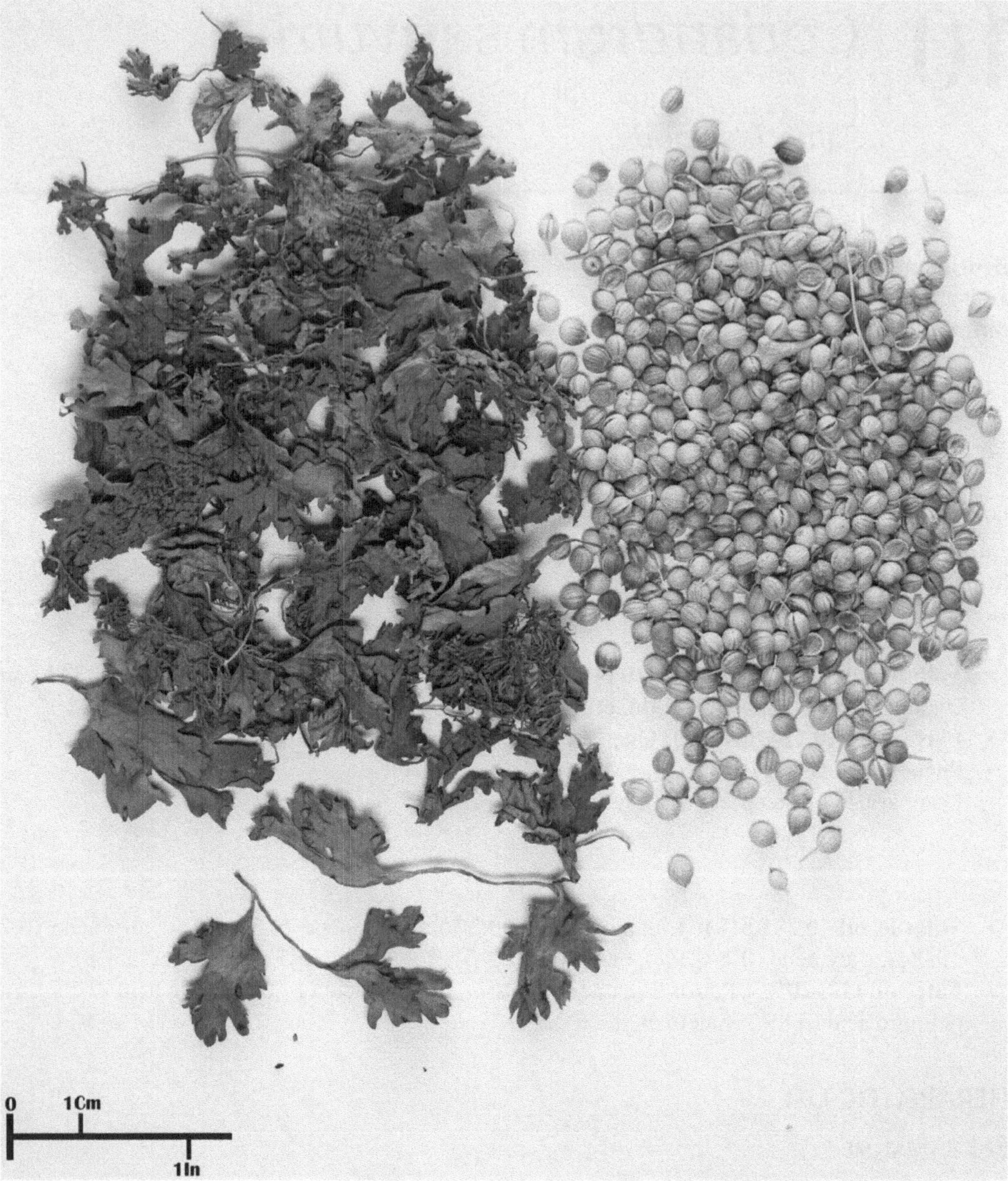

FIGURE 10.1 Coriander leaf (left) and fruit (right).

erysipelas. In combination with dried bread, it improves chronic ulcers, scabies, and itch and, in combination with barley flour, improves benign and hard tumors, topically.

Coriander fruit acts as brain, heart, and stomach tonic. Moreover, it relieves obsessive disorder, suppresses diarrhea, decreases semen volume, and improves urinary tract ulcers. Its maceration, concentrated extract or roasted fruits improves dysentery and gastroenteritis. In combination with grape juice, it increases semen volume and repels stomach worms. Topically, it stops ulcer bleeding and improves headache due to hot dystemperament. Its combination with honey and olive oil is useful for different skin pimples (Aghili Khorasani 1771; Avicenna 1025).

Current Evidence

Clinical Evidence

Dermatological disorders: In a double-blind RCT, daily consumption of 200 mg coriander fruit essential oil for 28 days reduced redness and itching induced by stinging stress. It also improved the perception of skin sensitivity and reactivity after 56 days of consumption (Kern et al., 2022). In another RCT, topical administration of ointment containing 6% coriander fruit essential oil twice daily for 28 days in 40 patients with mycosis showed highly significant improvement of the clinical signs of mycosis vs. placebo (Beikert et al., 2013).

Migraine headache: In a triple-blind RCT including 68 patients with migraine headache, administration of 15 mL coriander fruit syrup (100 mg ethanolic extract per 5 mL of syrup) three times a day during a month in intervention group vs. placebo group, in addition to 500 mg of sodium valproate per day, led to reduction in duration, severity and frequency of migraine headache (Kasmaei et al., 2016). In addition, after a 4-week follow-up, the probability of being migraine-free was significantly higher in all patients of the intervention group compared to placebo group, especially in patient less than 30 years of age (Mansouri et al., 2020).

Preclinical Evidence

Neurotoxicity: Oral administration of aqueous extracts of coriander at dose of 600 mg/kg for 60 days significantly reversed structural and functional variations in the cerebellar cortex and somatosensory cortex in lead-induced neurotoxicity in rats (Mustafa, 2021). In the same experimental model, oral administration of hydroalcoholic extract of coriander fruit at doses of 250 and 500 mg/kg for 7 days reversed lead-induced oxidative stress in different regions of rat brain (Velaga et al., 2014). In another animal study, administration of coriander leaves and stalks aqueous extract at dose of 360 mg/kg from 14th day of pregnancy to 14th day of lactation (corresponding 21 days of treatment) significantly improved spontaneous locomotor activity, palmar grip strength, balance, and motor coordination, as well as oxidative stress markers in behavioral tests in rat progeny after maternal exposure to methylmercury (Rodrigues et al., 2019).

Neuropathy: Oral administration of 50% hydroethanolic extract of coriander fruit at doses of 100, 200, and 400 mg/kg for 30 days, improved neuronal function by increasing mechanical thresholds, as well as hyperglycemia in STZ-induced diabetic neuropathic rats (Kajal and Singh, 2020).

Pain: Intraperitoneal single dose administration of 2.5 mg/kg coriander fruit essential oil in morphine-dependent mice, showed significant effects on morphine tolerance during the expression period and dependency (Barotyha et al., 2021). Intraperitoneal administration of ethyl acetate fractions of dichloromethane extracts of coriander leaves in mice at doses of 30, 100 or 300 mg/kg significantly decreased carrageenan-induced paw edema compared to control during the early phase of edema (Begnami et al., 2018).

Amnesia: Oral administration of coriander fruit extracts at three doses (100, 200, and 400 mg/kg) for 30 days led to memory boosting and regaining effects in scopolamine-induced rat model of amnesia (Kajal and Singh, 2020). Inhalation of coriander volatile oil 1% and 3% for 60 minutes period daily for 21 continuous days in beta-amyloid (1–42) rat model of Alzheimer's disease significantly decreased CAT activity and increased GSH level in the hippocampus compared to control group (Cioanca et al., 2014). The amnesic deficits (acquisition, retention and recovery) induced by scopolamine in rats was reversed dose dependently by oral administration of coriander fruit aqueous extract at doses of 100, 200, and 300 mg/kg for 5 consecutive days (Koppula and Choi, 2012).

Sedation: Administration of ethanolic extract of coriander fruit increased pentobarbital sodium-induced sleeping time at doses of 100, 150, and 200 mg/kg in comparison with control group in mice

(Alshahrani, 2016). Intraperitoneal administration of aqueous and hydroalcoholic extracts as well as the essential oil of coriander fruit at different doses of 100, 200, 400 and 600 mg/kg to male albino mice, prolonged pentobarbital-induced sleeping time compared to control group (Emamghoreishi et al., 2006). Interestingly, in the same experimental model, administration of higher doses of coriander hydroalcoholic extracts (250, 500, and 1,000 mg/kg) made no changes in sleep parameters compared to control group (Hajhashemi and Safaei, 2015).

Anxiety: Single dose intraperitoneal administration of 70% hydroethanolic extract of coriander leaves at doses of 200 and 400 mg/kg in mice, showed anxiolytic effects in a dose-dependent manner compared to control group (Harsha and Anilakumar, 2012). Oral administration of coriander fruit aqueous extract for 2 weeks at doses of 100, 200, and 400 mg/kg improved exploratory activity equivalent to diazepam as a standard drug in anxiety model induced by chronic restraint stress in mice. In addition, it restored monoamines and GABA levels to the respective baseline levels and reduced excitotoxic levels of glutamate in the hippocampus region (Sahoo and Brijesh, 2020). In another study, single dose oral administration of aqueous extract of coriander leaves at doses of 50, 100 and 200 mg/kg implied significant dose-dependent anxiolytic activity in the elevated plus maze test compared to negative control in mice (Latha et al., 2015). Anxiolytic-like property was also observed by intraperitoneal administration of aqueous extract of coriander fruit at doses of 25 mg/kg, and 50 mg/kg once daily for 10 days in elevated plus maze test (Ravindran et al., 2014). Moreover, inhalation of coriander volatile oil 1% and 3% for a 60-minute period daily for 21 continuous days increased anxiolytic/antidepressant-like behaviors in comparison to single dose interperitoneally injected diazepam at dose of 1.5 mg/kg (Cioanca et al., 2014). Intraperitoneal administration of aqueous extract of coriander fruit at doses of 50, 100 and 500 mg/kg demonstrated significant anxiolytic activity by reducing spontaneous activity and neuromuscular coordination (Emamghoreishi et al., 2005).

Myocardial damage: Oral administration of aqueous extract of coriander fruit 1 g/kg for 15 days as a treatment after, and as a pretreatment before isoproterenol-induced heart failure in rats improved the left ventricular functions and hemodynamic parameters (SBP and DBP, heart rate, and MAP) and increased baroreflex sensitivity. It also inhibited LPO, improved lipid profile, and downregulated the expression of endothelin receptors similar to simvastatin (10 mg/kg) (Dhyani et al., 2020). Cosupplementation of coriander fruit 80% methanolic extract at dose of 200 mg/kg by oral feeding for 8 weeks in high-cholesterol-diet-induced atherosclerosis in rats, alleviated pathophysiological alterations by decreasing TC, TAG, VLDL-C and LDL-C and increasing HDL-C (Patel et al., 2013). Oral pretreatment with methanolic extract of coriander fruit (200 and 300 mg/kg) for 30 days in isoproterenol-induced myocardial necrosis in rats, prevented myocardial infarction by inhibiting myofibrillar damage (Patel et al., 2012).

Testicular damage: Administration of aqueous extract of coriander fruit 25 mL/day for 42 days decreased testosterone level in mercury-induced toxicity in male rats (Abdel-Salam et al., 2018). However, concurrent daily administration of coriander ethanolic extract 250 mg/kg for 33 days increased testosterone level in lead-poisoned mice (Sharma et al., 2010).

Ulcerative colitis: Oral administration of 80% hydroethanolic extract of coriander fruit (500 and 1,000 mg/kg) and coriander essential oil (0.5 and 1 mL/kg) before colitis induction in rat model of acetic acid-induced acute colitis for 4 days, led to decrement colon weight, improvement of colon histopathology, and reduction of oxidative stress (Heidari et al., 2016).

Peptic ulcer: Pretreatment by aqueous suspension of coriander fruit at oral single dose of 500 mg/kg, was found to significantly reduce the gastric ulcers induced by necrotizing agents (ethanol, NaOH, NaCl). The plant could completely protect the histopathological changes in ethanol-treated rats, and restore gastric wall mucosa and nonprotein sulfhydryl groups in the gastric tissue. The anti-secretory activity of aqueous suspension of coriander was also demonstrated by intraduodenal administration, immediately after pylorus ligation (Al-Mofleh et al., 2006).

Dermatological effects: Topical application of 1% and 0.5% coriander 70% hydroethanolic extract for 7 consecutive days alleviated 2,4-dinitrochlorobenzene-induced contact dermatitis-like skin lesions in mice. Moreover, the Th2-mediated inflammatory cytokines, immunoglobulin E, TNF-α, IFN-γ, IL-1, IL-4, and IL-13, were significantly reduced (Park et al., 2014).

ADVERSE REACTIONS

TPM Literature

Coriander worsens respiratory diseases and if necessary, to reduce complications patients should consume soft-boiled eggs, quince syrup, and oxymel along with coriander. Excessive consumption of coriander, especially fresh leaves juice, induces amnesia, mental disorder, dizziness, dormancy, dimness of vision, dysphonia and decreases semen volume, erection, libido, and menstrual bleeding. In addition, the consumer smells coriander. For reducing and reversing side effects, after detoxifying, administration of soft-boiled egg yolk with pepper, salt and broth of fat chicken can be helpful (Aghili Khorasani 1771).

Current Evidence

Health risks or side effects are not reported upon proper administration of therapeutic dosages. There is a weak potential for sensitization (Gruenwald et al., 2007).

By topical administration of cream containing coriander fruit essential oil, irritating side effects like redness and itching was observed (Dastgheib et al., 2017).

CONTRAINDICATIONS

TPM Literature

None.

Current Evidence

None.

PREGNANCY AND LACTATION

TPM Literature

None.

Current Evidence

None.

DRUG INTERACTIONS

None.

METHOD OF ADMINISTRATION

TPM Literature

The juice of fresh leaves can be administered orally or topically. The dried leaves and fruits can be applied as powder, infusion, decoction, as well as maceration for oral or topical administration (Aghili Khorasani 1771).

Current Evidence

Powder, infusion, tincture and different extract of coriander fruit and leaves as well as essential oil of fruit can be used orally and topically (Gruenwald et al., 2007).

DOSAGE

The recommended daily dose for fruits and dried leaves is 3–5 g. The fresh leaves juice can be used up to 30 mL daily (Gruenwald et al., 2007; Aghili Khorasani 1771).

REFERENCES

Abdel-Salam AM, Al Hemaid WA, Afifi AA, et al. Consolidating probiotic with dandelion, coriander and date palm seeds extracts against mercury neurotoxicity and for maintaining normal testosterone levels in male rats. Toxicol Rep. 2018;5:1069–1077.

Aghili Khorasani MH 1771. *Makhzan-al-Adviah* (*The treasury of drugs*) (rewritten by Shams Ardakani MR, Rahimi R, Farjadmand F, 1st ed.). Tehran: Tehran University of Medical Sciences; 2009.

Al-Mofleh IA, Alhaider AA, Mossa JS, et al. Protection of gastric mucosal damage by *Coriandrum sativum* L. pretreatment in Wistar albino rats. Environ Toxicol Pharmacol. 2006;22(1):64–69.

Alshahrani AM. In vivo neurological assessment of sedative hypnotic effect of *Coriandrum sativum* L. seeds in mice. Int J Phytomed. 2016;8(1):113–116.

Avicenna 1025. *Al-Qanoon fi al-Tibb* (*The canon of medicine*) (rewritten by Masoudi A, ed.). Tehran: Almaei; 2015.

Barotyha E, Shafaroodi H, Asgarpanah J. Effect of the essential oil from coriander (*Coriandrum sativum* seeds) on morphine antinociception tolerance and withdrawal syndrome in mice. Farmacia. 2021;69(4):718–723.

Begnami AF, Spindola HM, Altgaltg R, et al. Antinociceptive and anti-edema properties of the ethyl acetate fraction obtained from extracts of *Coriandrum sativum* Linn. leaves. Biomed Pharmacother. 2018;103:1617–1622.

Beikert FC, Anastasiadou Z, Fritzen B, et al. Topical treatment of tinea pedis using 6% coriander oil in unguentum leniens: A randomized, controlled, comparative pilot study. Dermatology. 2013;226(1):47–51.

Cioanca O, Hritcu L, Mihasan M, et al. Inhalation of coriander volatile oil increased anxiolytic-antidepressant-like behaviors and decreased oxidative status in beta-amyloid (1–42) rat model of Alzheimer's disease. Physiol Behav. 2014;131:68–74.

Dastgheib L, Pishva N, Saki N, et al. Efficacy of topical *Coriandrum sativum* extract on treatment of infants with diaper dermatitis: A single blinded non-randomised controlled trial. Malaysian J Med Sci. 2017;24(4):97–101.

Dhyani N, Parveen A, Siddiqi A, et al. Cardioprotective efficacy of *Coriandrum sativum* (L.) seed extract in heart failure rats through modulation of endothelin receptors and antioxidant potential. J Diet Suppl. 2020;17(1):13–26.

Emamghoreishi M, Heidari-Hamedani G. Sedative-hypnotic activity of extracts and essential oil of Coriander seeds. Iran J Med Sci. 2006;31(1):22–27.

Emamghoreishi M, Khasaki M, Aazam MF. *Coriandrum sativum*: Evaluation of its anxiolytic effect in the elevated plus-maze. J Ethnopharmacol. 2005;96(3):365–370.

Gruenwald J, Brendler T, Jaenicke C. *PDR for herbal medicines*. Montvale: Thomson Reuters; 2007.

Hajhashemi V, Safaei A. Hypnotic effect of *Coriandrum sativum*, *Ziziphus jujuba*, *Lavandula angustifolia* and *Melissa officinalis* extracts in mice. Res Pharm Sci. 2015;10(6):477–484.

Harsha SN, Anilakumar KR. Effects of *Coriandrum sativum* extract on exploratory behaviour pattern and locomotor activity in mice: An experimental study. Int J Green Pharm. 2012;6(2):157–162.

Heidari B, Sajjadi SE, Minaiyan M. Effect of *Coriandrum sativum* hydroalcoholic extract and its essential oil on acetic acid-induced acute colitis in rats. Avicenna J Phytomed. 2016;6(2):205–214.

Kajal A, Singh R. *Coriandrum sativum* improve neuronal function via inhibition of oxidative/nitrosative stress and TNF-α in diabetic neuropathic rats. J Ethnopharmacol. 2020;263:112959.

Kasmaei HD, Ghorbanifar Z, Zayeri F, et al. Effects of *Coriandrum sativum* syrup on migraine: A randomized, triple-blind, placebo-controlled trial. Iran Red Crescent Med J. 2016;18(1):1–7.

Kern C, Gombert C, Roso A, Garcia C. Effect of the supplementation of virgin coriander seed oil on reducing reactivity in healthy women with sensitive skin: A randomized double-blind placebo-controlled pilot clinical study. Food Nutr Res. 2022;66:7730.

Koppula S, Choi DK. Anti-stress and anti-amnesic effects of *Coriandrum sativum* Linn. (Umbelliferae) extract: An experimental study in rats. Trop J Pharm Res. 2012;11(1):36–42.

Latha K, Rammohan B, Sunanda BPV, et al. Evaluation of anxiolytic activity of aqueous extract of *Coriandrum sativum* Linn. in mice: A preliminary experimental study. Pharmacognosy Res. 2015;7(suppl 1):S47–51.

Mahleyuddin NN, Moshawih S, Ming LC, et al. *Coriandrum sativum* L.: A review on ethnopharmacology, phytochemistry, and cardiovascular benefits. Molecules. 2021;27(1):209.

Mansouri S, Kazemi I, Baghestani AR, et al. Evaluating the effect of *Coriandrum sativum* syrup on being migraine-free using mixture models. Med J Islam Repub Iran. 2020;34:44.

Mustafa HN. Morphohistometric analysis of the effects of *Coriandrum sativum* on cortical and cerebellar neurotoxicity. Avicenna J Phytomed. 2021;11(6):589–598.

Park G, Kim HG, Lim S, et al. Coriander alleviates 2,4-dinitrochlorobenzene-induced contact dermatitis-like skin lesions in mice. J Med Food. 2014;17(8):862–868.

Patel D, Desai S, Gajaria T, et al. *Coriandrum sativum* L. seed extract mitigates lipotoxicity in RAW 264.7 cells and prevents atherogenic changes in rats. EXCLI J. 2013;12:313–334.

Patel D, Desai S, Gandhi HP, et al. Cardio protective effect of *Coriandrum sativum* L. on isoproterenol induced myocardial necrosis in rats. Food Chem Toxicol. 2012;50(9):3120–3125.

Ravindran A, Manohar VR, Rai M, et al. Chronic anxiolytic-like activity of aqueous extract of *Coriandrum sativum* seeds using elevated plus maze test in Swiss albino mice. Int J Pharm Pharm Sci. 2014;6(2):93–95.

Rodrigues KE, de Oliveira FR, Barbosa BRC, et al. Aqueous *Coriandrum sativum* L. extract promotes neuroprotection against motor changes and oxidative damage in rat progeny after maternal exposure to methylmercury. Food Chem Toxicol. 2019;133:110755.

Sahoo S, Brijesh S. Anxiolytic activity of *Coriandrum sativum* seeds aqueous extract on chronic restraint stressed mice and effect on brain neurotransmitters. J Funct Foods. 2020;68:103884.

Salem MA, Manaa EG, Osama N, et al. Coriander (*Coriandrum sativum* L.) essential oil and oil-loaded nano-formulations as an anti-aging potentiality via TGFβ/SMAD pathway. Sci Rep. 2022;12:6578.

Sharma V, Kansal L, Sharma A. Prophylactic efficacy of *Coriandrum sativum* (coriander) on testis of lead-exposed mice. Biol Trace Elem Res. 2010;136(3):337–354.

Velaga MK, Yallapragada PR, Williams D, et al. Hydroalcoholic seed extract of *Coriandrum sativum* (coriander) alleviates lead-induced oxidative stress in different regions of rat brain. Biol Trace Elem Res. 2014;159(1–3):351–363.

treatment of depression. The results showed that saffron administration was well comparable with fluoxetine (Khaksarian et al., 2019).

Cognitive impairment and dementia: Two meta-analyses of four and five RCTs, respectively, revealed that saffron significantly improves cognitive function measured by the Alzheimer's Disease Assessment Scale–Cognitive Subscale and Clinical Dementia Rating Scale–Sums of Boxes, compared to placebo. In addition, there was no significant difference between saffron and conventional medicine, as measured by cognitive scales such as Alzheimer's Disease Assessment Scale-Cog and Clinical Dementia Rating Scale–Sums of Boxes. Saffron nonsignificantly improved daily living function. The administered dose of saffron extract in three of the included RCTs was 30 mg/day, while one RCT administered saffron powder with a daily dose of 125 mg (Ayati et al., 2020; Avgerinos et al., 2020).

Oxidative stress: The results of a meta-analysis of seven RCTs indicated an association between saffron intake, mostly with a 30–100 mg/day of the products for a period of 4 weeks or longer, and a statistically significant decrease in MDA levels, as well as a significant increase in total antioxidant capacity. Saffron intake may have beneficial effects in improving oxidative stress in unhealthy patients (Morvaridzadeh et al., 2021).

Insomnia: The results of a meta-analysis on the effects of saffron supplementation on sleep quality among healthy adults, patients with insomnia or type 2 diabetes and patients under Methadone maintenance treatment showed that saffron improved Pittsburgh Sleep Quality Index, Insomnia Severity Index, and Restorative Sleep Questionnaire compared with placebo group. Intake of 100 mg/day saffron was observed to be more effective on improving sleep quality in subgroup analysis (Lian et al., 2022).

Respiratory problems: In a triple-blind RCT in 80 18–65-year-old patients with mild and moderate allergic asthma, daily administration of 100 mg saffron for 8 weeks could significantly reduce the hs-CRP ($p < 0.001$) and anti-HSP70 ($p < 0.001$) concentrations compared to the placebo group. Moreover, forced expiratory volume in first second, forced vital capacity, FEV1/FVC ratio and forced expiratory flow 25–75% were significantly increased in saffron in comparison to placebo group ($p < 0.05$) (Hosseini et al., 2018).

In another double-blind RCT in 80 patients with allergic asthma, saffron supplementation (100 mg/day dries for 8 weeks) improved the frequency of clinical symptoms of allergic asthma (frequency of the breath shortness during the day and night time, the use of salbutamol spray, waking up due to asthma symptoms and activity limitation) compared to the placebo ($p < 0.001$). Moreover, asthma severity almost significantly decreased in the saffron group ($p = 0.07$). It was also found that eosinophils and basophils levels were reduced in the saffron group ($p = 0.06$ and 0.05, respectively) (Zilaee et al., 2019).

Obesity and metabolic syndrome: The results of a meta-analysis of 14 RCTs found a significant reduction in TC and TAG following saffron intervention with a daily dosage of 30–450 mg of saffron, or 5–200 mg of crocin, and with a follow up of 1–12 weeks. A meta-regression analysis indicated that long-term saffron intake could increase HDL-C levels compared with placebo. No significant effect on weight and LDL-C levels was found (Rahmani et al., 2019). Another meta-analysis of 15 RCTs involving 1,139 participants investigated the effects of saffron supplementation, with a dose range of 15–100 mg/day of the products or 1 g of the plant added to tea, and with a treatment period of 4–12 weeks, on glycemic parameters, including FBS, FPI, HbA1c and QUICKI among both diabetic and nondiabetic patients. Saffron supplementation resulted in a significant decrease in FBS, HbA1c, FPI, and an increase in QUICKI compared to control. Saffron supplementation could not reduce HOMA-IR significantly (Sohaei et al., 2020).

In a meta-analysis of six RCTs evaluating the effect of saffron on serum TAG, TC, and FBG and of five studies for LDL-C and HDL-C, a significant reduction in TAG and TC levels, as well as a significant increase in HDL-C levels were reported; though, no significant effect was observed on LDL-C and FBS (Asbaghi et al., 2019). A meta-analysis of nine trials with 12 arms with 595 participants found that saffron consumption significantly reduced waist circumference and FBS. Subgroup analysis indicated that FBS was significantly decreased when intervention duration was longer than 12 weeks (Rahmani et al., 2020). Another meta-analysis of 25 RCTs reported a significant effect of saffron on the reduction of waist-to-hip ratio and FBS in patients with metabolic syndrome; however, its effect on body weight, BMI, waist circumference, and hip circumference was nonsignificant (Tahmasbi et al., 2022). Moreover, a clinical study in 60 obese diabetic men reported that administration of saffron (100 mg/day for 12 weeks) along with concurrent training (three times per week) has a significantly better effect on the improvement of TNF-α, hs-CRP, IL-6, IL-10, IL-1β, FBS, HbA1c, HOMA-IR, FPI, and body fat percentage compared with either saffron or exercise alone (Hooshmand Moghadam et al., 2022). In spite of heterogeneity of the included studies in different systematic reviews, saffron seems to have beneficial effects on metabolic syndrome and its complications, including obesity.

Hepatic dysfunction: A meta-analysis of nine RCTs showed that saffron supplementation significantly reduced serum ALT levels compared to placebo. However, saffron did not affect AST or ALP. No significant dose–response relationship between dosage and duration of saffron supplementation on serum levels of ALT, AST, and ALP was found (Mousavi et al., 2021). Contradictory to this, in another study of eight RCTs involving 463 participants, it was found that saffron intake was associated with a significant decrease in AST; whereas no significant effect on ALT and ALP levels was observed compared with placebo (Hasani et al., 2021). The daily dose range of saffron reported in these two studies was 15–100 mg; while clinical studies on the use of saffron for other indications have considered higher doses; thus, controversial results of these studies might be due to a low dose of saffron and considering the lack of adverse events in these studies, higher doses may be recommended for future studies.

Hypertension: The results of a meta-analysis of eight RCTs showed that saffron supplementation was associated with a significant decrease in SBP and DBP. Moreover, saffron supplementation reduced DBP in a nonlinear fashion, based on duration. However, the hypotensive effects of saffron were small and may not reach clinical importance (Setayesh et al., 2021). In an RCT on 48 elderly men with hypertension, saffron (200 mg daily) was administered alone or along with resistant training for 18 weeks. There was a significant decrease in SBP and endothelin-1, as well as an increase in adiponectin and NO compared with placebo and individual interventions (Hooshmand Moghadam et al., 2021). Also, saffron, concomitantly administered with resistant training, caused a significant reduction in MCP-1, IL-6, leptin, and resistin; though, no significant difference was observed between groups regarding hs-CRP, homocysteine, and TNF-α (Mojtahedi et al., 2022).

Sexual dysfunction: In a double-blind RCT in 62 male subjects with erectile dysfunction, daily administration of 30 mg saffron product for 6 weeks showed a significant improvement of International Index of Erectile Function questionnaire score compared with placebo (Najafabadi et al., 2022). In a meta-analysis of three RCTs, quantitative analysis showed that saffron with a dosage of 30–200 mg/day significantly improved all dimensions of Erectile Function questionnaire, including erectile function, orgasmic function, overall satisfaction, satisfaction with intercourse, and sexual desire (Maleki-Saghooni et al., 2018). Another meta-analysis of five studies comprising 173 participants receiving oral saffron with a similar dosage also showed a significant improvement of sexual dysfunction and its subscales (Ranjbar and Ashrafizaveh, 2019).

Glaucoma: A pilot double-blind, placebo-controlled RCT found that oral saffron supplementation (30 mg daily for 1 month) in combination with topical timolol 0.5% and dorzolamide 2% in patients with primary open angle glaucoma significantly reduced the intraocular pressure after 3 weeks compared with placebo. However, this effect was reversed after a 1-month wash-out period (Jabbarpoor Bonyadi et al., 2014).

Preclinical Evidence

Parkinson's disease: In a Drosophila model of rotenone-induced Parkinson's disease, saffron methanolic extract (containing 5.1 mg/mL crocin and 3.4 mg/mL safranal) significantly decreased rotenone-induced mortality, rescued the locomotor phenotype, and reduced oxidative stress markers in the head and body of flies. In addition, rotenone-induced mitochondrial dysfunctions and elevated acetylcholinesterase activity were attenuated by saffron (Rao et al., 2016). Saffron hydroethanolic extract (50 mg/kg, orally) prevented the increase in tyrosine hydroxylase levels in different parts of the brain of *Meriones shawi* affected by lead-induced dopaminergic and locomotor dysfunction. Moreover, saffron treatment of lead-treated animals attenuated locomotor impairment by 90% (Tamegart et al., 2019). Saffron also prevented α-synuclein aggregation and dissociated α-synuclein fibrils in a dose-dependent manner (IC_{50} = 0.656 μg/mL and EC_{50} = 4.17 μg/mL) (Inoue et al., 2018).

Antitussive effects: The ethanolic extract of saffron (100–800 mg/kg, intraperitoneally) reduced the number of citric acid-induced cough in guinea pigs (Hosseinzadeh and Ghenaati, 2006).

ADVERSE REACTIONS

TPM Literature

Common adverse effects of saffron intake are headache, nausea, dizziness, hypomania, and loss of appetite. Aniseed and oxymel can alleviate these adverse effects (Aghili Khorasani 1771).

Current Evidence

According to the findings of many RCTs, different oral doses of saffron powder ranging from 20 to 200 mg/day and duration between 10 days and 16 weeks has been reported to be well tolerated. However, mild headache, nausea, anxiety, and decreased appetite are side effects reported for saffron supplementation (Hausenblas et al., 2013; Ghaffari and Roshanravan, 2019). Saffron can be toxic and lethal when taken at higher concentration (more than 12 g); though, even doses higher than 5 g caused adverse reactions (Gruenwald et al., 2007; Ghaffari and Roshanravan, 2019). Saffron poisoning symptoms include vomiting, intestinal colic, nasal, intestinal and urogenital hemorrhage, dizziness, stupor, yellow skin and mucus membranes and central paralysis (Gruenwald et al., 2007).

CONTRAINDICATIONS

TPM Literature

None.

Current Evidence

Saffron intake above dietary levels should be cautiously in patients with diabetes, coagulation disorders, low blood counts, low blood pressure and allergy to saffron (Ulbricht et al., 2011).

PREGNANCY AND LACTATION

TPM Literature

Saffron should be avoided during pregnancy due to abortive effects (Gruenwald et al., 2007).

Current Evidence

Saffron should be avoided during pregnancy due to uterine stimulant effects (Gruenwald et al., 2007).

DRUG INTERACTIONS

Anticoagulants and antiplatelets: Coadministration of saffron extract (doses above dietary levels) with anticoagulants or antiplatelet drugs may inhibit platelet aggregation.
Antihypertensives: Concomitant use of saffron powder (doses ≥ 400 mg) with antihypertensive medicines may decrease standing SBP and mean arterial pressures (Ulbricht et al., 2011).

METHOD OF ADMINISTRATION

TPM Literature

For oral administration, dried stigma powder or infusion can be used. Saffron oil, prepared according to the instructions of TPM (an infusion of saffron powder boiled in fix oils such as olive and almond oils) is administered topically and for inhaling (Aghili Khorasani 1771).

Current Evidence

For oral administration, saffron infusion of aqueous extract or dry extract can be used (Blumenthal et al., 2000). Saffron oil or saffron essential oil mixed with a proper fix oil is administered topically or as massage oil.

DOSAGE

Evidence from clinical studies and meta-analysis recommends the oral doses of 20–200 mg/day of saffron stigma powder. The therapeutic dose should not exceed 1.5 g per day (Garnder and McGuffin, 2013). Various extracts with the equivalent dosage can be administered.

REFERENCES

Abu-Izneid T, Rauf A, Khalil AA, et al. Nutritional and health beneficial properties of saffron (Crocus sativus L): a comprehensive review. Crit Rev Food Sci Nutr. 2022;62(10):2683–2706.

Aghili Khorasani MH 1771. *Makhzan-al-Adviah* (*The treasury of drugs*) (rewritten by Shams Ardakani MR, Rahimi R, Farjadmand F, 1st ed). Tehran: Tehran University of Medical Sciences; 2009.

Asbaghi O, Soltani S, Norouzi N, et al. The effect of saffron supplementation on blood glucose and lipid profile: A systematic review and meta-analysis of randomized controlled trials. Complement Ther Med. 2019;47:102158.

Avgerinos KI, Vrysis C, Chaitidis N, et al. Effects of saffron (*Crocus sativus* L.) on cognitive function: A systematic review of RCTs. Neurol Sci. 2020;41:2747–2754.

Avicenna 1025. *Al-Qanoon fi al-Tibb* (*The canon of medicine*) (rewritten by Masoudi A, ed.). Tehran: Almaei; 2015.

Ayati Z, Yang G, Ayati MH, et al. Saffron for mild cognitive impairment and dementia: A systematic review and meta-analysis of randomised clinical trials. BMC Complement Med Ther. 2020;20(1):1–10.

Blumenthal M, Goldberg A, Brinckmann J. *Herbal medicine: Expanded Commission E monographs*. Newton, MA: Integrative Medicine Communications; 2000.

Ghaffari S, Roshanravan N. Saffron: An updated review on biological properties with special focus on cardiovascular effects. Biomed Pharmacother. 2019;109:21–27.

Gruenwald J, Brendler T, Jaenicke C. *PDR for herbal medicines*. Montvale: Thomson Reuters; 2007.

Hasani M, Malekahmadi M, Rezamand G, et al. Effect of saffron supplementation on liver enzymes: A systematic review and meta-analysis of randomized controlled trials. Diabetes Metab Syndr. 2021;15(6):102311.

Hausenblas HA, Saha D, Dubyak PJ, Anton SD. Saffron (*Crocus sativus* L.) and major depressive disorder: A meta-analysis of randomized clinical trials. J Integr Med. 2013;11(6):377–383.

Hooshmand Moghadam B, Eskandari M, Shabkhiz F, et al. Saffron (*Crocus sativus* L.) in combination with resistance training reduced blood pressure in the elderly hypertensive men: A randomized controlled trial. Br J Clin Pharmacol. 2021;87(8):3255–3267.

Hooshmand Moghadam B, Rashidlamir A, Attarzadeh Hosseini SR, et al. The effects of saffron (*Crocus sativus* L.) in conjunction with concurrent training on body composition, glycaemic status, and inflammatory markers in obese men with type 2 diabetes mellitus: A randomized double-blind clinical trial. Br J Clin Pharmacol. 2022;88(7):3256–3271.

Hosseini SA, Zilaee M, Shoushtari MH. An evaluation of the effect of saffron supplementation on the antibody titer to heat-shock protein (HSP) 70, hsCRP and spirometry test in patients with mild and moderate persistent allergic asthma: A triple-blind, randomized placebo-controlled trial. Respir Med. 2018;145:28–34.

Hosseinzadeh H, Ghenaati J. Evaluation of the antitussive effect of stigma and petals of saffron (*Crocus sativus*) and its components, safranal and crocin in guinea pigs. Fitoterapia. 2006;77(6):446–448.

Inoue E, Shimizu Y, Masui R, et al. Effects of saffron and its constituents, crocin-1, crocin-2, and crocetin on α-synuclein fibrils. J Nat Med. 2018;72(1):274–279.

Jabbarpoor Bonyadi MH, Yazdani S, Saadat S. The ocular hypotensive effect of saffron extract in primary open angle glaucoma: A pilot study. BMC Complement Med Ther. 2014;14(1):1–6.

Khaksarian M, Behzadifar M, Behzadifar M, et al. The efficacy of *Crocus sativus* (saffron) versus placebo and Fluoxetine in treating depression: A systematic review and meta-analysis. Psychol Res Behav Manag. 2019;12:297–305.

Lian J, Zhong Y, Li H, et al. Effects of saffron supplementation on improving sleep quality: A meta-analysis of randomized controlled trials. Sleep Med. 2022;92:24–33.

Maleki-Saghooni N, Mirzaeii K, Hosseinzadeh H, et al. A systematic review and meta-analysis of clinical trials on saffron (*Crocus sativus*) effectiveness and safety on erectile dysfunction and semen parameters. Avicenna J Phytomed. 2018;8(3):198–209.

Mojtahedi S, Hooshmand-Moghadam B, Rosenkranz S, et al. Improvement of inflammatory status following saffron (*Crocus sativus* L.) and resistance training in elderly hypertensive men: A randomized controlled trial. Exp Gerontol. 2022;162:111756.

Morvaridzadeh M, Agah S, Dulce Estêvão M, et al. Effect of saffron supplementation on oxidative stress parameters: A systematic review and meta-analysis of randomized placebo-controlled trials. Food Sci Nutr. 2021;9(10):5809–5819.

Mousavi SM, Mokhtari P, Asbaghi O, et al. Does saffron supplementation have favorable effects on liver function indicators? A systematic review and meta-analysis of randomized controlled trials. Crit Rev Food Sci Nutr. 2022;62(23):6315–6327.

Musazadeh V, Zarezadeh M, Faghfouri AH, et al. Saffron, as an adjunct therapy, contributes to relieve depression symptoms: An umbrella meta-analysis. Pharmacol Res. 2022;175:105963.

Najafabadi BT, Farsinejad M, Shokraee K, et al. Possible effects of saffron (*Crocus sativus*) in the treatment of erectile dysfunction: A randomized, double-blind, placebo-controlled trial. J Herb Med. 2022;32:100551.

Rahmani J, Bazmi E, Clark C, Nazari SS. The effect of saffron supplementation on waist circumference, HA1C, and glucose metabolism: A systematic review and meta-analysis of randomized clinical trials. Complement Ther Med. 2020;49:102298.

Rahmani J, Manzari N, Thompson J, et al. The effect of saffron on weight and lipid profile: A systematic review, meta-analysis, and dose–response of randomized clinical trials. Phytother Res. 2019;33(9):2244–2255.

Ranjbar H, Ashrafizaveh A. Effects of saffron (*Crocus sativus*) on sexual dysfunction among men and women: A systematic review and meta-analysis. Avicenna J Phytomed. 2019;9(5):419–427.

Rao SV, Yenisetti SC, Rajini PS. Evidence of neuroprotective effects of saffron and crocin in a Drosophila model of parkinsonism. Neurotoxicology. 2016;52:230–242.

Setayesh L, Ashtary-Larky D, Clark CC, et al. The effect of saffron supplementation on blood pressure in adults: A systematic review and dose-response meta-analysis of randomized controlled trials. Nutrients. 2021;13(8):2736.

Sohaei S, Hadi A, Karimi E, Arab A. Saffron supplementation effects on glycemic indices: A systematic review and meta-analysis of randomized controlled clinical trials. Int J Food Prop. 2020;23(1):1386–1401.

Tahmasbi F, Araj-Khodaei M, Mahmoodpoor A, Sanaie S. Effects of saffron (*Crocus sativus* L.) on anthropometric and cardiometabolic indices in overweight and obese patients: A systematic review and meta-analysis of randomized controlled trials. Phytother Res. 2022;36(9):3394–3414.

Tamegart L, Abbaoui A, Makbal R, et al. *Crocus sativus* restores dopaminergic and noradrenergic damages induced by lead in Meriones shawi: A possible link with Parkinson's disease. Acta Histochem. 2019;121(2):171–181.

Ulbricht C, Conquer J, Costa D, et al. An evidence-based systematic review of saffron (*Crocus sativus*) by the natural standard research collaboration. J Diet Suppl. 2011;8(1):58–114.

Zilaee M, Hosseini SA, Jafarirad S, et al. An evaluation of the effects of saffron supplementation on the asthma clinical symptoms and asthma severity in patients with mild and moderate persistent allergic asthma: A double-blind, randomized placebo-controlled trial. Respir Res. 2019;20(1):1–11.

12 *Drimia maritima* (L.) Stearn

Mahbubeh Bozorgi

Scientific name: *Drimia maritima* (L.) Stearn
Family: Asparagaceae
Common names:

- **English:** Squill, sea onion
- **Persian:** *'onṣol, 'eṣqīl, pīyāz-e daštī, pīyāz-e mūš*
- **Arabic:** *baṣal al-'unṣul, baṣal al-fār*

Medicinal part(s): Bulb (Figure 12.1)
Temperament (nature): Hot in the third degree and dry in the second degree
Major chemical constituents:

- **Bufadienolids (a type of cardiac glycosides):** Proscillaridin, scillaren A, scillarenin, scilliroside
- **Phenolic acids:** Caffeic acid, *p*-coumaric acid
- **Flavonoids:** Quercetin and taxifolin
- **Phytosterols:** Campesterol, stigmasterol (Bozorgi et al., 2017)

THERAPEUTIC USE

TPM Literature

Different types of squill have been mentioned in TPM literatures and the white and bright type of bulbs have been recommended for therapeutic purposes. It is useful in the form of roasted bulb or with honey/honey syrup for many neurological disorders including epilepsy, melancholia, headache and migraine, vertigo, palsy, trigeminal neuralgia, and dementia. It has been claimed to enhance eyesight and is used to prevent cataract. It is also beneficial in the form of oxymel for respiratory disorders including chronic cough and asthma. It is a gastric tonic and digestive aid and is recommended for treatment of liver disorders. It is useful for musculoskeletal diseases and sciatica. It is a lithotriptic and is used for dysuria. It is also beneficial for skin disorders including leprosy and alopecia areata (Aghili Khorasani 1771; Avicenna 1025).

Current Evidence

Clinical Evidence

Asthma: In a placebo-controlled RCT, effect of squill oxymel as an add-on treatment was investigated on 60 patients with moderate to severe persistent asthma. Patients were randomized to receive 10 mL of squill oxymel, simple oxymel, or placebo, twice a day for 6 weeks. Significant improvement in spirometry parameters was observed in the squill oxymel group compared to the other groups. The increases in FEV1, FEV1%, FEV1/FVC%, and MEF 25–75% during the intervention were

DOI: 10.1201/b22971-12

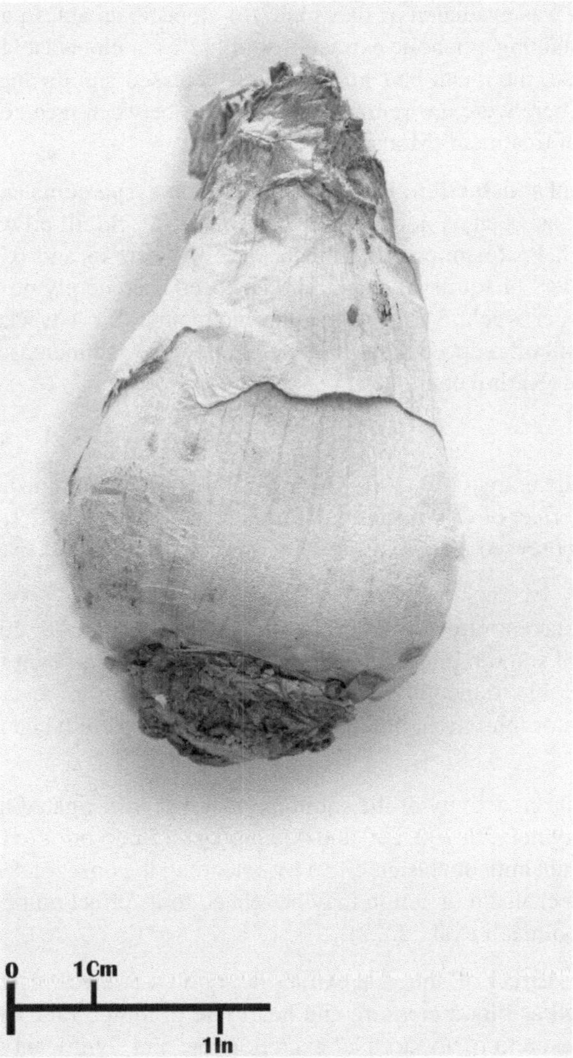

FIGURE 12.1 Squill bulb.

significantly higher in the squill oxymel group in comparison with the other groups. The clinical symptoms assessed by St George's Respiratory Questionnaire were significantly improved after intervention in both the squill oxymel and the simple oxymel groups (Nejatbakhsh et al., 2017).

COPD: Effect of squill oxymel as an add-on therapy in individuals with mild COPD was investigated in a triple-blinded RCT. Forty-two COPD patients were randomized to receive 10 mL of squill oxymel or placebo twice daily for eight weeks. As a result, patients who received squill oxymel showed a statistically significant increase in 6-minute walk test distance. Based on St. George's Respiratory Questionnaire variables, there was a significant difference between placebo and squill oxymel groups in the mean presymptom score and the mean postsymptom score (Mohammadi-Araghi et al., 2022).

Alopecia: Squill lotion was evaluated as hair tonic for alopecia areata. In a double-blind RCT, 42 patients used lotion containing ethanolic extract of squill (2%) or clobetasol lotion twice daily. After 12 weeks of intervention, the mean hair growth rates increased significantly in both squill group and clobetasol group. There were no significant differences between mean hair growth rates in two groups after 3 months of treatment (Moosavi et al., 2020).

Dyspareunia and sexual satisfaction: Effect of squill oil on dyspareunia and sexual satisfaction in 60 menopausal women has been explored in a triple-blind RCT. Squill oil was prepared by heating squill bulbs in olive oil. Postmenopausal women (age between 45 and 65 years) participated in this study. Three milliliters of squill oil or placebo has been used gently on the clitoris and vaginal opening for 2–3 times per week, 5 min before the intercourse for 4 weeks. As the result of this study, topical use of squill oil reduced painful sexual intercourse and increased sexual satisfaction in postmenopausal women (Karimi et al., 2021).

Preclinical Evidence

NAFLD: Squill ethanolic extract (50, 100, 150 mg/kg) was orally administered to rats for 2 weeks and compared with the effect of Chymostatin. Reduction in TAG, AST, ALT, and TC, as well as elevation of HDL-C was observed after treating with all concentrations of extract (Hadarbegi, 2015; Mahboubi et al., 2019).

Bronchospasm: The relaxant effect of squill extract (12.5, 25, 50, 100, 20, and 400 µg/mL) was examined on rat tracheal smooth muscle. Squill extract showed significant relaxant effect on these smooth muscles comparable to theophylline. Probable mechanisms are beta-2 adrenoceptor stimulation, muscarinic receptor inhibition, potassium opening, and calcium channels blocking (Kazemi Rad et al., 2021).

Convulsion: Anticonvulsant activity of the squill oxymel was investigated in albino mice. Animals orally received squill oxymel (50, 100, 200 and 400 mg/kg), 15 min prior to injection of PTZ. Squill oxymel showed significant anticonvulsant effect by extending the onset of seizures and reducing the duration of seizures. Mechanism of action may be related to its effect on benzodiazepine receptors on GABA complex (Abolmaali et al., 2022).

Cardiovascular effect: Effect of aqueous extract of squill was investigated on renal function of domestic rabbits, as well as blood pressure and heart rate of albino rats. Considerable increase in urine flow, total solute excretion, urinary Na^+ excretion rate and significant reduction in urinary K^+ excretion rate was observed in rabbits. The observed diuretic and natriuretic effects were similar to potassium sparing diuretic. A fall in blood pressure along with negative chronotropic effect was detected in rats (Dizaye et al., 2010).

ADVERSE REACTIONS

TPM Literature

There is a history of using this plant, especially its red type, to kill mice in different countries. In TPM literatures, raw squill is considered as a toxic plant and is used as a rodenticide and insect repellent. It has been mentioned that if squill is rubbed on the body in raw form, it can cause wounds.

Squill may be harmful for hot-tempered patients, especially for nervous system. It also causes headache and nausea and to reduce these side effects, it is better to be taken with sugar, rock candy, or oxymel. Fresh milk and fruit pastes are also recommended for detoxifying the body after taking extra amounts of unprocessed squill (Aghili Khorasani 1771).

Current Evidence

Common squill side effects are related to cardiac glycosides. Inhibition of Na^+/K^+–ATPase by cardiac glycosides results in inhibition of the active transport across the cell membranes. So, the concentrations of intracellular Na^+, extracellular K^+ and subsequently intracellular Ca^{2+} rise, which leads to increase in the contractility of myocardium. As a result, the cardiac output with reduction in heart rates increases. Marked hyperkalemia, conduction abnormalities, ventricular arrhythmias, nausea, vomiting, seizures, gastric irritation, and hypersensitivity reactions are considered as squill adverse reactions (Mahboubi et al., 2019). Vision disorders, confusion, psychosis, and hallucinations may also occur in case of overdose. Different forms of arrythmias are observed in squill overdose which can result in cardiac arrest and/or asphyxia (Gruenwald et al., 2007). However, maceration or boiling of squill in vinegar to prepare squill oxymel as a TPM dosage form from squill results in degradation of cardiac glycosides structure and so, these effects have not been reported for squill oxymel (Mahboubi et al., 2019; Bozorgi et al., 2017).

One case of death was reported in a 55-year-old man with a history of Hashimoto thyroiditis who took two squill bulbs orally to relieve arthritic pains (Tuncok et al., 1995)

CONTRAINDICATIONS

TPM Literature

It is stated that some types of this plant are fatal for humans. Based on TPM literature, squill should not be used without processing and modification methods (Aghili Khorasani 1771).

Current Evidence

Patients with cardiac disorders, impaired hepatic or renal functions, pregnant or lactating mothers, and children under 12 years should avoid using squill (Williamson et al., 2013). Squill is contraindicated in patients with hypokalemia, hypercalcemia, second-/third-degree atrioventricular block, Wolff-Parkinson-White syndrome, thoracic aortic aneurysm, hypertrophic cardiomyopathy, ventricular tachycardia, or carotid sinus syndrome (Gruenwald et al., 2007; Ulbricht, 2010).

PREGNANCY AND LACTATION

TPM Literature

Squill is contraindicated during pregnancy.

Current Evidence

Not recommended due to possible abortifacient effects (Ulbricht, 2010).

DRUG INTERACTIONS

D. maritima contains cardiac glycosides that can interact with long-term intake of corticosteroids, carbenoxolone calcium, digoxin, thiazides, loop diuretics, and laxatives due to its additive effects. Concomitant use with other drugs with arrhythmogenic properties such as quinidine, sympathomimetics, phosphodiesterase inhibitors, and methylxanthines increase the risk of arrythmias (Gruenwald et al., 2007; Ulbricht, 2010). It should be considered that processing methods of squill mentioned in TPM literatures aim to break down the chemical structure of cardiac glycosides in order to eliminate their pharmacological properties and adverse events from the final product (Mahboubi, 2019).

METHOD OF ADMINISTRATION

TPM Literature

Squill is usually used in medicinal formulations after processing. Roasting (backing) has been one of the squill processing methods suggested by TPM. For this purpose, squill bulb is usually covered with a layer of dough and is put in an oven at low heat to cook. Roasted squill alone or with honey has been used for oral or topical purposes. Other methods have been also mentioned for processing of squill. For example, dry or fresh bulbs were kept in vinegar for a long time and the obtained vinegar was used to prepare various syrups. Squill oxymel, which is prepared by boiling bulbs in vinegar and honey, has been one of the most widely used medicines in TPM. Dried and powdered squill have also been used to prepare different pills. Different oral dosage forms from squill like extracts, syrups, tinctures, vinegar, and oxymel have been mentioned in TPM references. Squill oil is obtained by boiling bulbs in olive oil and is usually used for topical purposes. In addition, other topical formulations like paste and lotions are also recommended for external use (Aghili Khorasani 1771).

Current Evidence

Squill is available as oxymel, as well as commercial liquid dosage forms (Gruenwald et al., 2007).

DOSAGE

There is insufficient evidence to recommend a dose for squill as it is usually consumed as processed dosage forms (Ulbricht, 2010). In some references, the daily dose for dried bulb, liquid extract, tincture, and vinegar has been mentioned as 180–600 mg or up to 2 mL of the liquid products (Gruenwald et al., 2007; Mahboubi et al., 2019).

REFERENCES

Abolmaali M, Motevalian M, Mehrzadi S, Shojaii A. Anticonvulsant effects of squill oxymel (a traditional formulation) in mice. Physiol Pharmacol. 2022;26(1):1–6.

Aghili Khorasani MH 1771. *Makhzan-al-Adviah* (*The treasury of drugs*) (rewritten by Shams Ardakani MR, Rahimi R, Farjadmand F, 1st ed). Tehran: Tehran University of Medical Sciences; 2009.

Avicenna 1025. *Al-Qanoon fi al-Tibb* (*The canon of medicine*) (rewritten by Masoudi A, ed). Tehran: Almaei; 2015.

Bozorgi M, Amin G, Shekarchi M, Rahimi R. Traditional medical uses of Drimia species in terms of phytochemistry, pharmacology and toxicology. J Tradit Chin Med. 2017;37(1):124–139.

Dizaye KF, Hamad BA. Cardiovascular studies of white squill (*Urginea maritima*) extract. Zanco J Med Sci. 2010;14(1):20–27.

Gruenwald J, Brendler T, Jaenicke C. *PDR for herbal medicines*. Montvale: Thomson Reuters; 2007.

Hadarbegi F. *Effect of extract of squill extract on nonalcoholic fatty liver*. Tehran: Islamic Azad University; 2015

Karimi F, Babazadeh R, Zojaji A, Jouya S. Squill oil for decreasing dyspareunia and increasing sexual satisfaction in menopausal women: A triple-blind randomized controlled trial. Avicenna J Phytomedicine. 2021;11(5):464–472.

Kazemi Rad H, Memarzia A, Amin F, Boskabady MH. Relaxant effect of *Urginea maritima* on tracheal smooth muscle mediated by the effect on beta-2 adrenergic, muscarinic receptors and calcium and potassium channels. Evid-Based Complement Altern Med. 2021;2021:1–9.

Mahboubi M, Mohammad Taghizadeh Kashani L, Mahboubi M. Squill (*Drimia maritima* L.) and its novel biological activity. Orient Pharm Exp Med. 2019;19(3):227–234.

Mohammadi-Araghi M, Eslaminejad A, Karegar-Borzi H, et al. An add-on treatment for moderate COPD with squill-Oxymel (a traditional formulation from *Drimia maritima* (L.) stearn): A pilot randomized triple-blinded placebo-controlled clinical trial. Evid-Based Complementary Altern Med. 2022;2022:5024792.

Moosavi ZB, Aliabdi M, Golfakhrabadi F, Namjoyan F. The comparison of therapeutic effect of clobetasol propionate lotion and squill extract in alopecia areata: A randomized, double-blind clinical trial. Arch Dermatol Res. 2020;312:173–178.

Nejatbakhsh F, Karegar-Borzi H, Amin G, et al. Squill oxymel, a traditional formulation from *Drimia maritima* (L.) Stearn, as an add-on treatment in patients with moderate to severe persistent asthma: A pilot, triple-blind, randomized clinical trial. J Ethnopharmacol. 2017;196:186–192.

Tuncok Y, Kozan O, Cavdar C, et al. *Urginea maritima* (squill) toxicity. J Toxicol Clin Toxicol. 1995;33(1):83–86.

Ulbricht CE. *Mosby's natural standard herb & supplement guide*. St. Louis: Elsevier; 2010.

Williamson E, Driver S, Baxter K (eds.). *Stockley's herbal medicines interactions*. London: Pharmaceutical Press; 2013.

13 *Echium amoenum* Fisch. & C.A.Mey.

Najmeh Sasani and Ehsan Amiri-Ardekani

Scientific name: *Echium amoenum* Fisch. & C.A.Mey.
Family: Boraginaceae
Common names:

- **English:** Red feathers, Echium
- **Persian:** *gāvzabān*
- **Arabic:** *lisān al-ṯaur*

Medicinal part(s): Flowers, leaves (Figure 13.1)
Temperament (nature): Hot and wet in the first degree
Major chemical constituents:

- **Phenolics:** Pyrogallol, salicylic acid, gallic acid, rosmarinic acid
- **Flavonoids:** Rutin, myricetin
- **Anthocyanins:** Cyanidin, delphinidin (Zannou et al., 2022)
- **Fatty acids:** γ-linolenic acid, α-linolenic acid, delta 6-fatty acryl desaturase, delta 8-sphingolipid desaturase (Farahmand et al., 2020)
- **Pyrrolizidine alkaloids:** Echimidine, echimidine isomer, 7-angeloyl retronecine, and 7-tigloyl retronecine (Azizi et al., 2018)

THERAPEUTIC USE

TPM Literature

E. amoenum is known as a mood-boosting and antidepressant plant and is used for meningitis, melancholy, panic disorder, fear, and generally psychological disorders due to melancholic dystemperament. Decoction of *E. amoenum* with rock candy (crystalized sugar), sugar, or honey is useful for roughness of trachea and chest, sore throat, cough, and dyspnea. Moreover, *E. amoenum* decoction with sugar is used for palpitation, icterus, nephrolithiasis, and bladder stone. For aphthous stomatitis of children, sprinkle its burnt flower powder on lesions relieves the oral cavity and tongue inflammation, and burning of the mouth. The aromatic water (distillate) is also recommended in different types of melancholic disorders (Aghili Khorasani 1771; Avicenna 1025).

Current Evidence

Clinical Evidence

PMS: In a double-blind RCT, 84 women with regular menstrual cycles suffering from PMS were randomized to receive either 150 mg of freeze-dried powder of *E. amoenum* decoction as a form of capsule three times a day or placebo from the 21st day of one cycle to the third day of the next cycle

DOI: 10.1201/b22971-13

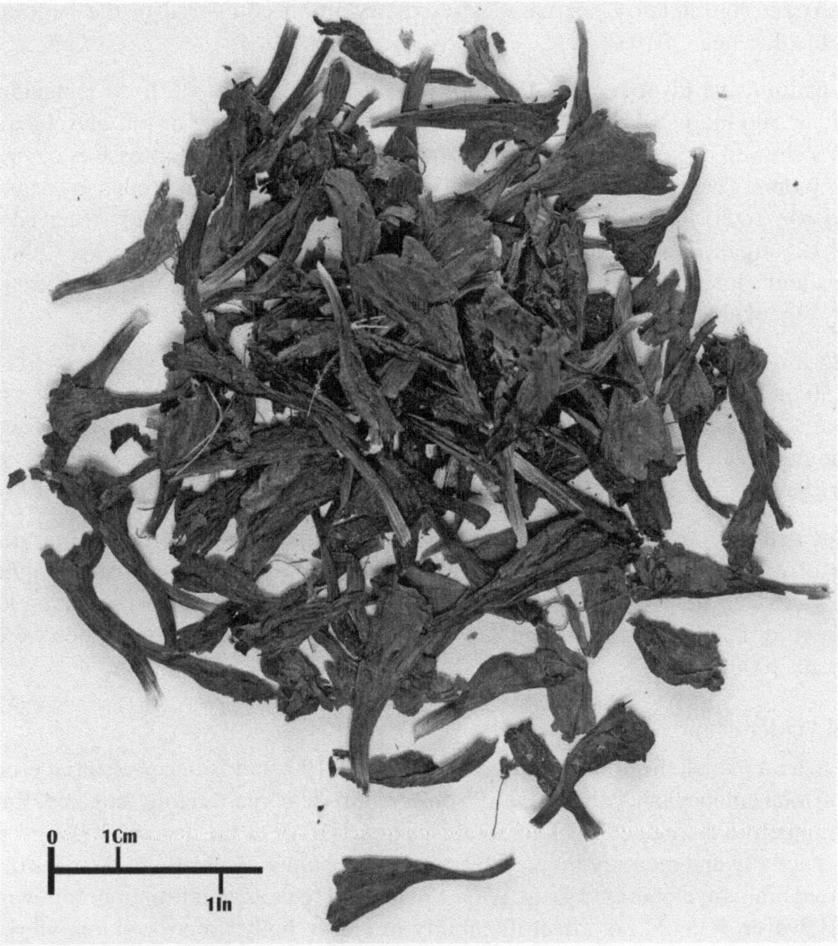

FIGURE 13.1 Red feathers flowers.

(10 days on aggregate) for two consecutive cycles. *E. amoenum* was more effective than a placebo in reducing the symptoms of PMS. The anxiety/tension and the tearful symptoms were the most important symptoms relieved with the positive impact of *E. amoenum* consumption (Farahmand et al., 2020).

Depression: In a 6-week double-blind RCT, 35 patients with mild to moderate major depressive disorder receive daily either placebo or 375 mg of *E. amoenum* dried aqueous extract (one oral capsule three times daily). In week 4, the extract showed a significant superiority over placebo in reducing depressive symptoms. The effect on anxiety was not significant. The most common adverse effect was headache; though, there was no significant difference between two groups regarding the incidence of adverse effects (Sayyah et al., 2006).

In another double-blind RCT, 72 menopausal women received 60 capsules of 500 mg *E. amoenum* ethanolic extract or fluoxetine for 8 weeks. A statistically significant improvement was observed in the mean score of depression in both groups in the fourth week of intervention vs. baseline values. No statistically significant difference was found between the two groups at the end of the study. Mean scores of depression in participants receiving *E. amoenum* ethanolic extract significantly decreased after intervention compared to the beginning of the study (Baghbadoranee, 2019).

Obsessive-compulsive disorder (OCD): In a 6-week double-blind RCT, 44 patients with OCD received either 500 mg per day of *E. amoenum* dried aqueous extract or placebo. In weeks 4 and 6, the extract showed a significant superiority over placebo in reducing obsessive, compulsive, and anxiety symptoms. There was no significant difference between the two groups in terms of adverse effects (Sayyah, 2009). In another double-blind RCT, 33 OCD patients daily received either four capsules of 125 mg of *E. amoenum* dried aqueous extract or placebo for 6 weeks. Although a marginally nonsignificant effect was observed in the fourth week, the effect was significant in week 6 without any remarkable adverse effect (Bargard, 2005).

Anxiety: In a double-blind RCT in 37 patients with generalized anxiety disorder (GAD), daily intake of 250 mg dried aqueous extract of *E. amoenum* or placebo, three times a day, as an add-on to fluoxetine (20 mg per day) for 8 weeks caused a significant anxiolytic activity. The difference between the two treatments was significant after 14 days with no difference in terms of observed side effects (Sayyah, 2012).

Antioxidant activity: In a before/after clinical trial, antioxidant properties of the decoction of the flowers of *E. amoenum* assessed among 38 healthy subjects who consume 7 mg/kg of dried decoction twice daily for 14 days. A significant reduction of blood lipid peroxidation level (LPO) and increment in blood total antioxidant capacity (TAC) and total thiol molecules were observed (Ranjbar et al., 2006).

Preclinical Evidence

Ischemia: In a rat model, the effect of different doses (50, 100, and 200 mg/kg, intraperitoneally) of *E. amoenum* total anthocyanin extract (ETAE) on cerebral ischemia were investigated. Rats received ETAE 30 min before the induction of cerebral ischemia. ETAE at the dose of 200 mg/kg improved spontaneous activity and memory induced by cerebral ischemia compared to the control group and also decreased brain myeloperoxidase activity, a marker of leukocyte infiltration, following cerebral ischemia. However, it could not affect the ability to climb, body proprioception, vibrissae touch, and brain water content. In addition, pretreatment with ETAE at higher doses significantly reduced ischemia-induced neuronal loss of the brain (Safaeian et al., 2015).

Alzheimer's disease: In a rat model of Alzheimer's disease, 5 and 50 mg/kg of lyophilized extracts of fresh *E. amoenum* petals were administered orally for 15 days. Treatment of nucleus basalis of Meynert (NBM) lesioned rats with 50 mg/kg extract significantly improved spatial memory. Moreover, this treatment decreased reactive oxygen species (ROS), LPO, and reduced acetylcholinesterase (AChE) enzyme activity accompanied by reduced degenerated cells in the hippocampus of NBM lesioned rats (Sadeghi et al., 2018b).

In another study, Wistar rats received *E. amoenum* extract (50, 75, and 100 mg/kg, intraperitoneally, daily for 21 days) 30 min before each scopolamine injection. *E. amoenum* extract in doses of 75 and 100 mg/kg, significantly increased the secondary latency and ameliorated scopolamine-induced motor incoordination in rotarod test. It also significantly increased the time spent in the open arms and reduced the time spent in the closed arms of elevated plus maze. Treatment of scopolamine-exposed rats with *E. amoenum* extract significantly increased TAC and reduced brain LPO (Rabiei and Setorki, 2018).

Parkinson's Disease: The effect of *E. amoenum* on Mn^{2+}-imposed toxicity was investigated in a rat model. The rats received 5 mg/kg of lyophilized extracts of fresh violet petals of *E. amoenum* orally before 15 mg/kg $MnCl_2$ intraperitoneal injection for 15 days. Results showed that oral administration of *E. amoenum* extract inhibited manganese neurotoxicity by oxidative stress attenuation and apoptosis reduction that led to improved depression like behavior. Plant extract also increased catecholamine content in Mn^{2+}-treated hippocampus (Sadeghi et al., 2018a).

Anxiety: In the elevated plus maze model of anxiety in mice, administration of 50 mg/kg of ethanolic extract of *E. amoenum* flowers accompanied by decreased spontaneous locomotor activity, indicating a sedative effect. Moreover, *E. amoenum* decreased ketamine-induced latency to sleep but did not affect the total duration of the sleep. At doses lower than 50 mg/kg, there was no significant changes in the behavior parameter that was measured on the elevated plus maze (Rabbani et al., 2004).

In another study, NMRI male mice were injected intraperitoneal with hydroalcoholic extract of *E. amoenum* (12.5, 25, and 50 mg/kg) or saline once each day for period of 7 days. No tolerance was developed to the anxiolytic effect of *E. amoenum* extract after 1 week treatment (Rabbani et al., 2011). In a rat model, *ad libitum* access to the tea of *E. amoenum* 0.3% (w/v), for a period of 24 h before the behavior test revealed that *E. amoenum* tea had anxiolytic effects in female rats; while had sedative effects in the male rats (Yousefi, 2016). Also, intraperitoneal administration of *E. amoenum* aqueous extract (62.5, 125, 250, and 500 mg/kg) revealed a mild to moderate anxiolytic effect in mice, and 125 mg/kg was the optimal dose (Shafaghi et al., 2002). In mice exposed to social isolation stress, intraperitoneal injection of hydroalcoholic extract of *E. amoenum* (50, 75, and 100 mg/kg) significantly reduced immobility in the forced swimming test. The extract (75 and 100 mg/kg) significantly increased the number of crossings in the center of the open field test. The time of staying in the open arms increased significantly in groups receiving the extract at 50, 75, and 100 mg/kg. Treatment with *E. amoenum* extract reduced the serum and brain tissue levels of nitric oxide (NO) and Malondialdehyde (MDA) in mice exposed to social isolation stress and enhanced serum and brain tissue TAC (Abdol and Setorki, 2020). *E. amoenum* hydroalcoholic extract (150 and 300 mg/kg) significantly ameliorated restraint stress-induced anxiety and depressive-like behaviors in mice. The extract significantly decreased serum corticosterone levels and also protein expression of neuroinflammatory markers in the hippocampus and prefrontal cortex subregions. Histopathological assessment showed no change in the liver of *E. amoenum*-treated groups (Nouri et al., 2019a).

Analgesic effect: Administration of *E. amoenum* methanolic extract (5, 10, 20, and 30 mg/kg, intraperitoneally) to male albino mice revealed that 10 mg/kg of extract had the highest analgesic activity in formalin and hot-plate test compared to the control group. The analgesic effect of extract was lower than morphine 2.5 mg/kg and aspirin 300 mg/kg in the chronic phase of pain in formalin test and in hot-plate test, as well (Heidari et al., 2006a).

Depression: Oral administration of 125 mg/kg aqueous extract of *E. amoenum* significantly increased serotonin and dopamine levels in the cerebrospinal fluid of reserpine-induced depression rats (Faryadian et al., 2014).

Blood pressure: Aqueous extract of *E. amoenum* at 400 and 600 mg/kg doses significantly increased blood pressure of rats in comparison with the control group and this effect was more significant after phenylephrine injection (Hamidi and Khaksari, 2011).

Liver enzymes: Administration of aqueous extract of *E. amoenum* flower (100, 200 or 400 mg/kg/day) significantly reduced serum levels of ALT and ALP in rats with no sign of hepatotoxicity (Zamansoltani et al., 2008).

Seizure: Administration of *E. amoenum* flowers methanolic extract (6.25 mg/kg, intraperitoneally) could significantly delay the onset of the seizure, decrease the severity, and mortality of seizure induced by picrotoxin in mice (Heidari et al., 2006b).

ADVERSE REACTIONS

TPM Literature

The plant is harmful for spleen and *Santalum album* L. can ameliorate its damage (Aghili Khorasani 1771).

Current Evidence

Aqueous extract of *E. amoenum* has not shown any adverse events at dose of 500–750 mg per day for 6–8 weeks during clinical studies (Baghbadoranee et al., 2019; Bargard et al., 2005; Sayyah et al., 2009; Sayyah et al., 2012). Histopathological assessment showed no changes in the liver of rats treated by *E. amoenum* hydroalcoholic extract (Nouri et al., 2019b).

Data about the potential of hepatotoxicity of *E. amoenum* is conflicting. Administration of aqueous extract of *E. amoenum* at doses of 100, 200 or 400 mg/kg/day for 2 weeks showed no sign of distinctive hepatotoxicity in rat model (Zamansoltani et al., 2008). However, in another study, *E. amoenum* extract caused hepatotoxicity and nephrotoxicity effects in dose and time-dependent manner in a mouse model. The extract (25, 12.5, 50 mg/kg, intraperitoneally) was administered for 28 days. There was a significant difference in the LPO in the liver of treated groups versus the control group. The significant difference was not observed in the levels of GSH of the liver of all groups. However, the levels of GSH of the kidney significantly decreased in the treated groups versus the control group. There was no significant difference in the liver enzymes, including ALP, ALT, and AST, between all groups. This indicates that damage increases with enhancing the time and concentrations of the extract. Biochemical analysis showed the creatinine and urea levels did not change in the treated groups versus the control group (Ghorbani et al., 2021).

E. amoenum did not cause significant damage to the heart tissue in mice model. Hepatotoxicity of consumption this plant should be considered at high doses (50 mg/kg) (Sadighara et al., 2019). Histopathological investigation showed high dose of *E. amoenum* may leads to the lesion in the brain tissue (Mohajer et al., 2019).

CONTRAINDICATIONS

TPM Literature

None.

Current Evidence

No data available. Because of the potential of hepatoxicity and nephrotoxicity, it is recommended to not be used in patients with liver and kidney disorders.

PREGNANCY AND LACTATION

TPM Literature

Due to emmenagogue properties, it should not be taken during pregnancy.

Current Evidence

None.

DRUG INTERACTIONS

None.

METHOD OF ADMINISTRATION

TPM Literature

The flowers are recommended as decoction and syrup for oral intake. Aromatic water (distillate) is also used orally. Sprinkle burnt powder on lesions is applied for oral conditions (Aghili Khorasani 1771).

Current Evidence

Powder, infusion, decoction, syrup, and aqueous extract are used orally.

DOSAGE

Up to 4 g per day of the flowers can be used for decoction/infusion (IHP Committee, 2003). A dose range of 250–500 mg per day of the freeze-dried aqueous extract for a period of 4–8 weeks are used in RCTs.

REFERENCES

Abdol N, Setorki M. Evaluation of antidepressant, antianxiolytic, and antioxidant effects of *Echium amoenum* L. extract on social isolation stress of male mice. Iran Red Crescent Med J. 2020;22(1):e97593.

Aghili Khorasani MH 1771. *Makhzan-al-Adviah* (*The treasury of drugs*) (rewritten by Shams Ardakani MR, Rahimi R, Farjadmand F, 1st ed.). Tehran: Tehran University of Medical Sciences; 2009.

Avicenna 1025. *Al-Qanoon fi al-Tibb* (*The canon of medicine*) (rewritten by Masoudi A, ed.). Tehran: Almaei; 2015.

Azizi H, Ghafari S, Ghods R, et al. A review study on pharmacological activities, chemical constituents, and traditional uses of *Echium amoenum*. Pharmacogn Rev. 2018;12(24):208–213.

Baghbadoranee PY. Comparison the effect of *Echium amoenum* extract with fluoxetine on depression in menopausal women: A double-blind randomized controlled trial. Asian J Pharm. 2019;13(3):271–275.

Bargard MS, Boostani H, Saiiah M, et al. Efficacy of aqueous extract of *Echium amoenum* L. in the treatment of mild to moderate obsessive-compulsive disorder. J Med Plants 2005;4(15):43–50.

Farahmand M, Khalili D, Ramezani Tehrani F, et al. Effectiveness of *Echium amoenum* on premenstrual syndrome: A randomized, double-blind, controlled trial. BMC Complement Med. 2020;20(1):1–9.

Faryadian S, Sydmohammadi A, Khosravi A, et al. Aqueous extract of *Echlum amoenum* elevate CSF serotonin and dopamine level in depression rat. Biomed Pharmacol J. 2014;7(1):137–142.

Ghorbani M, Araghi A, Shariatifar N, et al. The toxicity effect of *Echium amoenum* on the liver and kidney of mice. Curr Drug Discov Technol. 2021;18(4):548–553.

Hamidi EM, Khaksari M, Hojabri KH. The effects of aqueous extracts of *Echium amoenum* and *Citrus aurantiflia* on blood pressure and heart rate before and after phynelephrine injection in rat. J Kerman Univ Med Sci. 2011;18(4):349–357.

Heidari MR, Azad EM, Mehrabani M. Evaluation of the analgesic effect of *Echium amoenum* Fisch. & C.A. Mey. extract in mice: possible mechanism involved. J Ethnopharmacol. 2006a;103(3):345–349.

Heydari M, Mandegari A, Hosseini A, Vahedian M. Anticonvulsant effect of methanolic extract of Echium amoenum Fisch. and C.A. Mey. against seizure induced by picrotoxin in mice. Pak J Biol Sci. 2006b;9(4):772–776.

IHP Committee. *Iranian herbal pharmacopoeia (IHP)*. Tehran: Ministry of Health and Medical Education; 2003.

Mohajer A, Araghi A, Sadighara P. Oxidative stress and toxicity effect of *Echium amoenum* on mice brain. Comp Clin Path. 2019;28(2):397–401.

Nouri M, Farajdokht F, Torbati M, et al. A close look at *Echium amoenum* processing, neuroactive components, and effects on neuropsychiatric disorders. Galen Med. 2019a;8:e1559.

Nouri M, Farajdokht F, Torbati M, et al. Antidepressant and anxiolytic effect of *Echium amoenum* in restraint stress model: the role of neuroinflammation in the prefrontal cortex and hippocampus. Iran Red Crescent Med J. 2019b;21(10):e95438.

Rabbani M, Sajjadi SE, Khalili S. A lack of tolerance to the anxiolytic action of *Echium amoenum*. Res Pharm Sci. 2011;6(2):101–106.

Rabbani M, Sajjadi SE, Vaseghi G, Jafarian A. Anxiolytic effects of *Echium amoenum* on the elevated plus-maze model of anxiety in mice. Fitoterapia. 2004;75(5):457–464.

Rabiei Z, Setorki M. Effect of hydroalcoholic *Echium amoenum* extract on scopolamine-induced learning and memory impairment in rats. Pharm Biol. 2018;56(1):672–677.

Ranjbar A, Khorami S, Safarabadi M, et al. Antioxidant activity of Iranian *Echium amoenum* Fisch. & C.A. Mey flower decoction in humans: A cross-sectional before/after clinical trial. Evid-Based Complement Alternat Med. 2006;3(4):469–473.

Sadeghi L, Tanwir F, Babadi VY. Physiological and biochemical effects of *Echium amoenum* extract on Mn^{2+} -imposed Parkinson like disorder in rats. Adv Pharm Bull. 2018a;8(4):705–713.

Sadeghi L, Yousefi Babadi V, Tanwir F. Improving effects of *Echium amoenum* aqueous extract on rat model of Alzheimer's disease. J Integr Neurosci. 2018b;17(3–4):661–669.

Sadighara P, Araghi A, Tajdar-Oranj B, et al. The effect of borage (*Echium amoenum*) on the mouse heart and hematology parameters. Cardiovasc Hematol Disord Drug Targets. 2019;19(2):154–159.

Safaeian L, Tameh AA, Ghannadi A, et al. Protective effects of *Echium amoenum* Fisch. and C.A. Mey. against cerebral ischemia in the rats. Adv Biomed Res. 2015;4:107.

Sayyah M, Boostani H, Pakseresht S, Malaieri A. Efficacy of aqueous extract of *Echium amoenum* in treatment of obsessive-compulsive disorder. Prog Neuropsychopharmacol Biol Psychiatry. 2009;33(8):1513–1516.

Sayyah M, Sayyah M, Kamalinejad M. A preliminary randomized double blind clinical trial on the efficacy of aqueous extract of *Echium amoenum* in the treatment of mild to moderate major depression. Prog Neuropsychopharmacol Biol Psychiatry. 2006;30(1):166–169.

Sayyah M, Siahpoosh A, Khalili H, et al. A double-blind, placebo-controlled study of the aqueous extract of *Echium amoenum* for patients with general anxiety disorder. Iran J Pharm Res. 2012;11(2):697–701.

Shafaghi B, Naderi N, Tahmasb L, Kamalinejad M. Anxiolytic effect of *Echium amoenum* L. in mice. Iran J Pharm Res. 2002;1(1):37–41.

Yousefi M. Comparison of anxiolytic-like effects of *Echium amoenum* in the male and female rats. Der Pharma Chemica. 2016;8(18):35–39.

Zamansoltani F, Nassiri-Asl M, Karimi R, Mamaghani-Rad P. Hepatotoxicity effects of aqueous extract of *Echium amoenum* in rats. Pharmacologyonline. 2008;1:432–438.

Zannou O, Pashazadeh H, Ghellam M, et al. Extraction of anthocyanins from borage (*Echium amoenum*) flowers using choline chloride and a glycerol-based, deep eutectic solvent: Optimization, antioxidant activity, and in vitro bioavailability. Molecules. 2022;27(1):134.

14 *Foeniculum vulgare* Mill.

Mozhgan MehriArdestani

Scientific name: *Foeniculum vulgare* Mill.
Family: Apiaceae
Common names:

- **English:** Fennel
- **Persian:** *rāziyāne, bādiyān*
- **Arabic:** *rāziyānağ*

Medicinal part: Fruit, leaf, root (Figure 14.1)
Temperament (nature): Hot in the third degree and dry the in the first degree
Major chemical constituents:

- **Volatile oil:** Trans-anethole (80–90%), fenchone, estragole, α-pinene, camphene, *p*-cymene, myrcene, limonene, α- and β-phellandrene, terpinols, γ-fenchen
- **Hydroxycoumarins (minor):** Umbelliferone, scopoletin, osthenol, scoparin
- **Furocoumarins (minor):** Bergapten, columbianetin, psoralen, imperatorin, xanthotoxin, isopimpinellin
- **Flavonoids:** Glycosides of eriodictyol, quercetin, and kaempferol
- **Fatty oil:** Petroselinic acid and oleic acid (75–82.8%), linoleic acid, palmitic acid, stearic acid, myristic acid
- **Phenolic acids:** Caffeoylquinic acid: neochlorogenic acid, rosmarinic acid, chlorogenic acid, gallic acid, chlorogenic acid, caffeic acid, *p*-coumaric acid, ferulic acid-7-O-glucoside
- **Benzoisofuranone derivatives:** Miyabenol, trans-resveratrol-3-O-β-D-glucopyranoside, sinapyl glucoside, syringin-4-O-β-glucoside, 7α-hydroxycampesterol (Gruenwald et al., 2007; Rather et al., 2016; Al-Snafi, 2018)

THERAPEUTIC USE

TPM LITERATURE

The most used part of fennel is the fruits. Local application of fennel fruits and leaves as compress with the decoction or as an eyeliner improves eyesight and is effective in preventing cataract. If taken orally, it has a cleansing effect on the accumulated phlegm humor in GI tract and, consequently, antiemetic and antiflatulent properties. It is also a gastric tonic due to astringent effect and is helpful in stomach burning, abdominal cramps, and chronic diarrhea. Local application of warm fennel powder on children's stomachs can reduce colic pains and bloating. Oral consumption of fennel, especially if taken fresh, has potent galactagogue, as well as emmenagogue and diuretic properties. Decoction of fennel is known as a bioavailability enhancer which facilitates the oral absorption of other medicines into blood circulation. It is helpful in the treatment of hip and flank pain, as well. Moreover, it may be useful in the treatment of the stings of poisonous animals such as scorpions and bees (Aghili Khorasani 1771; Avicenna 1025).

DOI: 10.1201/b22971-14

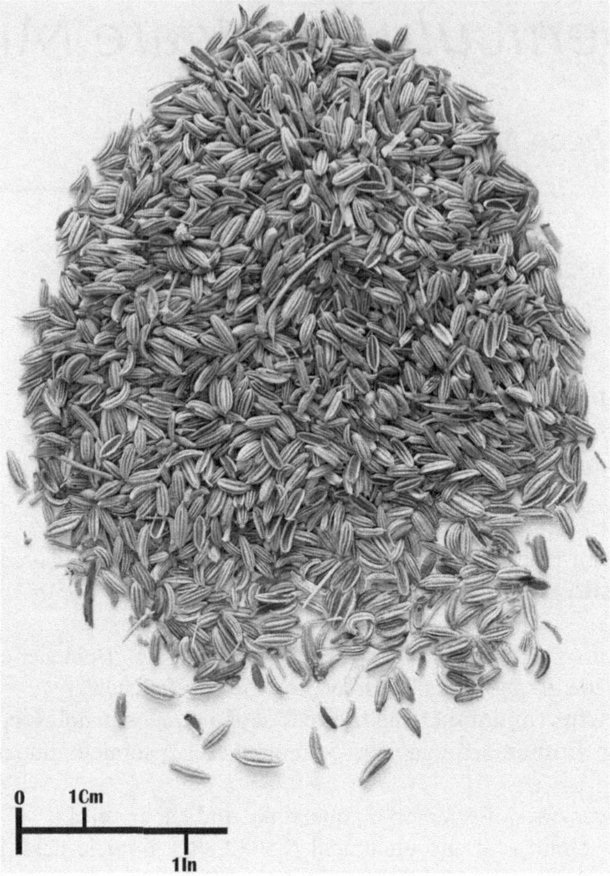

FIGURE 14.1 Fennel fruits.

Current Evidence

Clinical Evidence

Amenorrhea: In an RCT on women complained of menstrual cessation induced due to depot medroxyprogesterone acetate, patients were treated with fennel, oral contraceptive (LD) or placebo for 21 days. All participants received two placebo or fennel capsules (100 mg soft gel capsules, containing 30% w/w fennel essential oil, equal to 71–90 mg anethole) and one placebo or LD pill daily for 21 days. Significantly more women in the fennel and LD groups experienced menstrual bleeding compared to the placebo group. Mean amount of menstrual bleeding among those who experienced menstruation was significantly higher in the fennel group than both the LD and placebo groups. Also, women using fennel and LD were significantly more likely to have subsequent depot medroxyprogesterone acetate injection than those using placebo (Mohebbi-Kian et al., 2014).

Primary dysmenorrhea: In a systematic review and meta-analysis including 12 studies, it was revealed that fennel as oral drop or capsule, can significantly decrease the intensity of dysmenorrhea. The dose of 25–30 drops of 2% fennel preparations, or capsules containing 30–46 mg of fennel, 4–6 times per day were the routine dosage reported in RCTs. Also, comparison of fennel to mefenamic acid in six trials showed a statistically similar efficacy between these two interventions (Shahrahmani et al., 2021).

PCOS: In an RCT in 61 patients with PCOS, the effect of fennel fruit infusion along with dry cupping was compared with metformin. Fennel fruit was administered as an infusion of 5 g of the fruits, once a day except during menstruation; while metformin was administered 500 mg, three times daily. Patients in fennel group also received dry cupping from the seventh day of menstruation cycle, up to the 14th day. At the end of the 6-month intervention, fennel plus dry cupping was effective to regulate bleeding pattern with a similar efficacy to metformin; while the herbal intervention was more effective than metformin on the reduction of dysmenorrhea (Mokaberinejad et al., 2019). A double-blind RCT evaluated the effect of fennel essential oil capsule (46 mg), twice daily for a period of 12 weeks, in 30 students with PCOS. Considering ultrasonographic evaluation of ovarian cysts, hirsutism, BMI, and menstrual cycle, no significant difference was observed between the placebo group and fennel (Ghavi et al., 2019). Another RCT assessed the effect of fennel added to hypocaloric standard diet or hypocaloric high-protein diet on anthropometric and androgenic parameters in 64 cases with PCOS; however, 3 months of treatment with daily two soft gel capsules of fennel essential oil caused no additive antiobesity effect (Nadjarzadeh et al., 2021). The controversial results of these studies might be due to the difference in type of fennel preparation, sample size, and follow up period; thus, future studies are required to clarify the efficacy of fennel in PCOS.

Menopause: In an RCT on 60 postmenopausal women, fennel fruit ethanolic extract as a 5% vaginal cream was compared with a placebo cream regarding its effect on vaginal atrophy. The creams were administered 5 g per day for 8 weeks. The number of superficial cells and maturation vaginal index were significantly increased in the fennel group vs. control group at the end of the study. The number of intermediate and parabasal cells, as well as vaginal pH were significantly decreased in the fennel group compared to the control group (Yaralizadeh et al., 2016). Also, fennel cream was able to significantly improve sexual satisfaction in these women via reduction of dyspareunia due to vaginal dryness (Najar et al., 2015). Also, a meta-analysis on seven RCTs assessed the effect of fennel on menopause showed that despite the high risk of bias among these trials, most studies are in favor of the beneficial effects of fennel vs. placebo on menopausal symptoms. Most studies have used a dosage of 100 mg, three times daily, of fennel essential oil capsules (Lee et al., 2021).

Osteoarthritis: In a double-blind RCT including 66 women with osteoarthritis, fennel fruit extract with a dose of 800 mg per day was compared with placebo for 2 weeks. The patients completed the Western Ontario and McMaster Universities Osteoarthritis Index (WOMAC) questionnaire and VAS for pain intensity measurement before and after the intervention. A significant decrease was noted between the two groups in terms of pain, disability, total WOMAC score, and VAS variables. After comparing the pre- and postintervention, the variables mentioned above revealed a significant decline in both groups. The stiffness variable indicated a significant reduction in the fennel group (between baseline and study completion) after 2 weeks, but this decline was not significant in the placebo group, and was not significant either between the two groups (Alazadeh et al., 2020).

Hirsutism: In a double-blind RCT, 38 patients were treated with creams containing 1% or 2% of fennel fruit ethanolic extract, or placebo, twice daily for 12 weeks. Fennel cream could significantly and dose dependently decrease hair thickness and growth rate compared with placebo (Javidnia et al., 2003). Another RCT assessed the antihirsutism effects of fennel fruit ethanol extract as a 3% gel on 44 women with mild to moderate idiopathic hirsutism for 24 weeks which also reported a significant reduction of hair thickness vs. placebo (Akha et al., 2014).

Infantile colic: An RCT evaluated the effect of a fennel fruit oil emulsion (0.1%) on infantile colic including 125 infants with 2–12 weeks of age. The emulsion was administered orally before meals four times daily with a dose range of 5–20 mL for a period of 1 week. A significantly better relief of colic symptoms, i.e., decrease of cumulative crying to less than 9 hours per week, was observed upon treatment with fennel (65%) in comparison to placebo (23%) (Alexandrovich et al., 2003).

Prolactin level: To evaluate the effect of fennel on prolactin, 46 nursing mothers were administered with 3 g of fennel fruit powder, divided into six capsules daily for 15 days. Compared with the baseline levels, fennel could cause a significant rise in serum prolactin level (Honarvar et al., 2013).

PMS: Efficacy of fennel oil oral drop was evaluated in an RCT on 55 students with PMS. The patients were randomly divided into two groups, daily receiving 60 drops of 2% fennel essential oil or placebo in three divided doses, 3 days before and after menstruation. The severity of PMS symptoms, including anxiety, depression, excitement, and total clinical PMS symptoms was significantly reduced by fennel compared with placebo group (Delaram et al., 2011). In another RCT, 48 students with moderate or severe PMS were divided into four equal groups, administered with 2% fennel essential oil, aerobic exercise, fennel oil plus aerobic exercise, or placebo. The patients received 30 drops of fennel essential oil oral drop thrice daily, 3 days before and after menstrual cycle for two menstrual cycles. Aerobic exercise, fennel oil or fennel oil along with aerobic exercise groups significantly reduced PMS severity after first and second menstrual cycles, compared with placebo group. There was no significant difference in average of PMS symptoms among three groups after first and second menstrual cycles. Also, anxiety and depression were remarkably influenced after intervention with fennel plus exercise than fennel or exercise alone (Pazoki et al., 2016).

GI function recovery: In a surgeon-blinded RCT, 381 patients subjected to complex abdominal surgeries due to hepatobiliary, pancreatic, or gastric tumors were treated with heated fennel therapy alone or along with alimentary tract reconstruction, or placebo, alone or along with alimentary tract reconstruction. Fennel was administered as 500 g of the fruits heated in microwave, wrapped in a towel, and topically applied to the abdominal area, while the control group was treated with rice husk. The interventions started 6 h after the surgery and were repeated 6–8 times per day, each time lasting 15 min. The time to first flatus and first defecation and the fasting time were significantly less in the heated fennel therapy groups vs. controls. Abdominal distension was also significantly relieved in the experimental groups. Heated fennel therapy had no obvious beneficial effect on inflammatory markers, but improved the serum albumin level of the patients on day 9 after surgery. Among the patients with alimentary tract reconstruction, those in the fennel group had a clinically lesser hospital stay than those in the control group (Chen et al., 2020). In other study, 159 patients undergoing laparotomy for gynecological cancers were randomized to receive a cup of fennel tea or water. Fennel tea was prepared with 5 g of the fruits boiled with 130 mL of water, while patients in control group drank the equal quantity of water twice per day from the first morning after operation until the first flatus. The mean times to first flatus and defecation were significantly lower in fennel group compared with control group. Also, ileus symptoms had a lower frequency in patients treated with fennel tea compared to the control group (Ma et al., 2015).

Preclinical Evidence

Pain and Inflammation: The four extracts of aerial part of fennel, namely, hexane, methylene chloride, ethyl acetate, and methanolic extracts showed remarkable antinociceptive activity against acetic acid-induced nociception. Antinociceptive and anti-inflammatory activities were studied using the writhing method and Carrageenan-induced rat's paw edema in mice, respectively. The potent antinociceptive activity expressed by the methanolic (2,000 mg/kg) and ethyl acetate

(800 mg/kg) extracts can be attributed to the content of phenolic constituents. Also, the four extracts under investigation exhibited a significant anti-inflammatory activity (Nassar et al., 2010).

Glaucoma: The aqueous fruit extract of fennel demonstrated significant ocular hypotensive activity using water-loading and steroid-induced glaucoma model. This extract exhibited 17.49, 21.16, and 22.03% reduction of intraocular pressure in normotensive rabbits at 0.3%, 0.6%, and 1.2% (w/v) concentrations, respectively. A maximum mean difference of 31.20% was observed between vehicle-treated and extract-treated eyes in water-loading experimental animal model; while a maximum mean intraocular pressure lowering of 31.29% was observed in steroid-induced model of glaucoma (Agarwal et al., 2008).

Peptic ulcer: The aqueous extract of fennel showed remarkable antiulcerogenic effect against ethanol-induced gastric lesions in rats. This effect was highest and statistically significant in 300 mg/kg group vs. control group of animals. Additionally, aqueous extract of fennel significantly reduced the whole blood MDA levels; while significantly increased nitrite, nitrate, ascorbic acid, retinol, and beta-carotene levels (Birdane et al., 2007).

Antispasmodic activity: The antispasmodic activity of 2.5 and 10.0 mL/L of alcoholic extract of fennel were tested *ex vivo* in guinea pig ileum and using acetylcholine and histamine as spasmogens. An alcoholic extract of the fruits of fennel possesses antispasmodic activity, which inhibits the acetylcholine and histamine-induced guinea pig ileal contractions (Forster et al., 1980). In another study using metacholine-induced and KCl-induced contraction in guinea pig tracheal muscles, fennel essential oil, as well as the aqueous and ethanolic extracts were evaluated. While the essential oil and ethanolic extract had a significant spasmolytic effect on metacholine-induced contraction, aqueous extract was ineffective. On the other hand, the ethanolic extract and the essential oil were not significantly effective on the KCl-induced contraction, suggesting fennel to show its spasmolytic activity via potassium channel opening (Boskabady et al., 2004). Also, in isolated rat uterus, 50 μg/mL of fennel essential oil showed a significant antispasmodic effect on oxytocin-induced and prostaglandin-induced contraction (Ostad et al., 2001).

ADVERSE REACTIONS

TPM Literature

It is harmful for hot-tempered people and oxymel or sandalwood can ameliorate its damage. In addition, fennel is digested slowly and, in some cases, may weaken the stomach especially when it is taken with warm water (Aghili Khorasani 1771).

Current Evidence

Fennel oil has "generally recognized as safe" status for food use in the United States and side effects are not reported within therapeutic dosages of fennel products.

Rare cases of allergic reactions, such as atopic dermatitis and photosensitivity, are reported. Cross-sensitivity may appear in patients with a history of allergy to celery (Gruenwald et al., 2007).

Epileptic seizures, respiratory problems including hay fever, occupational rhinoconjunctivitis, and asthma have been reported with fennel oil.

Inhalation of essential oils of fennel resulted in 1.2–2.5-fold increase in relative sympathetic activity, representing low-frequency amplitude of SBP (Ulbricht, 2010). There is a report of premature thelarche and increased estradiol levels in girls with 5 months to 5 years of age who consumed 2 to 3 cups of fennel tea for a period of 4 months to 2 year (Gardner and McGuffin, 2013; Okdemir et al., 2014).

CONTRAINDICATIONS

TPM Literature

None.

Current Evidence

Fennel should not be consumed by individuals with a known allergy or hypersensitivity to other members of the Apiaceae family because of the chance of cross-sensitization.

Some references suggest estragole in fennel to be a procarcinogen (Ulbricht 2010); however, it does not mean a carcinogenic effect for fennel because the plant contains several other constituents which modify each other and the results of evaluations on a purified compound cannot be extrapolated to the plant extracts (Gori et al., 2012). It is better to use fennel for a maximum of 2 weeks (Gruenwald, 2007).

PREGNANCY AND LACTATION

TPM Literature

As it is an emmenagogue, it may induce bleeding during pregnancy and should be avoided during this period.

As it is a galactagogue, it can be used during lactation in the form of powder or decoction (Aghili Khorasani 1771).

Current Evidence

Fennel fruit is one of the most commonly used botanicals by nursing mothers, and it is also given to colicky infants (Gardner and McGuffin, 2013). There are no reports in the scientific literature of fennel oil being either safe or contraindicated during lactation (Mills et al., 2006). Fennel preparations (except infusion) are not recommended during pregnancy due to the emmenagogue properties (Gardner and McGuffin, 2013).

The use of fennel oil or alcoholic extract in breastfeeding mothers is not recommended due to lack of sufficient data. Oral intake of fennel for entire period of pregnancy results in shorter gestational age. Fennel essential oil reduced the limb bud differentiation from rat embryo (Mahboubi et al., 2019). Fennel essential oil significantly reduced the intensity of oxytocin and PGE2-induced contractions in the rat uterus and reduced the frequency of contractions induced by PGE2 (Mills et al., 2006).

DRUG INTERACTIONS

Fluoroquinolone antibiotics: Simultaneous use of fennel and ciprofloxacin may lead to decreased bioavailability of ciprofloxacin. Theoretically, fennel may also interfere similarly with other fluoroquinolone antibiotics.

Antiplatelets and anticoagulants: Fennel may increase the risk of bleeding when taken with antiplatelets, anticoagulants, or supplements that increase the risk of bleeding (*Ginkgo biloba*, garlic and saw palmetto) (Ulbricht, 2010).

METHOD OF ADMINISTRATION

TPM Literature

For the oral consumption of fennel, its decoction with water or its hydroalcoholic extract is used. Powdered fennel is recommended orally with or without water or sugar. Rubbing its powder to abdominal skin has been recommended for abdominal cramps. Intraocular use of its decoction has been applied for strengthening eyesight (Aghili Khorasani 1771).

Current Evidence

Crushed or ground fruits for teas, tea-like products, as well as other galenic preparations for internal use (Gruenwald et al., 2007).

DOSAGE

Adults (18 years and older): For ACE inhibitor-induced cough, 1–1.5 g of fennel fruit has been used up to three times daily. For dysmenorrhea, 25 drops of a 2% concentration of fennel fruit have been taken every 4 h for 5 days (Ulbricht, 2010). A general daily dose of 5-7 g can be considered for a maximum of 2 weeks (Gruenwald et al., 2007).
Children (younger than 18 years): For infantile colic (ages 2–12 weeks), 0.1% fennel fruit oil have been studied for 1 week (Ulbricht, 2010).

REFERENCES

Abbas A, Ikram R, Khan SS, et al. The fennel, *Foeniculum vulgare* incorporated diet shows anxiolytic potential: A pre-clinical study. Pak J Pharm Sci. 2019;32(4):1813–1819.

Afiat M, Amini E, Ghazanfarpour M, et al. The effect of short-term treatment with fennel on lipid profile in postmenopausal women: A randomized controlled trial. J Menopausal Med. 2018;24(1):29–33.

Agarwal R, Gupta SK, Agrawal SS, et al. Oculohypotensive effects of *Foeniculum vulgare* in experimental models of glaucoma. Indian J Physiol Pharmacol. 2008;52(1):77–83.

Aghili Khorasani MH 1771. *Makhzan-al-Adviah* (*The treasury of drugs*) (rewritten by Shams Ardakani MR, Rahimi R, Farjadmand F, 1st ed.). Tehran: Tehran University of Medical Sciences; 2009.

Akha O, Rabiei K, Kashi Z, et al. The effect of fennel (*Foeniculum vulgare*) gel 3% in decreasing hair thickness in idiopathic mild to moderate hirsutism: A randomized placebo controlled clinical trial. Caspian J Intern Med. 2014;5(1):26–29.

Alazadeh M, Azadbakht M, Niksolat F, et al. Effect of sweet fennel seed extract capsule on knee pain in women with knee osteoarthritis. Complement Ther Clin Pract. 2020;40:101219.

Alexandrovich I, Rakovitskaya O, Kolmo E, et al. The effect of fennel (*Foeniculum vulgare*) seed oil emulsion in infantile colic: A randomized, placebo-controlled study. Altern Ther Health Med. 2003;9(4):58–61.

Al-Snafi AE. The chemical constituents and pharmacological effects of *Foeniculum vulgare*: A review. IOSR J Pharm. 2018;8(5):81–96.

Avicenna 1025. *Al-Qanoon fi al-Tibb* (*The canon of medicine*) (rewritten by Masoudi A, ed.). Tehran: Almaei; 2015.

Birdane FM, Cemek M, Birdane YO, et al. Beneficial effects of *Foeniculum vulgare* on ethanol-induced acute gastric mucosal injury in rats. World J Gastroenterol. 2007;13(4):607.

Boskabady MH, Khatami A, Nazari A. Possible mechanism(s) for relaxant effects of *Foeniculum vulgare* on guinea pig tracheal chains. Pharmazie. 2004;59(7):561–564.

Chen B, He Y, Xiao Y, et al. Heated fennel therapy promotes the recovery of gastrointestinal function in patients after complex abdominal surgery: A single-center prospective randomized controlled trial in China. Surgery. 2020;168(5):793–799.

Delaram M, Jafari F. The effect of fennel on the pre-menstrual syndrome. Knowl Health. 2011;6:1–6.

Forster HB, Niklas H, Lutz S. Antispasmodic effects of some medicinal plants. Planta Med. 1980;40(4):309–319.

Gardner Z, McGuffin M. *Botanical safety handbook*. Boca Raton: Taylor & Francis; 2013.

Ghavi F, Taghizadeh M, Taebi M, Abdolahian S. Effect of *Foeniculum vulgare* essence on symptoms of polycystic ovarian syndrome (PCOS): A randomized double-blind, placebo-controlled trial. J Herb Med. 2019;17:100277.

Gori L, Gallo E, Mascherini V, et al. Can estragole in fennel seed decoctions really be considered a danger for human health? A fennel safety update. Evid-Based Complement Altern Med. 2012 (2012):860542.

Gruenwald J, Brendler T, Jaenicke C. *PDR for herbal medicines*. Montvale: Thomson Reuters; 2007.

Honarvar F, Tadayon M, Afshari P, et al. The effect of fennel on serum prolactin level in lactating women. Iran J Obstet Gynecol Infertil. 2013;16:18–24.

Javidnia K, Dastgheib L, Samani SM, Nasiri A. Antihirsutism activity of fennel (fruits of *Foeniculum vulgare*) extract: A double-blind placebo-controlled study. Phytomedicine. 2003;10(6–7):455–458.

Kim DH, Ahn YJ. Contact and fumigant activities of constituents of *Foeniculum vulgare* fruit against three coleopteran stored-product insects. Pest Manag Sci. 2001;57(3):301–306.

Lee HW, Ang L, Kim E, Lee MS. Fennel (*Foeniculum vulgare* Miller) for the management of menopausal women's health: A systematic review and meta-analysis. Complement Ther Clin Pract. 2021;43:101360.

Ma HW, Zhao JT, Zhao X. The effect of fennel tea drinking on postoperative gut recovery after gynecological malignancies operation. J Sichuan Univ (Med Sci Ed). 2015;46(6):940–943.

Mahboubi M. Fennel as valuable plant in management of women's health. J Menopausal Med. 2019;25(1):1–14.

Masoudzadeh SH, Mohammadabadi M, Khezri A, et al. Effects of diets with different levels of fennel (*Foeniculum vulgare*) seed powder on *DLK1* gene expression in brain, adipose tissue, femur muscle and rumen of Kermani lambs. Small Rumin Res. 2020;193:106276.

Mills E, Dugoua JJ, Perri D, and Koren G. *Herbal medicines in pregnancy and lactation: An evidence-based approach*. Toronto: Taylor & Francis; 2006.

Mohebbi-Kian E, Alizadeh-Charandabi SM, Bekhradi R. Efficacy of fennel and combined oral contraceptive on depot medroxyprogesterone acetate-induced amenorrhea: A randomized placebo-controlled trial. Contraception. 2014;90(4):440–446.

Mokaberinejad R, Rampisheh Z, Aliasl J, Akhtari E. The comparison of fennel infusion plus dry cupping versus metformin in management of oligomenorrhoea in patients with polycystic ovary syndrome: A randomised clinical trial. J Obstet Gynaecol. 2019;39(5):652–658.

Nadjarzadeh A, Ghadiri-Anari A, Ramezani-Jolfaie N, et al. Effect of hypocaloric high-protein, low-carbohydrate diet supplemented with fennel on androgenic and anthropometric indices in overweight and obese women with polycystic ovary syndrome: A randomized placebo-controlled trial. Complement Ther Med. 2021;56:102633.

Najar S, Yaralizadeh M, Abedi P, et al. Effect of fennel vaginal cream on dysparonia and sexual satisfaction among postmenopausal women: A double-blind randomized controlled trial. Iran J Obstet Gynecol Infertil. 2015;18(171):8–16.

Nassar MI, Aboutabl EA, Makled YA, et al. Secondary metabolites and pharmacology of *Foeniculum vulgare* Mill. Subsp. Piperitum. Rev Latinoam Quim. 2010;38(2):103–112.

Okdemir D, Hatipoglu N, Kurtoglu S, et al. Premature thelarche related to fennel tea consumption? J Pediatr Endocrinol Metab. 2014;27(1–2):175–179.

Ostad SN, Soodi M, Shariffzadeh M, et al. The effect of fennel essential oil on uterine contraction as a model for dysmenorrhea, pharmacology and toxicology study. J Ethnopharmacol. 2001;76(3):299–304.

Pazoki H, Bolouri G, Farokhi F, Azerbayjani MA. Comparing the effects of aerobic exercise and fennel on premenstrual syndrome. Middle East Fertil Soc J. 2016;21:61–64.

Rather MA, Dar BA, Sofi SN, Bhat BA, Qurishi MA. Foeniculum vulgare: A comprehensive review of its traditional use, phytochemistry, pharmacology, and safety. Arab J Chem. 2016;9:S1574–1583.

Shahrahmani H, Ghazanfarpour M, Shahrahmani N, et al. Effect of fennel on primary dysmenorrhea: A systematic review and meta-analysis. J Complemenr Integr Med. 2021;18(2):261–269.

Tanira MO, Shah AH, Mohsin A, et al. Pharmacological and toxicological investigations on *Foeniculum vulgare* dried fruit extract in experimental animals. Phytother Res. 1996;10(1):33–36.

Ulbricht CE. *Natural standard herb & supplement guide: An evidence-based reference*. St. Luis: Elsevier Mosby; 2010.

Yaralizadeh M, Abedi P, Najar S, et al. Effect of *Foeniculum vulgare* (fennel) vaginal cream on vaginal atrophy in postmenopausal women: A double-blind randomized placebo-controlled trial. Maturitas. 2016;84:75–80.

Yavangi M, Rabiee S, Nazari S, et al. Comparison of the effect of oestrogen plus *Foeniculum vulgare* seed and oestrogen alone on increase in endometrial thickness in infertile women. J Clin Diagn Res. 2018;12(1):1–4.

15 *Fumaria officinalis* L., *F. indica* (Hausskn.) Pugsley, *F. parviflora* Lam., *F. vaillantii* Loisel.

Roja Rahimi

Scientific name: *Fumaria officinalis* L., *F. indica* (Hausskn.) Pugsley, *F. parviflora* Lam., *F. vaillantii* Loisel.
Family: Papaveraceae
Common names:

- **English:** Fumitory, earth smoke
- **Persian:** *šāhtare*
- **Arabic:** *šāhtarağ, sulṭān al-baqūl, baqlat al-malik, šağarat al-damm*

Medicinal part(s): Aerial parts (Figure 15.1)
Temperament (nature): Moderate in hotness and coldness and dry in the second degree
Major chemical constituents:

- **Flavonoids:** Rutin, hyperoside
- **Hydroxycinnamic acid derivatives:** Caffeoylmalic acid
- **Isoquinoline alkaloids:** Fumarine, fumaricine, fumariline, fumaritine, fumarofine, cryptopine, aurotensine, stylopine, sinactine, sanguinarine
- **Organic acids:** Fumaric acid, chlorogenic acid, caffeic acid (Pharmacist's Letter, 2013; Gruenwald et al., 2007)

THERAPEUTIC USE

TPM Literature

Fumitory can excrete yellow bile, black bile, and phlegm from the body and thus, is blood purifier. Pouring its extract into eyes can improve eyesight. Application of its extract as mouthwash is useful for mucositis and gingivitis. It acts as a gastrointestinal tonic and can increase appetite. Moreover, when it is eaten with vinegar, it is useful for nausea and vomiting and can purge gastrointestinal tract from waste materials. It is also a liver tonic and useful for liver disorders. The extract of the fresh leaves with sugar is beneficial for purging gastrointestinal tract, liver disorders, as well as skin disease including eczema, pruritis, dandruff, and psoriasis. Fumitory is also applied topically for treatment of skin conditions. It is a diuretic, as well (Aghili Khorasani 1771; Avicenna 1025).

DOI: 10.1201/b22971-15

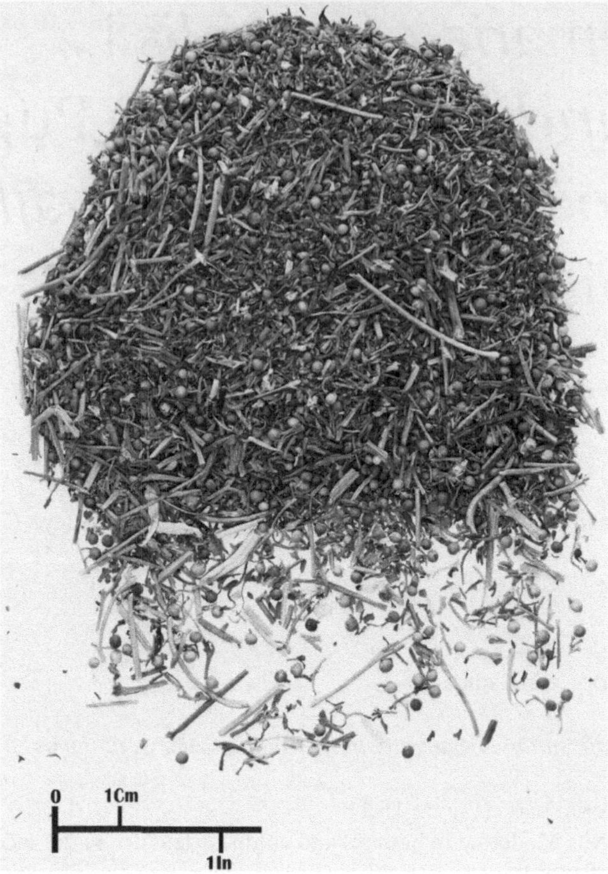

FIGURE 15.1 Fumitory aerial parts.

Current Evidence

Clinical Evidence

Skin disease: In a randomized double-blind, placebo-controlled study, applying cream from *F. parviflora* containing 4% alcoholic extract twice daily for 4 weeks reduced eczema area and severity index score in patients with chronic hand eczema (Jowkar et al., 2011). Administration of *F. parviflora* demonstrated beneficial effect on uremic pruritis. Hemodialysis patients with pruritus were randomly assigned to receive either *F. parviflora* powder (1 g per day) or a placebo for 8 weeks. The mean reduction in pruritus scores was significantly higher in the fumitory group than the placebo group. In addition, IFN-γ mean serum levels in the fumitory group significantly decreased and the mean serum IL-4 level was markedly increased in the fumitory group (Akrami et al., 2017). Four-week administration of syrup made from aqueous extract of *F. vaillantii* to patients with chronic urticaria showed similar effects to cetirizine syrup in urticaria activity score and chronic urticaria quality of life questionnaire. However, the efficacy of fumitory syrup is better that cetirizine 1 month after discontinuation of intervention (Eghbalian et al., 2018).

Biliary disorders: A double-blind placebo-controlled RCT was performed in a group of 30 patients with different biliary disorders (dyskinesia, cholecystitis, hepatopathy, cholelithiasis, postoperation cholecystectomy syndrome). Patients were taking three tablets containing 250 mg dried aqueous extract of fumitory for 28 days. The results showed reduction of symptoms especially fullness and flatulence in patients received fumitory tablets compared to placebo (Kopp, 1979).

Infantile colic: A double-blind RCT has been conducted on sixty 3–16-week-old newborns received 2.5 mL of placebo or fumitory extract. The length and frequency of crying periods and the number of times an infant would wake up due to colic pain were significantly decreased in fumitory group compared to placebo (Montaseri et al., 2013).

Preclinical Evidence

Gastrointestinal activity: Methanolic extract of *F. indica* in rats subjected to 1 hour daily unavoidable foot-shocks demonstrated the potent gastroprotective activity against chronic stress-induced ulcers which may be mediated by regulation of monoamine, corticosterone, and cytokine homeostasis (Shakya et al., 2016). Ethanolic extract of *F. indica* showed antisecretory activity in rat model of pyloric ligation-induced ulcer. GSH level, gastric wall mucus, and percentage protection of ulcer were significantly increased in absolute ethanol-induced ulcer model. Moreover, the extract revealed *in vitro* antacid activity (Chandra et al., 2015). The aqueous-methanol extract of *F. parviflora* showed prokinetic and laxative activities in mice and guinea pig at 30 and 100 mg/kg which is partially mediated through cholinergic pathways (Najeeb-ur-Rehman et al., 2012). The presence of cholinergic and calcium channel blockade constituents in fumitory may explain its beneficial effect in both constipation and diarrhea (Gilani et al., 2005).

Effects on liver: There are several studies on *Fumaria* spp. that demonstrate their hepatoprotective activity against hepatotoxicity, hepatic cancer, as well as hepatitis B and C virus (Jamaldeen et al., 2022).

Diuretic activity: A single dose of 250 mg/kg from *F. officinalis* revealed a strong increase in urinary volumetric excretion of saline-loaded rats, 24 h after the oral administration. Moreover, it increased the urinary excretion of sodium and potassium ions (Păltinean et al., 2017).

ADVERSE REACTIONS

TPM Literature

It is harmful for lung and chicory can ameliorate its damage (Aghili Khorasani 1771).

Current Evidence

Use of 250 mg dried water extract of fumitory for 28 days was tolerated and safe (Kopp, 1979). Applying cream from *F. parviflora* containing 4% alcoholic extract twice daily for 4 weeks caused side effects such as erythema and population (Jowkar et al., 2011). Nausea and stomach pain was reported following administration of aqueous extract of *F. vaillantii* (Eghbalian et al., 2018). Fumitory contains protopine alkaloids that may cause convulsion and death when ingested in large amounts (Pharmacist's Letter, 2013).

CONTRAINDICATIONS

TPM Literature

None.

Current Evidence

None.

PREGNANCY AND LACTATION

TPM Literature

None.

Current Evidence

The safety of fumitory during pregnancy and lactation has not been established. In view of lack of pharmacological and toxicity data, the use of fumitory during pregnancy and lactation should be avoided (Pharmacist's Letter, 2013).

DRUG INTERACTIONS

None.

METHOD OF ADMINISTRATION

TPM Literature

Fumitory powder or its decoction with sugar is used orally. Its powder is also applied topically as poultice for skin diseases (Aghili Khorasani 1771).

Current Evidence

It is used orally as powder or infusion. Also, it is used topically especially for skin diseases.

DOSAGE

Daily dose: 2–4 g daily in divided doses (Pharmacist's Letter, 2013).

REFERENCES

Aghili Khorasani MH 1771. *Makhzan-al-Adviah* (*The treasury of drugs*) (rewritten by Shams Ardakani MR, Rahimi R, Farjadmand F, 1st ed.). Tehran: Tehran University of Medical Sciences; 2009.

Akrami R, Hashempur MH, Tavakoli A, et al. Effects of *Fumaria parviflora* L on uremic pruritus in hemodialysis patients: A randomized, double-blind, placebo-controlled trial. Jundishapur J Nat Pharm Prod. 2017;12(3supp):e39744.

Al-Snafi AE. Constituents and pharmacology of *Fumaria officinalis*: A review. IOSR J Pharm. 2020;10(1):17–25.

Aoiadni N, Chiab N, Jdidi H, et al. The pyrethroid insecticide permethrin confers hepatotoxicity through DNA damage and mitochondria-associated apoptosis induction in rat: Palliative benefits of Fumaria officinalis. J Biochem Mol Toxicol. 2022;36(10):e23172.

Arbab AH, Parvez MK, Al-Dosari MS, Al-Rehaily AJ. In vitro evaluation of novel antiviral activities of 60 medicinal plants extracts against hepatitis B virus. Exp Ther Med. 2017;14(1):626–634.

Avicenna 1025. *Al-Qanoon fi al-Tibb* (*The canon of medicine*) (rewritten by Masoudi A, ed.). Tehran: Almaei; 2015.

Brice Landry K, Tariq S, Malik A, et al. *Berberis lyceum* and *Fumaria indica*: In vitro cytotoxicity, antioxidant activity, and in silico screening of their selected phytochemicals as novel hepatitis C virus nonstructural protein 5A inhibitors. J Biomol Struct Dyn. 2022;40(17):7829–7851.

Chandra P, Kishore K, Ghosh AK. Evaluation of antisecretory, gastroprotective and in-vitro antacid capacity of *Fumaria indica* in rats. J Environ Biol. 2015;36(5):1137–1142.

Eghbalian F, Esmaili N, Karimi M, et al. Comparison of the efficacy and tolerability of an oral dosage form made from *Fumaria vaillantii* versus cetirizinein management of chronic urticaria: A single-blind, randomized, clinical trial. Biomed Res Ther 2018, 5(6):2389–2401.

Gilani AH, Bashir S, Janbaz KH, Khan A. Pharmacological basis for the use of *Fumaria indica* in constipation and diarrhea. J Ethnopharmacol. 2005;96(3):585–589.

Gilani AH, Janbaz KH, Akhtar MS. Selective protective effect of an extract from *Fumaria parviflora* on paracetamol-induced hepatotoxicity. Gen Pharmacol. 1996;27(6):979–983.

Hussain T, Siddiqui HH, Fareed S, et al. Evaluation of chemopreventive effect of *Fumaria indica* against N-nitrosodiethylamine and CCl4-induced hepatocellular carcinoma in Wistar rats. Asian Pac J Trop Med. 2012;5(8):623–629.

Jamaldeen FN, Sofi G, Fahim MFM, et al. Shahatra (*F.parviflora* Lam): a comprehensive review of its ethnopharmacology, phytochemistry and pharmacology. J Ethnopharmacol. 2022;286:114839.

Jowkar F, Jamshidzadeh A, Mirzadeh Yazdi A, Pasalar M. The effects of *Fumaria parviflora* L extract on chronic hand eczema: A randomized double-blind placebo controlled clinical trial. Iran Red Crescent Med J. 2011;13:824–828.

Kopp H. Choleretsche Wirkung und Vertraeglichkeit von Chol-Kugeletten® bei Cholezystopathien. Therapiewoche. 1979;29:5645–5655.

Montaseri S, Pourarian S, Montaseri H. Effects of fumaria extract on colic pain in 3–16 weeks infants. Iran J Neonatol. 2013;4(2):10–15.

Najeeb-ur-Rehman MH, Al-Rehaily AJ, Mothana RA, Gilani AH. Species and tissue-specificity of prokinetic, laxative and spasmodic effects of *Fumaria parviflora*. BMC Complement Altern Med. 2012;12(1):1–8.

Păltinean R, Mocan A, Vlase L, et al. Evaluation of polyphenolic content, antioxidant and diuretic activities of six Fumaria species. Molecules. 2017;22(4):639.

Pharmacist's Letter. Natural Medicines Comprehensive Database. Stockton: Therapeutic Research Faculty, 2013.

Rathi A, Srivastava AK, Shirwaikar A, et al. Hepatoprotective potential of *Fumaria indica* Pugsley whole plant extracts, fractions and an isolated alkaloid protopine. Phytomedicine. 2008;15(6–7):470–477.

Shakya A, Soni UK, Rai G, et al. Gastro-protective and anti-stress efficacies of monomethyl fumarate and a *Fumaria indica* extract in chronically stressed rats. Cell Mol Neurobiol. 2016;36:621–635.

16 *Lavandula angustifolia* Mill., *Lavandula stoechas* L.

Seyede Nargess Sadati Lamardi

Scientific name: *Lavandula angustifolia* Mill., *Lavandula stoechas* L.
Family: Lamiaceae
Common name:

- **English:** French lavender (*L. stoechas*), English lavender (*L. angustifolia*)
- **Persian:** *'osṭoḫoddūs*
- **Arabic:** *anīs al-arwāḥ, mumsik al-'arwāḥ*

Medicinal part(s): Flower (Figure 16.1)
Temperament (nature): Hot in the first degree and dry in the second degree
Major chemical constituents:
L. angustifolia:

- **Volatile oil (0.5–9.62%):** Linalool (1.1–53.5%), linalyl acetate (4.2–56.70%), 1,8-cineole (0.31–44.4%), camphor (1.9–28%), lavandulyl acetate (1.2–15.9%), terpinene-4-ol (2–14.01%), α-terpineol (2–9.17%) (Akbar, 2018; Aprotosoaie et al., 2017; Moussi Imane et al., 2017; Śmigielski et al., 2013)
- **Phenolic compounds:** Apigenin, 7-methoxycoumarin, coumarin, methyl 2-hydroxy-3-(3,4-dihydroxyphenyl) propanoate, caffeic acid, methyl caffeate, 2-methoxyphenylpropionic acid, β-(4-hydroxyphenyl) lactic acid, methyl-2-hydroxy-3-(4-hydroxyphenyl) propanoate, methyl-3-(2-hydroxy-4-methoxyphenyl) propanoate, 4-hydroxybenzoic acid, 3,4-dihydroxybenzaldehyde, 3,4-dihydroxybenzoic acid, 2-hydroxycinnamic acid, 4-hydroxycinnamic acid (Yadikar et al., 2017)

L. stoechas:

Volatile oil (1–3%): Fenchone (3.06–75.50%), camphor (up to over 50%), and 1,8-cineole (20.29–34.4%), myrtenyl acetate (0.19–24.10%), 10s,11s-Himachala-3(12),4-diene (23.62%), cubenol (16.19%) (Özcan et al., 2018; Baali et al., 2018; Aprotosoaie et al., 2017; Baali et al., 2019)

THERAPEUTIC USE

TPM LITERATURE

Lavender is considered as a potent and specific cleanser of the brain from pathologic humors, especially black bile, in different forms of administration such as decoction, syrup, hot compress on the head, jam, or inhalation, and consequently, boosts brain power. Especially in the form of syrup, it

 DOI: 10.1201/b22971-16

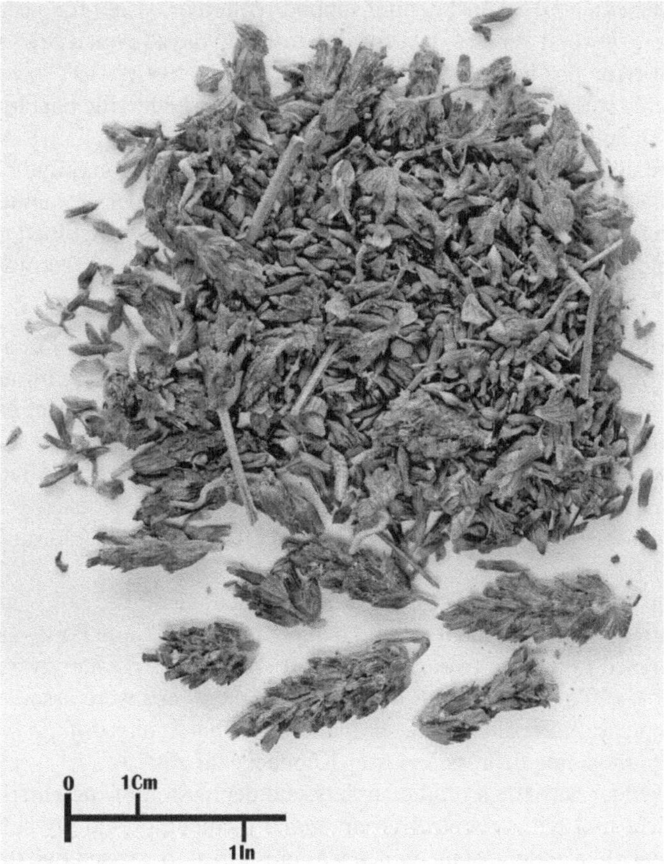

FIGURE 16.1 Lavender flower.

is one of the best treatments for a wide range of cold-tempered neurological disorders, such as melancholy, epilepsy and seizures, muscle twitching, insanity and amnesia, obsession, and depression. A mixture of lavender flowers with honey or sugar in the form of a thick jam is also considered as a potent antidepressant. Lavender decoction is a potent antitussive, can relieve the pain in ribs, and is useful in cough and cold. It is useful for lung, liver, spleen, and urinary tract diseases and infections. Fresh lavender extract, alone or with fresh lemon juice, is a tonic for the stomach (Aghili Khorasani 1771; Avicenna 1025).

Current Evidence

Clinical Evidence

Anxiety: In a systematic review and meta-analysis on 65 RCTs and 25 nonrandomized clinical studies, the efficacy of different doses and dosage forms of lavender on anxiety and anxiety-related conditions was evaluated. Most studies support the remarkable effects of lavender oil inhalation or massage on anxiety. A significant effect in diminishing anxiety levels was found in favor of the use of oral lavender essential oil (Silexan®) 80 mg per day for at least 6 weeks considering Hamilton Anxiety Scale or Zung Self-Rating Anxiety Scale. Generally, oral administration of lavender essential oil shows to be effective in the treatment of anxiety, whereas for inhalation there is only an indication of an effect of reasonable size, due to the heterogeneity of available studies (inhalation of a few drops of lavender essential oil on a neutral support [cotton or tissue] for a certain period of time [2–30 minutes] one to several times a day, for one-to-many days [even a few months]). Lavender essential oil administered through massage appears to be effective (2–10% lavender oil for 10–30 minutes), but available studies are not sufficient to determine whether the benefit is due to a specific effect of lavender (Donelli et al., 2019).

In another systematic review and meta-analysis on 22 RCTs, the anxiolytic effects of lavender aromatherapy with any form of application were evaluated. Lavender aromatherapy was found to have favorable effects on relieving self-rated anxiety, decreasing systolic blood pressure, heart rate, salivary cortisol, and chromogranin A levels; however, no significant effect was observed on diastolic blood pressure (Kang et al., 2019).

Depression: The efficacy of lavender on depression severity was assessed in a systematic review and meta-analysis of 17 RCTs. All routes of lavender administration, with any type of control group (placebo or active control) were included. Results showed significant efficacy of lavender in decreasing depression scores compared to the control group. Subgroup analysis proved that the effect of lavender was slightly more pronounced in participants with diagnosed depression, while its effect was statistically significant in patients having other diseases with simultaneous depressive symptoms. Also, the oral route was the most effective route of administration (Firoozeei et al., 2021).

A recent randomized, double-blind clinical trial evaluated the efficacy of *L. angustifolia* in comparison with fluoxetine for the treatment of mild to moderate depression. Forty-five adult outpatients were randomly assigned to receive two capsules of dried lavender powder every 12 h (1 g) or two capsules of fluoxetine (10 mg) every 12 h for 8 weeks. The groups were assessed by the Hamilton Rating Scale for Depression. Results of the study indicated that *L. angustifolia* has similar effects to fluoxetine on mild to moderate depression (Araj-Khodaei et al., 2020).

The effect of lavender herbal tea on the anxiety and depression of the elderly was evaluated in a single-blind clinical trial with a control group which included 60 elderly subjects. Intervention consisted of using 2 g of lavender teabag, which was prescribed to be used two times as decoction in the morning and night for 2 weeks. The results of this study indicated that consumption of lavender herbal tea can reduce depression and anxiety scores (Bazrafshan et al., 2020).

Pain: The effectiveness of lavender oil inhalation aromatherapy applied before dressing change on vital signs and pain levels of children with burns was tested in an RCT. A total of 108 children were studied in three groups: Lavender-15 Group inhaled lavender oil for 15 min before dressing, Lavender-60 Group inhaled lavender oil for 60 min before dressing, and control group inhaled jojoba (placebo) oil for 15 min before dressing. Pain levels and vital signs of the children were remeasured at the 1st and 30th minute after dressing. In postdressing measurements, the number of respirations, heart rate, mean arterial blood pressure and pain levels were lower in the lavender groups compared to the placebo group (Akgül et al., 2021).

Another RCT evaluated aromatherapy for postoperative abdominal pain in hospitalized patients. Study participants were randomized to receive either standard care or standard care and aromatherapy for postsurgical pain. In the aromatherapy group, one drop of lavender essential oil was topically applied to the back of the neck, temple, ear, wrist, or area of patient preference after medication and at random for pain. Of the 147 evaluable patients the use of aromatherapy showed no substantial benefit at improving pain scores or reducing medication use. A subgroup analysis of patients who received a regional nerve block for pain management; however, showed more than fivefold improvement in pain scores after the use of aromatherapy. The aromatherapy group used more medications at baseline, whereas 70% less medications were used by 24 h. Thus, aromatherapy helped in control of pain intensity for abdominal surgical patients (Welden et al., 2021).

In a double-blind RCT, the effect of the scent of lavender oil on pain in preterm infants during heel lancing was evaluated. Sixty-one premature babies (24–37 weeks of gestation) were enrolled in the study. Heart rate, oxygen saturation, and the baby's facial expression were recorded by a camera 3 min before the intervention, during the sampling, and 3 min after the procedure. There was a statistically significant difference between the two groups in terms of the Premature Infant Pain Profile-Revised during and after the sampling (Usta et al., 2021).

Insomnia: In a systematic review and meta-analysis of 19 clinical studies, the existing researches on aromatherapy with lavender oil as a treatment of insomnia were evaluated. The interventions comprising of all types of aromatherapies, including inhalation, massage, skin application. The comparisons included placebo or no intervention. The results showed that aromatherapy had a significant effect on improving sleep quality, regardless of the countries of origin of the patients. The inhalation group, rather than the massage group, had an obvious therapeutic effect, which may be due to the few numbers of studies using massage. In addition, different duration of the intervention does not seem to have a significant effect on the efficacy of aromatherapy (Tang et al., 2021).

Agitation in dementia: An RCT evaluated effectiveness of lavender essential oil on the agitated behavior of older people with and without dementia. Forty-nine nursing home residents with dementia and without dementia showing agitation participated in this study. Participants were randomized to a counterbalanced, repeated measures design experiment that tests the treatments lavender, lemon balm, and placebo (sunflower oil). Treatments were administered once daily for 2 weeks followed by a 2-week washout period before beginning the subsequent treatment. All participants trialed all three treatments over a 10-week period. Data were collected on the Neuropsychiatric Inventory (NPI) and Cohen-Mansfield Agitation Inventory (CMAI). Lavender was more effective in reducing CMAI physical nonaggressive behavior in patients with dementia. There was no reduction in agitation with treatments when compared to placebo independent of cognitive groups (Watson et al., 2019).

Preclinical Evidence

Alzheimer's disease: The effects of aqueous extract of *L. angustifolia* (50, 100 and 200 mg/kg) were assayed on spatial performance of beta amyloid (Aβ1–42)-induced Alzheimer's disease in rats. Administration of lavender extract for 20 days significantly improved the performance of control and Alzheimer's disease rats in Morris water maze, only at the dose of 200 mg/kg, as compared with their counterparts with vehicle treatment (Kashani et al., 2011). Histological observations revealed that the doses of 100 and 200 mg/kg markedly can eliminate the extent of Aβ aggregates in the hippocampus (Soheili et al., 2012). Furthermore, lavender extract (200 mg/kg) could reverse the direction of changes of some metabolites involved in Alzheimer's disease pathogenesis. The most significantly affected pathways belonged to carbohydrate and amino acid metabolism, including pantothenate and CoA metabolism, glyoxylate and dicarboxylate metabolism, alanine, aspartate and glutamate metabolism, cysteine and methionine metabolism (Oskouie et al., 2018).

Seizure: Anticonvulsant, sedative and antispasmodic activities of the hydromethanolic extract (70%) of *L. stoechas* flowers (400 and 600 mg/kg, intraperitoneally) was studied in mice. The higher dose of the extract significantly reduced the severity and increased the latency of PTZ-induced convulsions, as well as a reduction in lethality. Also, 600 mg/kg of *L. stoechas* extract exhibited sedative effect, as it prolonged the pentobarbital sleeping time in mice, with a potency similar to diazepam. In isolated rabbit jejunum preparations, *L. stoechas* caused a dose-dependent (0.1–1.0 mg/mL) relaxation of spontaneous contractions, possibly due to the blockade of calcium channels (Gilani et al., 2000).

The anti-epileptogenic and antioxidant activity of lavender hydroethanolic 70% extract (200, 400, and 800 mg/kg, intraperitoneally) on PTZ-induced seizures in mice model was evaluated. Administration of the extract every second day, 30 min before each PTZ injection was able to reduce seizure score of kindled mice and PTZ-induced mortality with a higher effectiveness vs. sodium valproate. A significant reduction of NO level was also observed in the brain tissues of the kindled mice (Rahmati et al., 2013).

ADVERSE REACTIONS

TPM Literature

It is harmful in people with hot and dry temperament and can cause thirst and nausea. This adverse effect is modified if taken with oxymel. It is said to be harmful to the lungs, and concomitant use with tragacanth and gum Arabic prevents this side effect (Aghili Khorasani 1771).

Current Evidence

No health hazards or side effects are reported upon administration of the therapeutic doses. The volatile oil possesses a weak potential for sensitization (Gruenwald et al., 2007). Allergic contact dermatitis, confirmed by patch testing, has been reported in individuals exposed to lavender essential oil (Aronson, 2008). In a systematic review and meta-analysis of the effects of lavender on anxiety, a limited number of studies reported adverse effects including headache, palpitations, infection, and gastrointestinal disturbances (eructation, diarrhea, breath odor, and dyspepsia), none of which were serious side effects (Donelli et al, 2019).

CONTRAINDICATIONS

TPM Literature

None.

Current Evidence

None.

PREGNANCY AND LACTATION

TPM Literature

None.

Current Evidence

A study in 1935 reported that lavender stimulated uterine contractions in isolated pregnant guinea pig uterus. No other information on the safety of lavender in pregnancy was identified (Gardner and Mcguffin, 2013).

DRUG INTERACTIONS

Selective serotonin reuptake inhibitors: A case report demonstrated a possible association between lavender tea, sertraline and the manifestation of moderate serotonin toxicity with objective clinical features (Seet and Rotella, 2021).

Oral contraceptives: A placebo-controlled, cross-over RCT on 24 healthy fertile women reported that an oral dose of 160 mg per day of lavender oil (Silexan) has no drug interaction with an oral contraceptive containing ethinyl estradiol (0.03 mg) and levonorgestrel (0.15 mg) (Heger-Mahn et al., 2014).

METHOD OF ADMINISTRATION

TPM Literature

Lavender can be used in various medicinal forms such as fresh extract, pills, oils, and oxymel, as well as extract, aromatic water, cooked, and concoction.

For neurological disorders, lavender is used as a form of syrup or jam. For lung, liver, spleen, and kidney diseases is used as drinking decoction. For forgetfulness lavender can be used as warm compress on the head and for relieving joint pain is used as poultice as well as incense to its cooked (Aghili Khorasani 1771).

Current Evidence

The whole drug is used for infusion, as an extract, and as a bath additive. The essential oil can be used via inhalation or topical massage in aromatherapy.

DOSAGE

Infusion: 1–2 teaspoons (5–10 g) of drug per cup of warm water, it can be administered one cup three times daily.
Lavender oil: 1–4 drops (about 20–80 mg), e.g., on a sugar cube.
External use as bath additive: 20–100 g of drug for a 20 L bath (Gruenwald et al., 2007; Blumenthal et al., 2000).

REFERENCES

Aghili Khorasani MH 1771. *Makhzan-al-Advіah* (*The treasury of drugs*) (rewritten by Shams Ardakani MR, Rahimi R, Farjadmand F, 1st ed.). Tehran: Tehran University of Medical Sciences; 2009.

Akbar S. *Handbook of 200 medicinal plants: A comprehensive review of their traditional medical uses and scientific justifications*. Cham: Springer; 2018.

Akgül EA, Karakul A, Altın A, et al. Effectiveness of lavender inhalation aromatherapy on pain level and vital signs in children with burns: A randomized controlled trial. Complement Ther Med. 2021;60:102758.

Aprotosoaie AC, Gille E, Trifan A, et al. Essential oils of *Lavandula genus*: A systematic review of their chemistry. Phytochem Rev. 2017;16:761–799.

Araj-Khodaei M, Noorbala AA, Yarani R, et al. A double-blind, randomized pilot study for comparison of *Melissa officinalis* L. and *Lavandula angustifolia* Mill. With fluoxetine for the treatment of depression. BMC Complement Med Ther. 2020;20(1):1–9.

Aronson JK. *Meyler's side effects of herbal medicines*. Oxford: Elsevier; 2008.

Avicenna 1025. *Al-Qanoon fi al-Tibb* (*The canon of medicine*) (rewritten by Masoudi A, ed.). Tehran: Almaei; 2015.

Baali F, Boumerfeg S, Napoli E, et al. Chemical composition and biological activities of essential oils from two wild Algerian medicinal plants: *Mentha pulegium* L. and *Lavandula stoechas* L. J Essent Oil-Bear. Plants. 2019;22(3):821–837.

Bazrafshan MR, Jokar M, Shokrpour N, Delam H. The effect of lavender herbal tea on the anxiety and depression of the elderly: A randomized clinical trial. Complement Ther Med. 2020;50:102393.

Blumenthal M, Goldberg A, Brinckmann J. *Herbal medicine: Expanded Commission E monographs*. Ann Arbor: Integrative Medicine Communications; 2000.

Donelli D, Antonelli M, Bellinazzi C, et al. Effects of lavender on anxiety: A systematic review and meta-analysis. Phytomedicine. 2019;65:153099.

Firoozeei TS, Feizi A, Rezaeizadeh H, et al. 2021. The antidepressant effects of lavender (*Lavandula angustifolia* Mill.): A systematic review and meta-analysis of randomized controlled clinical trials. Complement Ther Med. 2021;59:102679.

Gardner Z, McGuffin M. *Botanical safety handbook*. Boca Raton: CRC Press; 2013.

Gilani A, Aziz N, Khan M, et al. Ethnopharmacological evaluation of the anticonvulsant, sedative and antispasmodic activities of *Lavandula stoechas* L. J Ethnopharmacol. 2000;71(1–2):161–167.

Gruenwald J, Brendler T, Jaenicke C. *PDR for herbal medicines*. Montvale: Thomson Reuters; 2007.

Heger-Mahn D, Pabst G, Dienel A, et al. No interacting influence of lavender oil preparation silexan on oral contraception using an ethinyl estradiol/levonorgestrel combination. Drugs R&D. 2014;14(4):265–272.

Kang HJ, Nam ES, Lee Y, Kim M. How strong is the evidence for the anxiolytic efficacy of lavender? Systematic review and meta-analysis of randomized controlled trials. Asian Nurs Res. 2019;13(5):295–305.

Kashani MS, Tavirani MR, Talaei SA, Salami M. Aqueous extract of lavender (*Lavandula angustifolia*) improves the spatial performance of a rat model of Alzheimer's disease. Neurosci Bull. 2011;27(2):99–106.

Moussi Imane M, Houda F, Said Amal AH, et al. Phytochemical composition and antibacterial activity of Moroccan Lavandula angustifolia Mill. J Essent Oil-Bear Plants. 2017;20(4):1074–1082.

Oskouie AA, Yekta RF, Tavirani MR, et al. *Lavandula angustifolia* effects on rat models of Alzheimer's disease through the investigation of serum metabolic features using NMR metabolomics. Avicenna J Med Biotechnol. 2018;10(2):83.

Rahmati B, Khalili M, Roghani M, Ahghari P. Anti-epileptogenic and antioxidant effect of *Lavandula officinalis* aerial part extract against pentylenetetrazol-induced kindling in male mice. J Ethnopharmacol. 2013;148(1):152–157.

Seet HR, Rotella JA. Moderate serotonin toxicity precipitated by a possible interaction between lavender tea and sertraline. Emerg Med Australas. 2021;33(5):947–948.

Śmigielski KB, Prusinowska R, Krosowiak K, Sikora M. Comparison of qualitative and quantitative chemical composition of hydrolate and essential oils of lavender (*Lavandula angustifolia*). J Essent Oil Res. 2013;25(4):291–299.

Soheili M, Tavirani MR, Salami M. Clearance of amyloid beta plaques from brain of Alzheimeric rats by *Lavandula angustifolia*. Neurosci Med. 2012;3(4):26193.

Tang Y, Gong M, Qin X, et al. The therapeutic effect of aromatherapy on insomnia: A meta-analysis. J Affective Dis. 2021;288:1–9.

Usta C, Tanyeri-Bayraktar B, Bayraktar S. Pain control with lavender oil in premature infants: A double-blind randomized controlled study. J Altern Complement Med. 2021;27(2):136–141.

Watson K, Hatcher D, Good A. A randomised controlled trial of lavender (*Lavandula angustifolia*) and lemon balm (*Melissa officinalis*) essential oils for the treatment of agitated behaviour in older people with and without dementia. Complement Ther Med. 2019;42:366–373.

Welden LMS, Leatherland P, Schitter MB, et al. Abdominal surgical patients randomized to aromatherapy for pain management. J Perianesth Nurs. 2021;36(3):291–299. e293.

Yadikar N, Bobakulov KM, Eshbakova KA, Aisa HA. Phenolic compounds from Lavandula angustifolia. Chem Nat Comp 2017;53(20):1–3.

17 *Glycyrrhiza glabra* L.

Zahra Memariani and Reihaneh Moeini

Scientific name: *Glycyrrhiza glabra* L.
Family: Fabaceae
Common names:

- **English:** Licorice, liquorice, sweet wood, glycyrrhiza
- **Persian:** *šīrīn bayān, mahak*
- **Arabic:** *'irq al-sūs, sūs*

Medicinal part(s): Dried roots and the rhizome with roots (Figure 17.1)
Temperament (nature): Hot in the second degree and dry in the first degree
Major chemical constituents:

- **Triterpene saponins (3–15%):** Glycyrrhetic acid derivatives, glycyrrhizin (18β-glycyrrhetic acid salts) and derivatives, glabric acid, glabrolide, uralenic acid
- **Flavonoids:** Liquiritigenin and isoliquiritigenin glycosides, such as liquiritin, isoliquiritin, liquiritin apioside, and licuraside
- **Isoflavonoids:** Formononetin, glycyrrhisoflavone, glabridin, glabrene, glabrol, 3-hydroxyglabrol
- **Cumestan derivatives:** Glycyrol, isoglycyrol
- **Hydroxycoumarins:** Glycycoumarin, licopyranocoumarin, herniarin, umbelliferone, liqcoumarin
- **Steroids:** Sterols, including stigmasterol, β-sitosterol
- **Volatile oil (trace):** Eugenol, anethole, estragole, hexanoic acid (Gruenwald et al. 2007; Husain et al., 2021)

THERAPEUTIC USE

TPM Literature

Use of licorice powder on eyelids and eyelashes strengthens eyesight and helps eliminate chronic yellowing of the sclera and is used to treat pterygium as well. For oral intake, the root is used in forms of pure powder, infusion or decoctions, and concentrated extract of its decoction (black licorice). In addition to being a neurotonic, its administration is prescribed for various types of neurological problems, including headaches. It is highly recommended for respiratory system disorders, such as burning sensation, dryness and inflammation of the throat, hoarseness, shortness of breath, asthma, and cough. Both forms, especially the infusion, are prescribed for gastritis. Licorice is also introduced to suppress thirst and as a laxative, carminative, anticolic, and antihemorrhoid medication. It is recommended to be added to purgative decoctions and liver medicines in order to improve their bioavailability and decrease their side effects. Its diuretic effects make it useful as a remedy for decreasing dysuria and improving bladder ulcers. Licorice is also used as an emmenagogue to

DOI: 10.1201/b22971-17

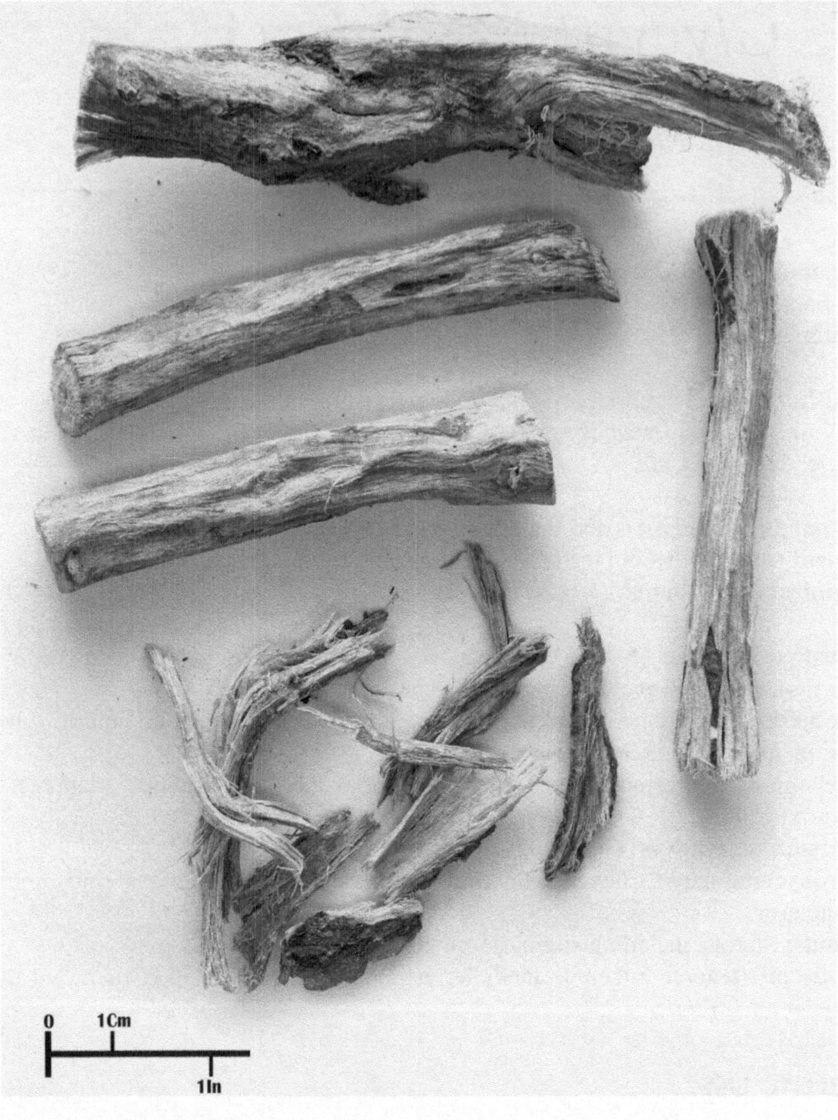

FIGURE 17.1 Licorice root.

induce menstruation. Consumed with fennel and sugar, it has been introduced as an effective purifier and can cure chronic fever and refresh skin.

Licorice poultice in combination with honey and wax is recommended for paronychia. Frequent topical usage of its poultice with pure water can improve psoriasis too. Its extract also is used for wound healing (Aghili Khorasani 1771; Avicenna 1025).

Current Evidence

Clinical Evidence

Atopic eczema: In a placebo-controlled RCT on 90 patients with mild to moderate atopic dermatitis, topical gels containing 1% and 2% licorice methanolic extract could reduce the scores of erythema, edema and itching over 2 weeks in a dose-dependent manner (Saeedi et al., 2003).

Melasma: In a double-blind RCT on 18 patients, the effectiveness of a combined product containing licorice extract (licorice extract, 4-ethoxybenzaldehyde, tetrahexyldecyl ascorbate, niacinamide, ethyl linoleate, hexylresorcinol, and retinol) in reducing hyperpigmentation due to UV radiation compared to 4% hydroquinone cream was evaluated. It was found that at the end of the study, the product resulted in a significant decrease in pigmentation compared to the baseline and a greater increase in skin brightness compared to 4% hydroquinone (Makino et al., 2013).

Biochemical and metabolic effects: A systematic review and meta-analysis including 26 RCTs showed that licorice consumption significantly led to reduction of BW and consequently BMI of the patients. Significant increase in the DBP was also detected. The results of secondary outcomes show the hepatoprotective effects of licorice with significant reduction of ALP, GGT and BUN and increase of Na^+ (Luís et al., 2018). Moreover, the results of one RCT on 110 individuals with hypercholesterolemia showed that after one year consumption of 0.2 g per day of ethanolic extract of licorice root, a significant reduction was observed in TC, LDL-C, and carotid intima media thickness, as well as SBP and DBP vs. placebo group (Fogelman et al., 2016).

Parkinson's disease: In a placebo-controlled RCT in 78 Parkinson's disease patients, licorice syrups with a dose of 5 mL (containing 136 mg of licorice extract), twice a day could significantly improve Unified Parkinson's rating scale, daily activities, and tremor after 6 weeks compared to placebo. After 4 months, better motor test and rigidity scores were observed (the total duration of study was 6 months). No significant changes in BP, FBS, or electrolyte abnormality were observed (Petramfar et al., 2020).

Acute conjunctivitis: Licorice extract drop was effective in acute conjunctivitis according to results of an old clinical study on 50 patients. The subsidence of acute clinical signs and symptoms started from fourth day onwards in 25 patients who received licorice drop and the complete symptoms disappearance took 5–7 days. These results were comparable with results of using chloramphenicol drop as the standard treatment (Srinivas, 1986).

Dry eye disease: In a multicenter, open-label, pilot RCT, 28 days administration of 2.5% eye drops of glycyrrhizin twice daily in 37 adult patients with moderate dry eye disease led to improvement in 71.6% of them, evident from significant improvements of tear break-up time and Schirmer scores (Burillon et al., 2018).

Oral mucositis: A double-blind RCT on 60 patients with radiotherapy-induced oral mucositis showed that a mucoadhesive licorice product (containing 0.18 mg of licorice root extract) has a similar efficacy to triamcinolone for the management of the condition (Ghalayani et al., 2017).

Aphthous stomatitis: In a double-blind RCT on 70 subjects with recurrent aphthous stomatitis, effects of diphenhydramine solution and diphenhydramine containing 5% hydroethanolic extract of licorice were assessed. Participants were asked to swish 3 mL of either solution around their mouth for about 3 minutes four times a day until the complete oral lesions' disappearance. Licorice-containing product showed a significantly better effect on the average pain scores and the average duration of wound healing (Akbari et al., 2020). Another RCT in 54 subjects with aphthous ulcer also confirmed the effect of licorice mouthwash (40 g of the root boiled in 1 L of water) on the reduction of ulcer pain considering VAS, compared with placebo (Liu et al., 2022). A systematic review and meta-analysis of six RCTs showed that topical application of licorice with 1–5% concentration for 4–8 days can significantly reduce aphthous pain, ulcer size, and healing (Dorsareh et al., 2023).

Xerostomia: In one RCT which compared the effect of pure water mouthwash, licorice mouthwash, and no mouthwash on xerostomia and unstimulated whole saliva flow rate among 122 hemodialysis patients, licorice mouthwash (8.34 g of licorice concentrate in 500 mL of pure water) increased unstimulated salivary flow rate significantly and about four times more than the water. Moreover, it significantly improved the scores of the Summated Xerostomia Inventory in contrast to pure water. Both pure water and licorice mouthwash improved the objective measure of salivary flow rate; though, only the licorice mouthwash provided subjective relief of xerostomia (Yu et al., 2016).

Dental caries: In a systematic review of six studies, licorice was found to reduce the number of *Streptococcus mutans* in children's mouths and to prevent dental caries. It could limit the fall of pH on biofilm and prevent acidic environment that increases the risk of dental caries. Furthermore, licorice in lollipop form is well accepted by children (Tharakan et al., 2020). Another study showed a single rinse of the mouth with licorice ethanolic extract (350 mg/10 mL) had an MIC of 2.15 ± 0.91 in comparison to 3.14 ± 2.02 of 0.2% for chlorhexidine which had no significant statistical difference (Kumar et al., 2020).

Peptic ulcer and *H. pylori* infection: A double-blind RCT of 60 patients with abdominal pain or dyspepsia and peptic ulcer, gastritis, or duodenitis in upper endoscopy and *H. pylori* positivity showed using 380 mg of licorice tablet twice daily for 14 days instead of bismuth subsalicylate in standard treatment led to a better eradication of *H. pylori* (Momeni et al., 2014). Another study showed that adding 380 mg licorice twice daily to clarithromycin-based triple regimen for 2 weeks resulted in improvement of outcomes in 120 patients with *H. pylori* infection. The eradication of *H. pylori* was 83% in clarithromycin-based regimen plus licorice compared to 62.5% in clarithromycin-based regimen alone (Hajiaghamohammadi et al., 2016). On the contrary, a previous study on 40 peptic ulcer patients with *H. pylori* infection demonstrated that replacing bismuth by licorice in quadruple standard therapy led to poorer results vs. standard quadruple therapy. However, finally it was introduced as an acceptable treatment (Rahnama et al., 2013).

Functional dyspepsia: In one double blinded RCT with sample size of 50 patients, a flavonoid-rich extract of licorice (GutGard) in dose of 75 mg twice daily for 30 days improved severity symptoms (using seven-point Likert scales) and quality of life (using the short form Nepean Dyspepsia Index) of patients with functional dyspepsia (Raveendra et al., 2012).

Depression: In an RCT in hospitalized patients with major depression disorder, 12 cases were treated with a licorice extract (containing 7–8% of glycyrrhizin), 700 mg twice daily, as an adjuvant to conventional therapy, compared with 55 cases who were only treated with conventional therapy. Considering Hamilton Depression Rating Scale, 2 weeks of treatment with licorice showed a significantly better therapeutic response vs. control group, especially in patients with lower SBP. Inhibition of 11-beta-hydroxysteroid-dehydrogenase type 2 by glycyrrhizin seems to be the underlying mechanism and thus, licorice may be effective in a specific subtype of depression (Murck et al., 2020).

NAFLD: In a double-blind RCT on 66 patients with NAFLD, administration of one capsule containing 2 g aqueous licorice root extract (equivalent to 400 mg of glycyrrhizic acid) per day for 2 months caused significant reductions in ALT and AST compared with placebo (Hajiaghamohammadi et al., 2012). Another RCT in 60 women with NAFLD showed that 12-week intake of 1 g licorice extract could significantly decrease ALT, FPI, HOMA-IR, MDA, and liver steatosis (observed in ultrasonography) in comparison to placebo (Rostamizadeh et al., 2022).

Cough and sore throat: Licorice is approved by Commission E for cough and bronchitis (Gruenwald et al., 2007). Results of a double-blind, placebo-controlled RCT in 70 patients with chronic cough indicated that intake of a pastille containing 240 mg licorice, three times daily, for 2 weeks significantly reduced cough severity score in comparison to placebo using the Leicester Cough Questionnaire (Ghaemi et al., 2020). In an RCT on 144 patients subjected to tracheal intubation for operation, different concentrations of a licorice solution (0.25, 0.5, or 1 g in 30 mL of water), gargling for 30 seconds 5 min before induction of anesthesia were evaluated regarding their effect on sore throat. The 1 g/30 mL concentration led to a significant reduction in the incidence and intensity of sore throat at rest and during swallowing without having adverse effects, as well as the incidence of cough after extubation compared with lower doses (Honarmand et al., 2016). Another RCT also reported the antitussive effects of licorice lozenge containing 97 mg licorice extract vs. sugar candy in 100 smokers undergoing tracheal intubation for operation (Gupta et al., 2013).

Acute sinusitis: One case report study reported symptom relieving in a patient with acute sinusitis after 3 days of administration of 12–15 drops of a 2,000-mg tincture of *G. glabra* twice a day (Martin et al., 2018).

Allergic rhinitis: In a controlled RCT in 60 patients with allergic rhinitis, administration of a licorice nasal irrigation (3 mg/mL of lyophilized aqueous extract) once daily for 1 month showed a significant improvement in rhinorrhea, olfactory disturbance nasal pruritus and blockage, sneezing, and postnasal discharge using VAS score, in comparison to both normal saline and nasal corticosteroids (Chang et al., 2021).

Menopause: In a multicenter double-blind RCT, daily administration of three capsules containing 330 mg licorice extract in comparison to placebo in 90 menopausal women complaining of hot flash significantly decreased frequency and severity of hot flashes over the 8 weeks of intervention and the effect continued for 2 weeks after the end of treatment duration (Nahidi et al., 2012).

Wound: According to a placebo-controlled RCT in 50 patients with second-degree burn wound, topical treatment with a hydrogel containing 5% licorice hydroethanolic extract for 2 weeks showed a significant improvement in inflammation, redness, burning sensation, and pain of the wounds, as well as a faster healing rate compared with placebo (Zabihi et al., 2023).

Preclinical Evidence

Wound: Licorice hydroethanolic extract administration, both topically and orally, showed remarkable wound healing effects. Licorice alcoholic extract modulated cutaneous wound healing in rats by increasing SOD, GSH, Gpx, total and differential leucocyte counts, and neutrophil phagocytosis and reducing MDA. Moreover, complete re-epithelialization with increasing collagen synthesis was detected in histopathological findings. Indeed, licorice extract supplementation led to acceleration of wound healing by increasing angiogenesis and collagen deposition through upregulation of TGF-β, VEGF and bFGF gene expression levels compared with the control group (Assar et al., 2021).

Melasma: Licorice extract (0.1 mg) was added to tranexamic acid (2.2 mg) in dissolving microneedles preparation for melasma therapy in guinea pigs. Patch preparations used in melasma spots (every 3 days, for 8 h each time) for 3 weeks significantly decreased melanin deposition in guinea pigs (Xing et al., 2021).

Neuronal injury: 50 and 100 mg/kg of roasted licorice played a neuroprotective role against hypoxia and ischemic damage in the gerbil hippocampus. In roasted licorice-treated animals, approximately 66–71% of CA1 pyramidal cells in the ischemic hippocampus were stained with cresyl violet compared to the control group, while no significant change was detected in nonroasted groups. In addition, Cu, Zn-SOD (SOD1) activity, and protein levels were more preserved in ischemic animals of the roasted licorice-treated group compared to the control group (Hwang et al., 2006).

Memory: Oral administration of four doses (75, 150, 225, and 300 mg/kg) of aqueous extract of *G. glabra* root for 6 weeks enhanced the memory according to results of the Morris water maze,

Hebb–William maze, and elevated plus maze tests. Moreover, administration of 150 and 225 mg/kg doses of *G. glabra* also reversed diazepam-induced amnesia (Chakravarthi and Avadhani, 2013). Furthermore, oral administration of 150 mg/kg/day of *G. uralensis*, *G. glabra*, and SW (a new variety produced through interbreeding between *G. uralensis* and *G. glabra*) extract to mice with LPS-induced cognitive impairment significantly restored spatial and objective recognition memory (Cho et al., 2018).

Sleep: Licorice ethanolic extract could increase the sleep induction effect of pentobarbital in mice in a dose-dependent manner. Also, it increased non-REM sleep, especially at 250 and 500 mg/kg doses, without decreasing delta activity, possibly via interaction with $GABA_A$ receptors (Cho et al., 2012).

Cough: Licorice was introduced as one of the two most effective antitussive medicinal herbs in coughs induced by citric acid according to results of one comparative review study (Saadat et al., 2018). Based on the results of one animal study using the phenol red secretion model and classical ammonia-induced cough model in mice, licorice aqueous and ethanolic extracts at 200 mg/kg decreased cough frequency by 25–59% and liquiritin apioside and liquiritin (at 50 mg/kg; intragastrically) were introduced as licorice major expectorant and antitussive compounds with antitussive effects via both peripheral and central mechanisms (Kuang et al., 2018).

Nephrotoxicity: *G. glabra* root hydroethanolic extract, 200 mg/kg orally for 12 days ameliorated the gentamicin-induced nephrotoxicity in mice (Nassan et al., 2021). Another study with similar method also revealed that licorice aqueous extract was effective in both protection and treatment for gentamicin-induced acute tubular necrosis in rats through reduction of BUN, creatinine, uric acid, LPO, and total peroxides, as well as elevation of TAC and GSH (Aksoy et al., 2012).

ADVERSE REACTIONS

TPM Literature

It may be harmful to kidneys and spleen. For decreasing the side effects for kidney and spleen, using with damask rose and tragacanth is recommended, respectively (Aghili Khorasani 1771).

Current Evidence

There are variety of adverse effects such as cardiac dysfunction, edema, and HTN reported with high doses (400 mg per day) of glycyrrhizic acid (correspond to about 200 g licorice roots). Consumption of licorice in amounts of 50–200 g per day (equivalent to 75–540 mg per day of glycyrrhizinic acid) can lead to a significant increase in blood pressure (Wang et al., 2013).

The mineralocorticoid effects of licorice are well known. In long-term (more than 4 weeks) therapeutic doses and/or intake of high amount, consumption of licorice can reduce potassium and sodium retention. Most cases of licorice-related side effects have been reported following excessive consumption of licorice candy which can lead to temporary paralysis, vision loss, sodium and fluid retention, high blood pressure, and decreased serum aldosterone levels. Licorice-related potassium depletion leads to tachycardia, rhabdomyolysis, myopathy, and hypokalemic paralysis. These adverse effects are primarily associated to the function of the glycyrrhizin compound (Gruenwald et al., 2007; Wang et al., 2013).

No side effects have been reported with licorice at doses less than 50 g per day for less than 6 weeks.

In some people who are very sensitive, consuming 100 mg of glycyrrhizin per day (approximately 50 g of licorice) may cause side effects. Most people who take 400 mg daily experience side effects. A 12-week clinical trial of glycyrrhizin in women showed no side effects at a dose of 2 mg/kg glycyrrhizin per day, equivalent to approximately 6 g of licorice (Gruenwald et al., 2007).

CONTRAINDICATIONS

TPM Literature

None.

Current Evidence

There are certain conditions that may prevent an individual from taking licorice, such as allergy to licorice, any constituents of that, or any herbs of the Fabaceae (Leguminosae) family (Ulbricht, 2010), chronic hepatitis, cholestatic liver disease, cirrhosis of the liver, renal impairments, diabetes, HTN, arrhythmias, hypertonia, low blood potassium, congestive heart failure (Gruenwald et al., 2007; Gardner and McGuffin, 2013).

Chronic consumption (even low dose) and using excessive amounts of licorice has been contraindicated for patients taking cardiac glycosides (ESCOP, 2003; Delbò, 2013). It should not be used in individuals using thiazide diuretics, corticosteroids, and stimulant laxatives (ESCOP, 2003).

PREGNANCY AND LACTATION

TPM Literature

None.

Current Evidence

There is not enough evidence to support the safety of licorice during pregnancy and lactation. Therefore, it is not recommended in pregnancy and breastfeeding (Gardner and McGuffin, 2013; Delbò, 2013).

DRUG INTERACTIONS

Antihypertensives: Licorice seems to reduce the effects of antihypertensive drugs (Williamson et al., 2013). In cases of loop diuretics and thiazides diuretics, it may have additive effect in potassium depletion.

Laxatives: If licorice is consumed in large amounts with laxatives, it may exacerbate potassium depletion.

Corticosteroids: According to its mineralocorticoid activity, glycyrrhizin in licorice increases plasma levels of hydrocortisone and prednisolone and potentiates the effects of hydrocortisone. Although this interaction may not apply to other corticosteroids, it is best to monitor concomitant use of licorice and corticosteroids, especially in the case of long-term use or high doses of licorice (Williamson et al., 2013; Gardner and McGuffin, 2013).

Coumarin anticoagulants: It has been suggested that licorice potentially increase the effect of warfarin (Williamson et al., 2013); while in a recent case, sudden decrease in INR values was reported after the ingestion of hard-boiled candy licorice by an old female patient treated with phenprocoumon (Marcumar®), a coumarin oral anticoagulant similar to warfarin. This may be explained by the effect of licorice and its constituents on the pharmacokinetics of phenprocoumon (Roemer et al., 2021).

Cardiac glycosides: High doses of licorice might induce hypokalemia, which is related to potential digitalis toxicity (Devang et al., 2021). Generally, licorice has been contraindicated for patients taking cardiac glycosides including digoxin (ESCOP, 2003; Delbò, 2013).

METHOD OF ADMINISTRATION

TPM Literature

Its usable part is mostly peeled root which is used in two forms: infusion and concentrated extract of its decoction (black licorice). Its poultice in combination with honey and wax or with pure water is prescribed for skin disorders. Its extract also is used for wound healing. Topical usage of its powder on eyelids and eyelashes also is recommended (Aghili Khorasani 1771).

Current Evidence

Roots in powder or comminuted form, dry extracts for infusions, decoctions, liquid or solid preparations for internal consumption (Gruenwald et al., 2007).

To prepare an infusion, 1–1.5 g of the comminuted roots should be added to cold water and heated until it boils and then, should be removed from the heat, or the boiling water should be poured over the drug and brew for 10–15 min (Gruenwald et al., 2007).

DOSAGE

The average dose is 2–10 g per day (Delbò, 2013), or 5–15 g of the root (correspondent to 200–600 mg glycyrrhizin). Its tea can be taken one cup after meals. Licorice should not to be used for more than 6 weeks (Gruenwald et al., 2007).

REFERENCES

Aghili Khorasani MH 1771. *Makhzan-al-Adviah* (*The treasury of drugs*) (rewritten by Shams Ardakani MR, Rahimi R, Farjadmand F, 1st ed.). Tehran: Tehran University of Medical Sciences; 2009.

Akbari N, Asadimehr N, Kiani Z. The effects of licorice containing diphenhydramine solution on recurrent aphthous stomatitis: A double-blind, randomized clinical trial. Complement Ther Med. 2020; 50:102401.

Aksoy N, Dogan Y, Iriadam M, et al. Protective and therapeutic effects of licorice in rats with acute tubular necrosis. J Ren Nutr. 2012;22(3):336–343.

Assar DH, Elhabashi N, Mokhbatly AA, et al. Wound healing potential of licorice extract in rat model: Antioxidants, histopathological, immunohistochemical and gene expression evidences. Biomed Pharmacother. 2021; 143:112151.

Avicenna 1025. *Al-Qanoon fi al-Tibb* (*The canon of medicine*) (rewritten by Masoudi A, ed.). Tehran: Almaei; 2015.

Burillon C, Chiambaretta F, Pisella PJ. Efficacy and safety of glycyrrhizin 2.5% eye drops in the treatment of moderate dry eye disease: Results from a prospective, open-label pilot study. Clin Ophthalmol. 2018; 12:2629–2636.

Chakravarthi KK, Avadhani R. Beneficial effect of aqueous root extract of *Glycyrrhiza glabra* on learning and memory using different behavioral models: An experimental study. J Nat Sci Biol Med. 2013;4(2):420–425.

Chang GH, Lin YS, Hsu KH, et al. Nasal irrigation with *Glycyrrhiza glabra* extract for treatment of allergic rhinitis: A study of in vitro, in vivo and clinical trial. J Ethnopharmacol. 2021; 275:114116.

Cho MJ, Kim JH, Park CH, et al. Comparison of the effect of three licorice varieties on cognitive improvement via an amelioration of neuroinflammation in lipopolysaccharide-induced mice. Nutr Res Pract. 2018;12(3):191–198.

Cho S, Park JH, Pae AN, et al. Hypnotic effects and GABAergic mechanism of licorice (*Glycyrrhiza glabra*) ethanol extract and its major flavonoid constituent glabrol. Bioorg Med Chem. 2012;20(11):3493–3501.

Delbò RM. *Assessment report on* Glycyrrhiza glabra *L. and/or* Glycyrrhiza inflata *Bat. and/or* Glycyrrhiza uralensis *Fisch., radix*. Amsterdam: European Medicines Agency; 2013.

Devang N, Adhikari P, Nandini M, et al. Effect of licorice on patients with HSD11B1 gene polymorphisms: A pilot study. J Ayurveda Integr Med. 2021;12(1):131–135.

Dorsareh F, Vahid-Dastjerdi G, Bouyahya A, et al. Topical Licorice for Aphthous: A Systematic Review of Clinical Trials. Iran J Med Sci. 2023;48(5):437–447.

ESCOP. *The scientific foundation for herbal medicinal products: Liquiritiae radix (liquorice root)*. 2nd ed. New York: Thieme; 2003.

Fogelman Y, Gaitini D, Carmeli E. Antiatherosclerotic effects of licorice extract supplementation on hypercholesterolemic patients: Decreased CIMT, reduced plasma lipid levels, and decreased blood pressure. Food Nutr Res. 2016;60(1):30830.

Gardner Z, McGuffin M. *Botanical safety handbook*. Boca Raton: Taylor & Francis; 2013.

Ghaemi H, Masoompour SM, Afsharypuor S, et al. The effectiveness of a traditional Persian medicine preparation in the treatment of chronic cough: A randomized, double-blinded, placebo-controlled clinical trial. Complement Ther Med. 2020; 49:102324.

Ghalayani P, Emami H, Pakravan F, Nasr Isfahani M. Comparison of triamcinolone acetonide mucoadhesive film with licorice mucoadhesive film on radiotherapy-induced oral mucositis: A randomized double-blinded clinical trial. Asia Pac J Clin Oncol. 2017;13(2): e48–56.

Gruenwald J, Brendler T, Jaenicke C. *PDR for herbal medicines*. Montvale: Thomson Reuters; 2007.

Gupta D, Agrawal S, Sharma JP. Effect of preoperative licorice lozenges on incidence of postextubation cough and sore throat in smokers undergoing general anesthesia and endotracheal intubation. Middle East J Anaesthesiol. 2013;22(2):173–178.

Hajiaghamohammadi AA, Zargar A, Oveisi S, et al. To evaluate of the effect of adding licorice to the standard treatment regimen of *Helicobacter pylori*. Braz J Infect Dis. 2016;20(6):534–538.

Hajiaghamohammadi AA, Ziaee A, Samimi R. The efficacy of licorice root extract in decreasing transaminase activities in non-alcoholic fatty liver disease: A randomized controlled clinical trial. Phytother Res. 2012;26(9):1381–1384.

Honarmand A, Safavi M, Arani AS, Shokrani O. The efficacy of different doses of liquorice gargling for attenuating postoperative sore throat and cough after tracheal intubation. Eur J Anaesthesiol. 2016;33(8):595–596.

Husain I, Bala K, Khan IA, Khan SI. A review on phytochemicals, pharmacological activities, drug interactions, and associated toxicities of licorice (*Glycyrrhiza* sp.). Food Front. 2021;2(4):449–485.

Hwang IK, Lim SS, Choi KH, et al. Neuroprotective effects of roasted licorice, not raw form, on neuronal injury in gerbil hippocampus after transient forebrain ischemia. Acta Pharmacol Sin. 2006;27(8):959–965.

Kuang Y, Li B, Fan J, et al. Antitussive and expectorant activities of licorice and its major compounds. Bioorg Med Chem. 2018;26(1):278–284.

Kumar A, Kumar T, Jha A, et al. Cariostatic efficacy of aqueous and ethanolic extracts of liquorice in the schoolchildren: In vivo comparative study. J Contemp Dent Pract. 2020;21(5):575–579.

Lim, T.K. *Edible medicinal and non-medicinal plants*, vol. 1. New York: Springer Science & Business Media; 2012.

Liu HL, Hsu PY, Chung YC, et al. Effective licorice gargle juice for aphthous ulcer pain relief: A randomized double-blind placebo-controlled trial. Pak J Pharm Sci. 2022;35(5):1321–1326.

Luís Â, Domingues F, Pereira L. Metabolic changes after licorice consumption: A systematic review with meta-analysis and trial sequential analysis of clinical trials. Phytomed. 2018; 39:17–24.

Makino ET, Mehta RC, Banga A, et al. Evaluation of a hydroquinone-free skin brightening product using in vitro inhibition of melanogenesis and clinical reduction of ultraviolet-induced hyperpigmentation. J Drugs Dermatol. 2013;12(3): s16–20.

Martin BR, Reshamwala G, Short M. Treatment of a woman with *Glycyrrhiza glabra* for acute sinusitis: A case report. J Chiropr Med. 2018;17(4):268–274.

Momeni A, Rahimian G, Kiasi A, et al. Effect of licorice versus bismuth on eradication of *Helicobacter pylori* in patients with peptic ulcer disease. Pharmacognosy Res. 2014;6(4):341.

Murck H, Lehr L, Hahn J, et al. Adjunct therapy with *Glycyrrhiza glabra* rapidly improves outcome in depression: A pilot study to support 11-beta-hydroxysteroid dehydrogenase type 2 inhibition as a new target. Front Psychiatry. 2020;11:605949.

Nahidi F, Zare E, Mojab F, Alavi-Majd H. Effects of licorice on relief and recurrence of menopausal hot flashes. Iran J Pharm Res. 2012;11(2):541–548.

Nassan MA, Soliman MM, Aldhahrani A, et al. Ameliorative impacts of *Glycyrrhiza glabra* root extract against nephrotoxicity induced by gentamicin in mice. Food Sci Nutr. 2021;9(7):3405–3413.

Ottenbacher R, Blehm J. An unusual case of licorice-induced hypertensive crisis. S D Med. 2015;68(8):346–349.

Petramfar P, Hajari F, Yousefi G, et al. Efficacy of oral administration of licorice as an adjunct therapy on improving the symptoms of patients with Parkinson's disease: A randomized double blinded clinical trial. J Ethnopharmacol. 2020;247:112226.

Rahnama M, Mehrabani D, Japoni S, et al. The healing effect of licorice (*Glycyrrhiza glabra*) on *Helicobacter pylori* infected peptic ulcers. J Res Med Sci. 2013;18(6):532–533.

Raveendra KR, Srinivasa V, Sushma KR, et al. An extract of *Glycyrrhiza glabra* (GutGard) alleviates symptoms of functional dyspepsia: A randomized, double-blind, placebo-controlled study. Evid-Based Complement Altern Med. 2012;2012: 216970.

Roemer HC, Kunz L, Botzenhardt S. The influence of excessive consumption of liquorice on phenprocoumon (Marcumar®): A case report. J Int Med Res. 2021;49(11):3000605211049649.

Rostamizadeh P, Asl SM, Far ZG, et al. Effects of licorice root supplementation on liver enzymes, hepatic steatosis, metabolic and oxidative stress parameters in women with nonalcoholic fatty liver disease: A randomized double-blind clinical trial. Phytother Res. 2022;36(10):3949–3956.

Saadat S, Shakeri F, Boskabady MH. Comparative antitussive effects of medicinal plants and their constituents. Altern Ther Health Med. 2018;24(4):36–49.

Saeedi M, Morteza-Semnani K, Ghoreishi MR. The treatment of atopic dermatitis with licorice gel. J Dermatolog Treat. 2003;14(3):153–157.

Srinivas, C. *Glycyrrhiza glabra* in acute conjunctivitis. Ancient Sci Life. 1986;5(3):151–153.

Stargrove MB, Treasure J, McKee DL (eds). *Herb, nutrient, and drug interactions: Clinical implications and therapeutic strategies*. St. Louis: Mosby Elsevier; 2008.

Thandar Y, Gray A, Botha J, Mosam A. Topical herbal medicines for atopic eczema: A systematic review of randomized controlled trials. Br J Dermatol. 2017;176(2):330–343.

Tharakan AP, Pawar M, Kale S. Effectiveness of licorice in preventing dental caries in children: A systematic review. J Indian Soc Pedod Prev Dent. 2020;38(4):325–331.

Ulbricht CE. Mosby's Natural Standard Herb & Supplement Guide. St. Louis: Massachusetts: Elsevier; 2010.

Wang X, Zhang H, Chen L, et al. Liquorice, a unique "guide drug" of traditional Chinese medicine: A review of its role in drug interactions. J Ethnopharmacol. 2013;150(3):781–790.

Williamson E, Driver S, Baxter K (eds.). *Stockley's herbal medicines interactions*. London: Pharmaceutical Press; 2013.

Xing M, Wang X, Zhao L, et al. Novel dissolving microneedles preparation for synergistic melasma therapy: Combined effects of tranexamic acid and licorice extract. Int J Pharm. 2021;600:120406.

Yu IC, Tsai YF, Fang JT, et al. Effects of mouthwash interventions on xerostomia and unstimulated whole saliva flow rate among hemodialysis patients: A randomized controlled study. Int J Nurs Stud. 2016;63:9–17.

Zabihi M, Hatefi B, Ardakani ME, et al. Impact of licorice root on the burn healing process: A double-blinded randomized controlled clinical trial. Complement Ther Med. 2023;73:102941.

18 *Malva sylvestris* L., *Malva neglecta* Wallr.

Roodabeh Bahramsoltani and Mehdi Sabet Jahromi

Scientific name: *Malva sylvestris* L., *Malva neglecta* Wallr.
Family: Malvaceae
Common names:

- **English:** Common mallow, high mallow (*M. sylvestris*), dwarf mallow (*M. neglecta*)
- **Persian:** *panīrak*, *ẖeyrū*
- **Arabic:** *ẖubbāzī*

Medicinal part(s): Flowers, leaves, seeds (Figure 18.1)
Temperament (nature): Cold in the first degree, wet in the first degree
Major chemical constituents:

- **Anthocyanins:** Malvin, malvidin, delphinidin
- **Flavonoids:** Quercetin, myricetin, apigenin, kaempferol, genistein
- **Organic acids:** Citric acid, oxalic acid, malonic acid, malic acid
- Mucilage (5–12%) (Gruenwald et al., 2007; Pinela et al., 2016)

THERAPEUTIC USE

TPM Literature

The smashed leaves of mallow are recommended topically for the treatment of eye injuries. Chewing the fresh leaves has soothing effects on mouth ulcers such as aphthous stomatitis. In oral intake, it is a mild laxative and increases breastmilk production. The decoction sweetened with sugar can be used for cough and hoarseness (dysphonia). It is also useful for painful spleen and bladder, dysuria, jaundice, and skin diseases secondary to liver malfunction such as some types of eczema due to its detoxifying effects on liver. The leaves may be boiled in water and the filtrate can be used as sitz bath. This is a drug delivery method to vagina and rectum and in this way, mallow is used for the treatment of some uterine problems and as an emollient for anusitis. The dried leaves powder is used for scalp wounds and scaling. Also, if the powdered leaves are mixed with butter and applied topically on body, it acts as an insect repellent. Smashed leaves are used for bone fracture, swellings, and bee sting. Fresh buds and leaves of the plant are also cooked with poultry meat as a food (Aghili Khorasani 1771; Avicenna 1025).

Seeds have therapeutic indications similar to the leaves; however, they are not widely available in the herbal market. The seeds have a higher amount of mucilage; thus, they are more effective for cough, dysphonia, and rhinitis. They can be added to formulations containing pungent spices to prevent burning sensation. Also, they can be used for intestinal ulcers and stomach burning. The seeds, individually or in combination with barley flour, can be topically applied for swellings and insect bites (Aghili Khorasani 1771).

DOI: 10.1201/b22971-18

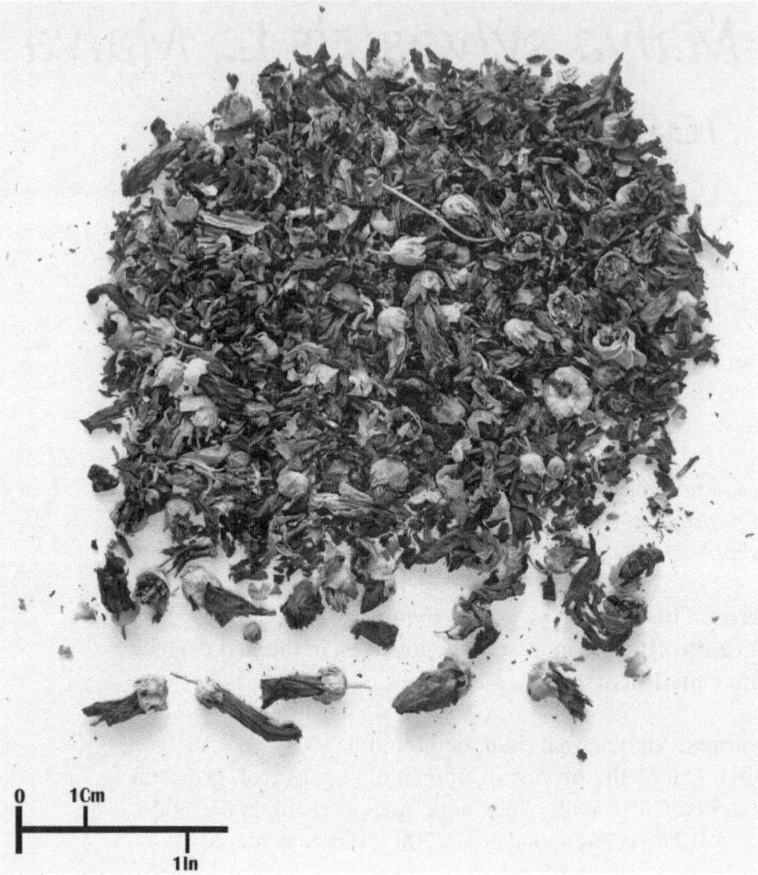

FIGURE 18.1 High mallow flower.

Current Evidence

Clinical Evidence

Cough and bronchitis: Flowers and leaves of high/dwarf mallow are approved for cough, bronchitis, and throat inflammation by Commission E (Blumenthal et al., 2000).

Constipation: Flower aqueous extract of high mallow is clinically assessed for its laxative effects. In a double-blind, placebo-controlled RCT, high mallow syrup was administered equal to a dose of 1 g of extract per day in 110 patients with functional constipation. After 4 weeks of intervention, there was a significant decrease in hard stool formation, sense of incomplete evacuation, need for manual maneuvers, and straining during defecation, as well as an increase in the number of defecations (Elsagh et al., 2015).

Radiotherapy-induced adverse effects: Due to soothing effects considered for mallow in TPM, researchers have assessed whether the plant is effective for the management of radiotherapy-induced oral mucositis and xerostomia. The formulation was designed as a 1:1 mixture of high mallow and marshmallow flower powders in 4 g sachets which should be brewed with 250 mL of boiling water for 10 min and then swallowed, three times daily. A primary triple-blind, placebo-controlled pilot RCT showed the beneficial effects of this formula in 23 patients with head and neck cancer who underwent radiotherapy. The intervention began from the beginning of radiotherapy up to 2 weeks after the last radiotherapy session for total of 7 weeks. The herbal mixture could significantly reduce mouth pain scale compared with the placebo (Rezaeipour et al., 2017). A larger study on 62 patients compared the effect of this formula with an artificial saliva as the control drug. After 4 weeks of treatment, patients in the intervention group had a lower degree of mouth dryness in comparison to those received the artificial saliva. Also, patients' preference, assessed with VAS, was toward the herbal intervention (Ameri et al., 2016). Regarding the quality of life, European Organization for Research and Treatment of Cancer Quality of Life Questionnaire–Head and Neck Module was considered. Accordingly, significant improvements were observed in swallowing, speech, and dry mouth scores in comparison to the control (artificial saliva); however, this difference was not statistically significant in case of difficulty in mouth opening, sticky saliva, cough, pain, senses, eating, and social contacts (Heydarirad et al., 2017). Additionally, this herbal preparation was administered with the same treatment regimen in patients with prostate cancer suffering from radiotherapy-induced acute proctitis. In a double-blind, placebo-controlled, multicenter RCT, 65 patients were enrolled to receive one of the interventions from the beginning of a 3-week course of radiotherapy until 2 weeks after the last radiotherapy session (total of 5 weeks). Based on the assessments using VAS, diarrhea and anal burning were significantly reduced upon treatment with the herbal preparation. There was no significant difference between groups regarding radiation toxicity considering Radiation Therapy Oncology Group scale (Moeini et al., 2018).

Dermatological problems: In an RCT, 50 patients with hand eczema were treated with either 4% high mallow extract in eucerin, or placebo. The ointment was applied as a fingertip, twice daily, for 6 weeks. A significant improvement was observed in all evaluated scores including dryness, itching, erythema, edema, excoriation, lichenification, and oozing in comparison to the placebo (Barikbin et al., 2010). Another RCT assessed the effect of 5% high mallow flower aqueous extract in eucerin for the treatment of atopic dermatitis in pediatrics. Total of 50 patients, aged between 6 months and 12 years were randomly treated with either mallow cream or placebo, twice daily, for 4 weeks. In comparison to placebo, a significant improvement was achieved by high mallow cream regarding skin thickening score, redness score, and total Scoring Atopic Dermatitis (Meysami et al., 2021).

Preclinical Evidence

Constipation: In a rat model of loperamide-induced constipation, aqueous extract of high mallow leaves was orally administered with the daily doses of 100, 200, and 400 mg/kg for 5 days. The extract demonstrated a significant dose-dependent improvement of gastric emptying, intestine transit time, food intake, and frequency of defecation, as well as a decrease in stool dehydration. Colic hydrogen peroxide level and lipid peroxidation were also reduced upon treatment with the extract (Jabri et al., 2017).

Colitis: Different extracts of aerial parts of high mallow, including aqueous, ethanol, and *n*-hexane extracts, as well as purified polysaccharides of the plant were assessed in acetic acid-induced colitis in rats. All preparations were administered orally with a dose of 200 mg/kg. Results showed a significant improvement in macroscopic and microscopic scores of rats treated with the aqueous extract and polysaccharides, when administered before disease induction (prophylactic administration); while the effect was lower for the ethanol and *n*-hexane extracts which suggests hydrophilic compounds and especially, polysaccharides to be responsible for the ulcer-healing properties of this plant (Hamedi et al., 2016).

Inflammation: Fractionated ethanol extract of high mallow leaves was evaluated in carrageenan-induced inflammation by intraperitoneal and subplantar injection in paw in mice with an oral dose range of 3–30 mg/kg. Among fractions with different polarities, the aqueous fraction showed the best effect on the reduction of neutrophil migration, paw edema, and IL-1β and was determined as the most effective treatment. Also, *in vitro* evaluations showed the inhibitory effects of this fraction on the osteoclastogenic activities in RAW264 cells which is in line with TPM claims regarding the bone repair activity of the plant; however, the level of evidence is still too low to extrapolate to clinical settings (Benso et al., 2016).

Wounds: A cream containing 1% flower aqueous extract was topically applied, two times a day, for 10 days on cut wounds involving superficial fascia in mice. Wound healing was significantly improved with respect to inflammatory cells, keratinization, fibrosis, and scar formation in comparison to negative control (Afshar et al., 2015). In another study, wound healing properties of 5% and 10% flower hydroethanolic extract in cream base was evaluated in a rat model of second-degree burn wound. After 35 days of treatments, both creams showed a significant improvement in wound closure and fibroblast proliferation; as well as a remarkable decrease in irritation and macrophage infiltration in comparison to negative control. No significant difference was observed between the effect of 5% and 10% creams (Nasiri et al., 2015). Flower extract of high mallow, prepared using diethyl ether as solvent, was formulated as a 5.6% cream and assessed in a full-thickness excision wound model in diabetic rats. Upon 18 days of treatment, a significant improvement of wound closure was observed, along with fewer inflammation and necrosis, as well as better formation of collagen fibers (Pirbalouti et al., 2010). There is also an *in vivo* study on the wound healing properties of *M. neglecta* in rat model of excision wound. Hydromethanolic extract of the leaves were incorporated into ointment base with 10%, 15%, and 20% concentrations which were topically applied once a day until the complete wound closure. A dose-dependent increase in wound healing rate and re-epithelialization was observed with the herbal treatment (Saleem et al., 2020).

ADVERSE REACTIONS

TPM Literature

Since the plant is wet-tempered, it can cause indigestion in long-term use and in people with cold and wet temperament; thus, in these cases, it is better to be taken with hot-tempered electuaries such as those containing pepper and cumin, or with pickled vegetables. Fruit pastes, such as quince paste, can also decrease the side effects of mallow due to their tonic effects on stomach (Aghili Khorasani 1771; Avicenna 1025).

Current Evidence

Topical use up to 5% concentration of the extract in human and 20% concentration in animals caused no side effects (Meysami et al., 2021; Saleem et al., 2020).

Oral use up to the dose of 6 g per day of the flower powder caused no side effects in human (Heydarirad et al., 2017).

CONTRAINDICATIONS

TPM Literature

None.

Current Evidence

None.

PREGNANCY AND LACTATION

TPM Literature

It is contraindicated during pregnancy. It can be used orally during lactation to increase milk production (Aghili Khorasani 1771).

Current Evidence

None.

DRUG INTERACTIONS

Conventional drugs should be taken at least 1 hour prior or several hours after the intake of mallow since the high mucilage content of the plant may affect the absorption of other medicines (Gardner and McGuffin, 2013).

METHOD OF ADMINISTRATION

TPM Literature

For oral administration, as a syrup may be prepared by boiling the leaves with sugar. The leaves can also be added to poultry meat. The leaves can be chewed for oral ulcers.

For topical administration, the dried or fresh plant material can be used as a poultice.

For vaginal or rectal administration, plant material can be infused in boiling water and the filtered solution is poured in a large bowl, then, the patient should sit in the bowl so that the solution reaches the vagina (Aghili Khorasani 1771; Avicenna 1025).

Current Evidence

For oral administration, the plant material should be mixed with cold water and boiled for 10 min (Gruenwald et al., 2007).

DOSAGE

Flowers/leaves: 5 g daily (Gruenwald et al., 2007).

REFERENCES

Afshar M, Ravarian B, Zardast M, et al. Evaluation of cutaneous wound healing activity of *Malva sylvestris* aqueous extract in BALB/c mice. Iran J Basic Med Sci. 2015;18(6):616–622.

Aghili Khorasani MH 1771. *Makhzan-al-Adviah* (*The treasury of drugs*) (rewritten by Shams Ardakani MR, Rahimi R, Farjadmand F, 1st ed). Tehran: Tehran University of Medical Sciences; 2009.

Ameri A, Heydarirad G, Rezaeizadeh H, et al. Evaluation of efficacy of an herbal compound on dry mouth in patients with head and neck cancers: A randomized clinical trial. J Evid-Based Complement Altern Med. 2016;21(1):30–33.

Avicenna 1025. *Al-Qanoon fi al-Tibb* (*The canon of medicine*) (rewritten by Masoudi A, ed.). Tehran: Almaei; 2015.

Barikbin B, Maarefat A, Rahgoshai R, et al. *Malva sylvestris* in the treatment of hand eczema. Iranian J Dermatol. 2010;13(4):131–134.

Benso B, Franchin M, Massarioli AP, et al. Anti-inflammatory, anti-osteoclastogenic and antioxidant effects of Malva sylvestris extract and fractions: In vitro and in vivo studies. PLoS One. 2016;11(9):e0162728.

Blumenthal M, Goldberg A, Brinckmann J. *Herbal medicine: Expanded Commission E monographs*. Ann Arbor: Integrative Medicine Communications; 2000.

Elsagh M, Fartookzadeh MR, Kamalinejad M, et al. Efficacy of the *Malva sylvestris* L. flowers aqueous extract for functional constipation: A placebo-controlled trial. Complement Ther Clin Pract. 2015;21(2):105–111.

Gardner Z, McGuffin M. *Botanical safety handbook*. Boca Raton: Taylor & Francis; 2013.

Gruenwald J, Brendler T, Jaenicke C. *PDR for herbal medicines*. Montvale: Thomson Reuters; 2007.

Hamedi A, Rezaei H, Azarpira N, et al. Effects of *Malva sylvestris* and its isolated polysaccharide on experimental ulcerative colitis in rats. J Evid-Based Complement Altern Med. 2016;21(1):14–22.

Heydarirad G, Rezaeizadeh H, Choopani R, et al. Efficacy of a traditional Persian medicine preparation for radiation-induced xerostomia: A randomized, open-label, active-controlled trial. J Integr Med. 2017;15(3):201–208.

Jabri MA, Wannes D, Hajji N, et al. Role of laxative and antioxidant properties of *Malva sylvestris* leaves in constipation treatment. Biomed Pharmacother. 2017;89:29–35.

Meysami M, Hashempur, MH, Kamalinejad M, Emtiazy M. Efficacy of short term topical *Malva sylvestris* L. cream in pediatric patients with atopic dermatitis: A randomized double-blind placebo-controlled clinical trial. Endocr Metab Immune Disord Drug Targets. 2021;21(9):1673–1678.

Moeini R, Farhan F, Mofid B, et al. The effect of the combination of *Malva sylvestris* L. and *Althaea digitata* Boiss. on prevention of acute radiation proctitis in patients with prostate cancer. J Herb Med. 2018;12:16–22.

Nasiri E, Hosseinimehr SJ, Azadbakht M, et al. Effect of *Malva sylvestris* cream on burn injury and wounds in rats. Avicenna J Phytomed. 2015;5(4):341–354.

Pinela J, Barros L, Antonio AL, et al. Quality control of gamma irradiated dwarf mallow (*Malva neglecta* Wallr.) based on color, organic acids, total phenolics and antioxidant parameters. Molecules. 2016;21(4):467.

Pirbalouti AG, Azizi S, Koohpayeh A, Hamedi B. Wound healing activity of *Malva sylvestris* and *Punica granatum* in alloxan-induced diabetic rats. Acta Pol Pharm. 2010;67(5):511–516.

Rezaeipour N, Jafari F, Rezaeizadeh, et al. Efficacy of a Persian medicine herbal compound (*Alcea digitata* Alef and *Malva sylvestris* L.) on prevention of radiation induced acute mucositis in patients with head and neck cancer: A pilot study. Int J Cancer Manag. 2017;10(9):e8642.

Saleem U, Khalid S, Zaib S, et al. Phytochemical analysis and wound healing studies on ethnomedicinally important plant *Malva neglecta* Wallr. J Ethnopharmacol. 2020;1(249):112401.

19 *Matricaria chamomilla* L.

Arman Zargaran

Scientific name: *Matricaria chamomilla* L. (syn. *Matricaria recutita* L.)
Family: Asteraceae
Common names:

- **English:** Chamomile, German chamomile
- **Persian:** *bābūne*
- **Arabic:** *bābūnağ*

Medicinal part(s): Flowers (Figure 19.1)
Temperament (nature): Hot in the second degree and dry in the first degree
Major chemical constituents:

- **Essential oil:** (−)-α-bisabolol, sesquiterpenes and proazulenes (e.g., matricarin and matricin). During steam distillation, by the effect of heating, matricin in chamomile oil would be converted to chamazulene, that has blue color
- **Flavonoids:** Apigenin, luteolin, quercetin, rutin
- **Coumarins:** Umbelliferone, herniarin and its methyl ether (Williamson et al., 2013)

THERAPEUTIC USE

TPM Literature

Chamomile is a tonic for brain, nervous system, and sexual desire. Oral intake or topical application of chamomile infusion or oil is helpful to relieve headaches and catarrh. Chewing chamomile flowers is helpful for healing oral ulcers. If administered as an ophthalmic drop, it alleviates eye pain and conjunctivitis. It is also helpful in asthma and chest pain. Due to spasmolytic properties, oral chamomile is helpful in visceral pains, colic, and oliguria. Due to diuretic effect, it can be beneficial for urinary stones. Oral chamomile infusion and its sitz bath is emmenagogue and thus, is used for the treatment of amenorrhea. It can also facilitate natural vaginal delivery, as well as placenta expulsion. Furthermore, chamomile is a galactagogue and diaphoretic agent. It is an antifatigue agent and also can ease inflammation in topical or systemic administration. Also, it was used for jaundice.

Chamomile oil, prepared in sesame oil based on TPM instructions is mentioned to be used topically and orally in fevers. Its topical application is also recommended for joint pain, back pain, gout, and local inflammations (Aghili Khorasani 1771; Avicenna 1025).

Current Evidence

Clinical Evidence

Anxiety and depression: A placebo-controlled RCT in 93 patients with GAD showed that long-term (26 weeks) and short-term (8 weeks) administration of 500 mg of chamomile extract (three

DOI: 10.1201/b22971-19

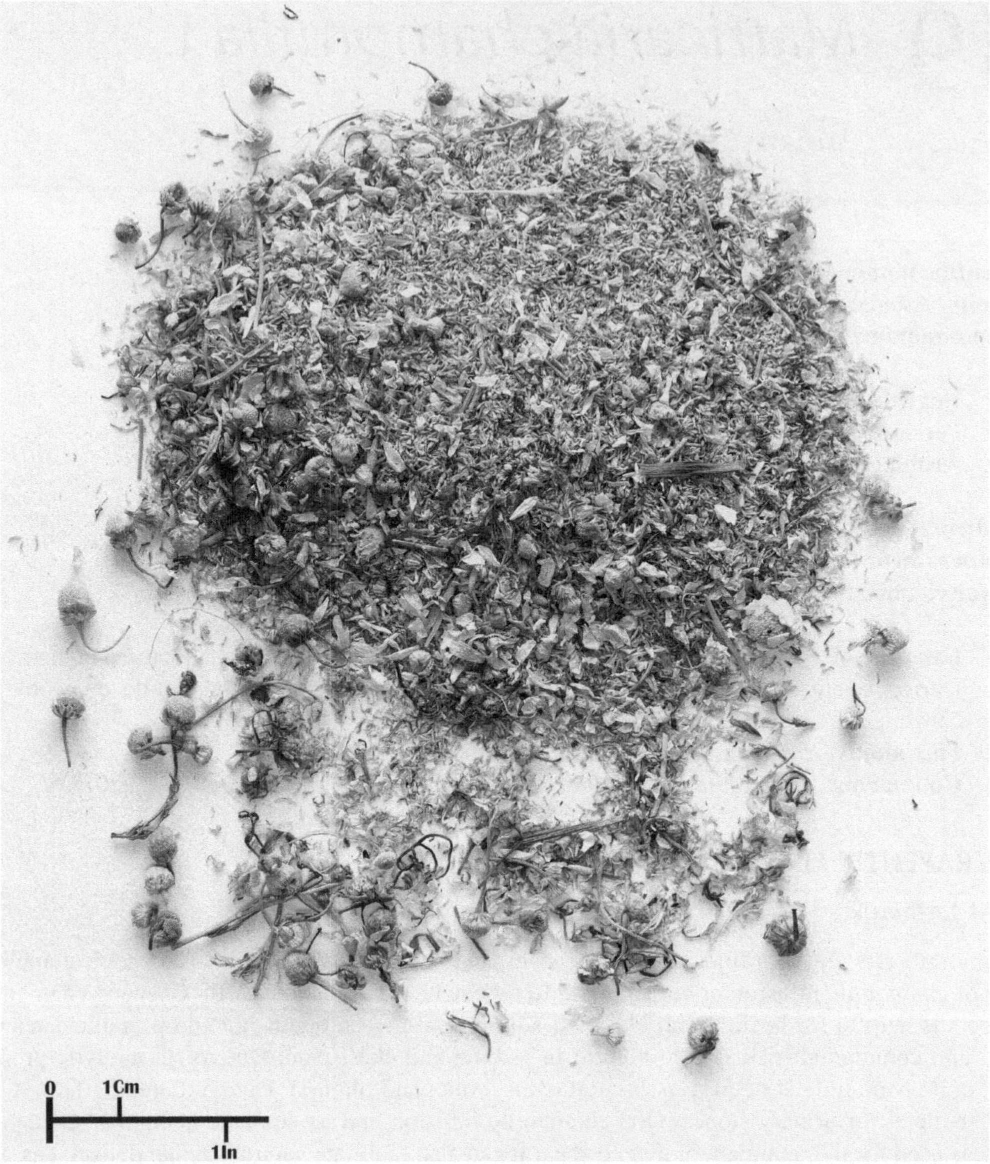

FIGURE 19.1 Chamomile flower.

times daily) can reduce moderate to severe GAD symptoms; but did not reduce rate of relapse (Mao et al., 2016; Keefe et al., 2016). Furthermore, it was reported that in the subjects with GAD and comorbid depression, there is a meaningful antidepressant effect by chamomile in addition to the anxiolytic activity, considering Hamilton rating scores for depression and anxiety, as well as Beck inventory scales for depression and anxiety (Amsterdam et al., 2020). In another clinical study by the same team, a modest anxiolytic effect was demonstrated for chamomile extract on 61 patients with mild to moderate GAD (Amsterdam et al., 2009). Also, in another study on 57 patients, anxiolytic and antidepressant effect of chamomile was demonstrated based on Hamilton Depression Rating score (Amsterdam et al., 2012). Aside from oral intake, an RCT in 183 elderlies showed than

1-month inhalation of 1.5% chamomile essential oil has a significant effect on the improvement of anxiety and depression symptoms (Ebrahimi et al., 2022). In a clinician guideline for the treatment of psychiatric disorders with phytoceuticals published in 2022, chamomile is not recommended as monotherapy for GAD; however, it may be effective if it is used in combination with other psychoactive herbs (Sarris et al., 2022).

Wound: In an RCT on 72 patients with peristomal skin lesions, effectiveness of twice-daily application of a topical chamomile solution (6 g/150 mL boiled water as a compress for 1 hour) was assessed to relieve itching and inflammation which caused a significantly faster wound repair vs. 1% hydrocortisone during 4 weeks of treatment (Charousaei et al., 2011).

Migraine headache: In a double-blind, placebo-controlled, crossover RCT on 72 patients having migraine without aura, efficacy of a topical oleogel made by chamomile oil based on TPM instructions was evaluated. Rubbing 2 mL of the oleogel on temporal area, forehead, and behind the ears upon migraine attack caused a significant reduction of pain considering VAS (Zargaran et al., 2018).

Mastalgia: In a double-blind RCT in 60 patients with mastalgia, 8-week supplementation with chamomile extract (five drops of a commercial extract, three times daily) showed a significant effect on the reduction of pain vs. placebo considering VAS and breast pain chart (Saghafi et al., 2018).

Musculoskeletal pain: Chamomile oil, prepared based on the TPM instructions, showed a significant analgesic effect upon topical use (three times daily for 3 weeks) in 99 patients with knee osteoarthritis. According to this RCT, chamomile oil was significantly better than both placebo and 1% diclofenac topical gel as the control drug, so that the patients needed fewer intake of acetaminophen for pain control (Shoara et al., 2015). In another RCT in 90 prehospital emergency technicians with low back pain, a similar treatment pattern using topical chamomile oil caused a significant reduction of pain and improvement of daily activities vs. placebo at the second week of intervention, but not at the end of the third week (Shirzad-Siboni et al., 2022). Also, in a before-after evaluation of 24 patients with knee osteoarthritis, 15 minutes soft prolonged massage with 20 mL of chamomile oil (every other day) for 20 days was significantly effective to reduce pain considering VAS and knee osteoarthritis outcome score (Islam et al., 2021).

Dysmenorrhea: A systematic review on seven RCTs proposed that the oral chamomile with a daily dose range of 750–2,400 mg from 2 days before to 1 day after menstruation or during the first 3 days of menstruation for at least two cycles could be beneficial for reducing pain and menstrual bleeding in primary dysmenorrhea (Niazi and Moradi, 2021).

PMS: In a double-blind RCT in 90 female subjects, chamomile ethanolic extract with a 300 mg daily dose showed a significant improvement in psychological pains of PMS vs. mefenamic acid (control drug); though, no difference was observed in physical symptoms (Sharifi et al., 2014). Another RCT in 118 cases with moderate to severe PMS also showed that daily 750 mg of chamomile powder for 8 days has a significant effect on the psychological, physical, and overall PMS symptoms vs. placebo (Najafi Mollabashi et al., 2021).

PCOS: In a placebo-controlled RCT on 80 patients with PCOS, oral supplementation with chamomile (370 mg, three times daily) for 3 months caused a significant decrease in testosterone level; though, no significant difference was observed in case of dehydroepiandrosterone sulfate, LH/FSH ratio, and lipid parameters (Heidary et al., 2018).

Lactation: A case report showed a remarkable increase in the amount of milk production, along with breast tension, in a nursing mother 4–6 hours after oral consumption of a chamomile infusion (1–3 g of chamomile, 1.5–2 L per day) from third to sixth month postpartum (Silva et al., 2018).

Menopause: According to a placebo-controlled RCT in 96 postmenopausal women, 5% chamomile vaginal gel administered as 1 g per night (every night for 2 weeks, followed by two nights per week for 10 weeks) could significantly improve sexual function based on the female sexual function index with a nearly similar efficacy to conjugated estrogen vaginal cream (Bosak et al., 2022).

Carpal tunnel syndrome: According to two RCTs in 86 patients with mild to moderate and 26 patients with severe carpal tunnel syndrome, 4-week topical application of chamomile oil, prepared based on TPM instructions, could be an adjuvant treatment along with splint which showed significant improvements in pain and function in both groups of patients (Hashempour et al., 2017; Hashempour et al., 2015).

Oral mucositis: A systematic review evaluated the effect of chamomile mouthwash on chemotherapy-induced oral mucositis including six papers, of which four RCTs showed significant alleviating properties. Chamomile extract with a concentration range of 1–2.5% and daily administration of one to four times during chemotherapy can be recommended for the primary and secondary prevention of oral mucositis (de Lima Dantas et al., 2022). A more recent RCT in 45 patients under chemotherapy showed that a 3% chamomile topical oral gel used three times daily for 3 weeks, alone or in combination with conventional care (topical antifungal, anti-inflammatory, and analgesic agents), can significantly reduce the onset and severity of oral mucositis (Elhadad et al., 2022). Also, in a double-blind phase II RCT in 40 patients undergoing allogenic hematopoietic stem cell transplantation, 1% chamomile mouthwash could reduce the incidence, intensity, and duration of mucositis (Braga et al., 2015).

Radiodermatitis: According to an RCT in 48 patients under radiotherapy due to head and neck cancer, a topical gel containing 8.35% chamomile extract (three times daily for the whole duration of radiotherapy) could delay the onset and decrease the severity of dermatitis in comparison to urea cream (Ferreira et al., 2020). In another phase II RCT, 54 breast cancer patients receiving radiotherapy were topically treated with either chitosan-coated chamomile microparticles or placebo. Chamomile microparticles caused a lower severity, pain, and pruritus, as well as a better skin recovery (Garbuio et al., 2022). Also, an uncontrolled trial in 43 patients under radiotherapy due to head and neck cancer showed that a compress with chamomile infusion (10 g flower in 400 mL of water), three times daily for 20 minutes, caused a considerable regression of the dry desquamation and prevention of moist desquamation (Meneses et al., 2022).

Nausea and vomiting: In a controlled RCT in 65 women under chemotherapy for breast cancer, addition of 1 g daily of chamomile extract from 5 days before to 5 days after chemotherapy to the routine antiemetic drugs was effective to reduce the frequency of vomiting, but ineffective on the severity of nausea (Sanaati et al., 2016).

Enuresis in children: Using topical chamomile oil for 8 weeks decrease the frequency of nocturia in children with monosymptomatic nocturnal or daytime enuresis according to a clinical study (Sharifi et al., 2017).

Infantile colic: In a placebo-controlled RCT on 74 infants with colic, 2-week application of chamomile oil, prepared based on the TPM instructions, on the abdominal area of infants (three times daily) showed a significant decrease in crying time and improvement of sleep duration in comparison to liquid paraffin (Salehipoor et al., 2019).

Type 2 diabetes: A systematic review considering five clinical trials reported significant effect of chamomile (2.5–10 g daily as tea) compared with placebo on the improvement of FBS and lipid parameters of type 2 diabetic patients by 4–12 weeks of administration. Two studies with treatment durations of 8 and 12 weeks also showed a significant reduction of HbA1c. Furthermore, one RCT reported a lower level of hs-CRP and TNF-α by chamomile (Hajizadeh-Sharafabad et al., 2020).

Insomnia: In an RCT on 34 patients, 270 mg of oral chamomile extract twice daily for 28 weeks showed a modest benefit on daytime functioning and mixed benefits on sleep diary measures in patients with chronic primary insomnia (Zick et al., 2011). Another RCT including 60 elderlies evaluated the effect of chamomile extract capsules (200 mg twice daily for 28 days) on the sleep quality which showed a significant improvement vs. placebo (Adib-Hajbagheri and Mousavi, 2017). Also, an RCT in 80 postnatal women revealed that intake of chamomile tea (2 g of flower infused for 10–15 minutes in 300 mL of boiled water) for 2 weeks can significantly decrease physical symptoms-related sleep inefficiency and depression symptoms compared with control group (no intervention); however, this difference did not remain significant at the end of the fourth week, showing a short-term efficacy for chamomile tea at the evaluated dose (Chang and Chen, 2016).

Labor: An RCT on 80 post-term pregnant women showed that daily intake of 3 g of chamomile for 1 week, can significantly stimulate labor vs. placebo (Gholami et al., 2016). Another RCT in 130 primipara women used chamomile essential oil inhalation in first stage of delivery. A significant decrease in the intensity of contractions and a better satisfaction was reported in the intervention group vs. control; however, no difference was observed in duration and number of contractions (Heidari-Fard et al., 2018). Also, in a placebo-controlled RCT, inhalation of 5% chamomile essential oil for 15–20 minutes three times after cesarean section resulted in a significant pain reduction based on VAS (Zardosht et al., 2021).

Rhinosinusitis: In a placebo-controlled RCT on 74 patients with chronic rhinosinusitis, a nasal drop of chamomile hydroethanolic extract in normal saline or sesame seed oil (as placebo) was administered three times daily for 3 weeks which showed a significant improvement of Lund-Mackay score in clinical symptoms, paranasal CT scan, and endoscopic nasal evaluations in comparison to placebo (Nemati et al., 2021). An RCT on a group of 123 patients with allergic rhinitis under treatment with nasal mometasone evaluated a nasal spray of chamomile extract in isotonic seawater (Kamillosan® Ocean Nasal Spray) which was administered twice daily for 4 weeks. A significantly better improvement in symptoms as measured by Sino-Nasal Outcome Test 22 and nasal mucociliary clearance time was observed by chamomile (Atar et al., 2022).

Gingivitis: In an RCT in 55 patients with gingivitis and chronic periodontitis, administration of a mouthwash containing 5% chamomile ethanolic extract twice a day for 15 days exhibited a significant improvement in gingival bleeding index, similar to chlorhexidine (Batista et al., 2014).

Phlebitis: In 40 patients admitted to CCU ward and under treatment with intravenous amiodarone, a placebo-controlled RCT showed that a topical chamomile ointment (1.5% chamomile extract), applied three times daily for 3 days, can significantly reduce the number of patients developed phlebitis. The chamomile ointment also delayed the onset of phlebitis (Sharifi-Ardani et al., 2017).

Preclinical Evidence

PCOS: A study on rats with PCOS showed that chamomile hydroethanolic extract (25, 50, 75 mg/kg, intraperitoneally for 10 days) can increase dominant follicles and LH secretion causes, along with improvement in endometrial tissue arrangements (Farideh et al., 2010). Also, in estradiol valerate-induced PCOS in rats, chamomile ethanolic extract (75 mg/kg) for 1 month could reduce PCOS-related kidney damage via reduction of serum urea, testosterone, LPO, and apoptosis, as well as improvement of endogenous antioxidants (Alahmadi et al., 2021).

Skin disorders: A study on rats showed that nanoemulgel containing chamomile and olive oils has significant effect on treating atopic dermatitis (El-Salamouni et al., 2020). Martins et al. showed that chamomile preparation in comparison to corticosteroids has faster wound healing effect in rat model (Martins et al., 2009).

Systematic inflammation: Several animal studies confirmed the anti-inflammatory effect of chamomile essential oil and extract with a focus on the reduction of CRP, TNF-α, and ILs (Mihyaoui et al., 2022). In an animal study in mice, chamomile methanolic extract (800 mg/kg) could control gastrointestinal helminthiasis due to *Heligmosomoides polygyrus* and decrease associated inflammation and oxidative stress (Hajaji et al., 2019). In STZ-induced diabetes in rabbits, oral administration of chamomile essential oil (25, 50, and 100 mg/kg/day) for 3 weeks showed a significant decrease in FBS, NF-κB, and NLRP3 proteins (Saghahazrati et al., 2020).

Oral ulcer: In a group of rats with ALX-induced diabetes and traumatic oral ulcers, application of a topical 10% chamomile ointment for 10 days caused complete healing of ulcers similar to triamcinolone ointment via reduction of TNF-α and epithelial cells apoptosis (Oliveira et al., 2016).

ADVERSE REACTIONS

TPM Literature

It could be harmful for pharynx and to prevent this side effect; it is better to be taken with honey and pomegranate (Aghili Khorasani 1771)

Current Evidence

Chamomile is often considered as a safe medicinal herb. Rare cases of anaphylactic reactions are reported by internal use of chamomile tea. Contact dermatitis and allergic conjunctivitis are reported due to applying chamomile eye washes (Aronson, 2008). There is also a possibility of drowsiness and sedation; thus, caution should be considered upon driving or other tasks which need alertness. Cross-sensitivity may occur in subjects allergic to other plants of the Asteraceae family (Ulbricht, 2010).

CONTRAINDICATIONS

TPM Literature

None.

Current Evidence

Using chamomile in the persons who have hypersensitivity to Astreaceae family is contraindicated (Aronson, 2008). Anaphylactic shock and contact dermatitis are reported (Gardner and McGuffin, 2013).

PREGNANCY AND LACTATION

TPM Literature

Due to emmenagogue properties, chamomile is not recommended during pregnancy.

Current Evidence

Due to stimulant effects on uterine, chamomile should be avoided in pregnancy. There are no definite data on the use of chamomile in lactation (Ulbricht, 2010).

DRUG INTERACTIONS

Coumarin anticoagulants: There is only one report on using chamomile causes bleeding in a patient who used warfarin (Williamson et al., 2013).

Benzodiazepines and barbiturates: Chamomile contains phytochemicals that can bind to benzodiazepine and GABA receptors in the brain and cause some sedative effects and may increase the effects of sedative drugs. So, if chamomile is administered with sedative drugs including benzodiazepines and barbiturates, driving or other tasks which need alertness should be avoided (Srivastava et al., 2010).

METHOD OF ADMINISTRATION

TPM Literature

Chamomile infusion and decoction are recommended orally. Macerated solution is used for topical application and as sitz bath. Chamomile oil, prepared in sesame oil as base, can be used topically (Aghili Khorasani, 1771).

Current Evidence

In oral administration, the flower powder, extract, tea, and tincture are used. In topical use, warm compress and oil can be used. The essential oil may be used via inhalation for aromatherapy.

DOSAGE

In oral use, up to 3 g of the chamomile flower may be taken as infusion. A tea can be taken 3–4 times per day (Gruenwald et al., 2007). In topical use, 1.5 cup of water may be mixed with 2 g of the plant and the infusion can be used as a warm compress (Skidmore-Roth, 2009).

REFERENCES

Adib-Hajbaghery M, Mousavi SN. The effects of chamomile extract on sleep quality among elderly people: A clinical trial. Complement Ther Clin Pract. 2017;35:109–114.

Aghili Khorasani MH 1771. *Makhzan-al-Adviah* (*The treasury of drugs*) (rewritten by Shams Ardakani MR, Rahimi R, Farjadmand F, 1st ed.). Tehran: Tehran University of Medical Sciences; 2009.

Alahmadi AA, Alahmadi BA, Wahman LF, El-Shitany NA. Chamomile flower extract ameliorates biochemical and histological kidney dysfunction associated with polycystic ovary syndrome. Saudi J Biol Sci. 2021;28(11):6158–6166.

Amsterdam JD, Li QS, Xie SX, Mao JJ. Putative antidepressant effect of chamomile (*Matricaria chamomilla* L.) oral extract in subjects with comorbid generalized anxiety disorder and depression. J Altern Complement Med. 2020;26(9):815–821.

Amsterdam JD, Li Y, Soeller I, et al. A randomized, double-blind, placebo-controlled trial of oral *Matricaria recutita* (chamomile) extract therapy of generalized anxiety disorder. J Clin Psychopharmacol. 2009;29(4):378–382.

Amsterdam JD, Shults J, Soeller I, et al. Chamomile (*Matricaria recutita*) may have antidepressant activity in anxious depressed humans: An exploratory study. Altern Ther Health Med. 2012;18(5):44–49.

Aronson JK. *Meyler's side effects of herbal medicines*. Oxford: Elsevier; 2008.

Atar Y, Karaketir S, Aydogdu I, et al. Comparison of isotonic seawater nasal spray containing chamomile liquid extract and other isotonic seawater nasal washing solutions for allergic rhinitis. Ann Otol Rhinol Laryngol. 2022;131(4):427–434.

Avicenna 1025. *Al-Qanoon fi al-Tibb* (*The canon of medicine*) (rewritten by Masoudi A, ed.). Tehran: Almaei; 2015.

Zardosht R, Basiri A, Sahebkar A, Emami SA. Effect of chamomile oil on cesarean section pain in primiparous women: A randomized clinical trial. Curr Rev Clin Exp Pharmacol. 2021;16(4):369–374.

Zargaran A, Borhani-Haghighi A, Salehi-Marzijarani M, et al. Evaluation of the effect of topical chamomile (*Matricaria chamomilla* L.) oleogel as pain relief in migraine without aura: A randomized, double-blind, placebo-controlled, crossover study. Neurol Sci. 2018;39(8):1345–1353.

Zick SM, Wright BD, Sen A, Arnedt JT. Preliminary examination of the efficacy and safety of a standardized chamomile extract for chronic primary insomnia: A randomized placebo-controlled pilot study. BMC Complement Altern Med. 2011;11(1):1–8.

20 *Melissa officinalis* L.

Behjat Javadi

Scientific name: *Melissa officinalis* L.
Family: Lamiaceae
Common names:

- **English:** Lemon balm
- **Persian:** *bādranğbūyeh, bādrangbūyeh*
- **Arabic:** *turunğān, mufarraḥ al-qalb*

Medicinal part(s): Flowers, leaves, seeds (Figure 20.1)
Temperament (nature): Hot and dry in the second degree
Major chemical constituents:

- **Polyphenols:** *Cis*- and *trans*-rosmarinic acid isomers, caffeic acid derivatives
- **Flavonoids:** Luteolin, naringin, and hesperidin
- **Volatile compounds:** Geranial, neral, citronellal, and geraniol
- **Triterpenes:** Ursolic acid and oleanolic acid (Gruenwald et al., 2007)

THERAPEUTIC USE

TPM Literature

Lemon balm leaves are exhilarant, cardiac and gastric tonic, mild sedative, memory enhancer, antidote for toxic mushrooms, and wound disinfectant. It is used orally for a variety of mental and CNS diseases including anxiety, depression, psychosis, obsession, dementia, epilepsy, stroke, tremor, paralysis, migraine, vertigo, and syncope. It is also recommended for the treatment of asthma, fevers, hiccups, joint inflammation, and pain. Chewing the leaves is used to remove halitosis. Oral intake of lemon balm is helpful for the relief of GI cramps, ulcers, and is stomach tonic in case of cold/wet dystemperament. The decoction can be used as a sitz bath for amenorrhea (Aghili Khorasani 1771; Avicenna 1025).

Current Evidence

Clinical Evidence

Sleeping disorders: Lemon balm intake is approved by Commission E for the treatment of nervous sleeping disorders (Blumenthal et al., 2000). The British Herbal Pharmacopoeia has recommended the plant as a sedative (Willoughby and Mills, 1996).

Gastrointestinal problems: Lemon balm intake is approved by Commission E for the treatment of functional gastrointestinal complaints (Blumenthal et al., 2000).

Anxiety: The results of a systematic review and a meta-analysis of six RCTs published up to 2020 showed that lemon balm significantly improved mean anxiety and depression scores compared with

DOI: 10.1201/b22971-20

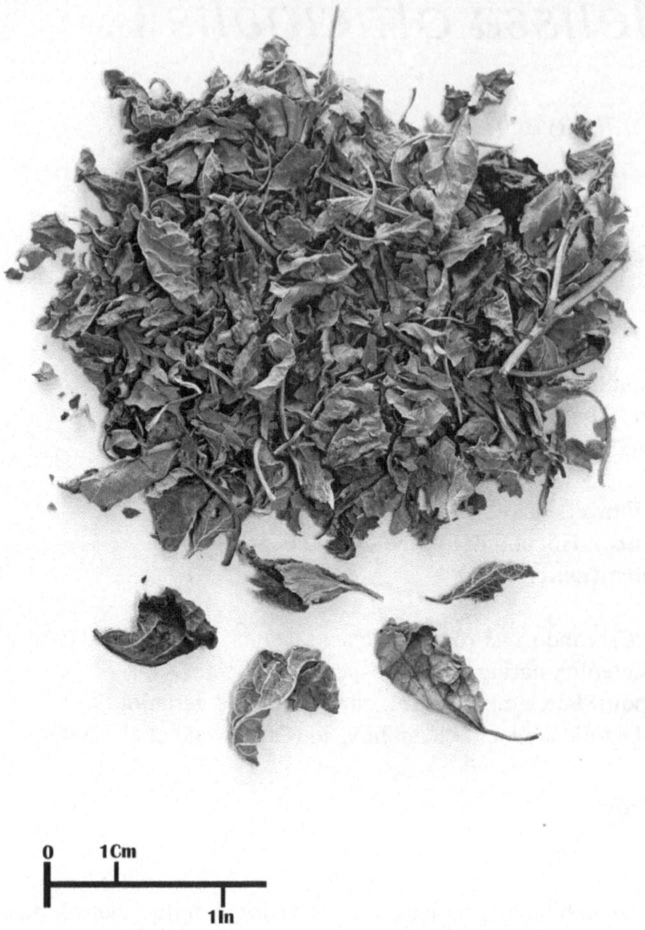

FIGURE 20.1 Lemon balm aerial parts.

the placebo. The plant was mostly administered with an oral dose of 300–600 mg of the extract, or 1–1.5 g of the plant powder. A minimum duration of 5–7 days is required to observe anxiolytic effects; whereas antidepressant properties need a longer period of time, between 10 days to 8 weeks, to appear (Ghazizadeh et al., 2021).

Cognition and memory deficit: Several RCTs have shown the effects of lemon balm in the treatment of Alzheimer's disease and cognitive deficit. A double-blind, placebo-controlled RCT investigated the effects of topical application of lemon balm essential oil on the agitation behavior of patients with severe dementia. Faces and arms were massaged with essential oil twice a day for a period of 4 weeks. The results showed that 60% of patients receiving essential oil and 14% of patients in the placebo group experienced a 30% reduction of Cohen-Mansfield Agitation Inventory score. Overall improvements in agitation were 35% in patients receiving essential oil and 11% in those treated with placebo. The quality of life of patients in the essential oil group was also improved significantly (Ballard et al., 2002). Another RCT investigating the effects of lemon balm on cognition and mood of healthy humans showed that acute administration of the ethanolic extract (600 mg) can modulate mood and cognitive performance (Kennedy et al., 2002). Similarly, a 16-week placebo-controlled RCT on 42 patients with mild to moderate Alzheimer's disease demonstrated reduction of agitation and improvement in cognitive and behavioral functions after administration of hydroalcoholic extract of lemon balm (60 drops per day) containing 500 µg citral per milliliter (Akhondzadeh et al., 2003). In a double-blind, placebo-controlled, 24-week RCT, 23 patients with mild Alzheimer's disease-related dementia received lemon balm extract (500 mg of rosmarinic acid daily) rich in rosmarinic acid or placebo. The mean Neuropsychiatric Inventory Questionnaire score improved by 0.5 point in the lemon balm group and worsened by 0.7 point in the placebo group between the baseline and 24-week visit, indicating a significant difference (Noguchi-Shinohara et al., 2020). Furthermore, the same dosage was assessed in a 96-week RCT in 323 elderlies without dementia which demonstrated a preventive effect on cognitive decline in a subgroup of patients without hypertension (Noguchi-Shinohara et al., 2023).

Cardiometabolic disorders: A systematic review and meta-analysis of seven RCTs investigated the effect of oral use of lemon balm on several cardiometabolic outcomes. The plant powder was mostly administered with 1–3 g per day and for 2–3 months. The results showed that lemon balm intake was only associated with a reduced TC and a reduced SBP (Heshmati et al., 2020). Another meta-analysis of four RCTs with 244 participants showed that lemon balm significantly lowered TC, LDL-C, HbA1c, and SBP with a dose range of 350–3,000 mg per day and a treatment period of 2–3 months (Liao et al., 2021).

Oxidative stress: A single-arm clinical trial was performed to evaluate the improving effects of lemon balm infusion on oxidative stress in 55 radiology staff. The plant was administered as an infusion of 1.5 g/100 mL hot water, twice daily, for 30 days. The results showed a significant improvement in plasma levels of SOD, CAT, and Gpx, as well as reduction of plasma DNA damage, lipid peroxidation, and MPO activity vs. baseline (Zeraatpishe et al., 2011).

Viral infections: Two clinical studies, a multicenter study involving 115 patients and another subsequent double-blind placebo-controlled RCT involving 116 patients, showed a topical cream containing 1% dried extract of lemon balm was significantly active against HSV infections. The studies demonstrated that early initiation of the treatment can result in a maximum efficacy (Wölbling and Leonhardt, 1994). Also, the British Herbal Pharmacopoeia recommended the plant as a topical antiviral (Willoughby and Mills, 1996).

Pain and inflammation: A single-blind RCT investigated the effects of lemon balm extract on alleviating moderate to severe postpartum pain in 110 women receiving either lemon balm leaf dried hydroethanolic extract capsules (395 mg) or mefenamic acid (250 mg) every 6 h for 24 h postpartum. The severity of pain between groups was not significantly different within one and two hours postpartum, but different at hour three and thereafter, with pain lower in the lemon balm group at all time points (Dastjerdi et al., 2019).

Dysmenorrhea: In a double-blind RCT, 110 students (18–25 years old) with dysmenorrhea received lemon balm ethanolic extract (330 mg) or placebo three times a day at first 3 days of menstrual cycles for 2 months. In the second cycle, the pain severity was significantly lower in lemon balm-treated patients vs. placebo group (Mirabi et al., 2017). A follow-up, double-blind, placebo-controlled RCT on 90 patients (16–26 years old) with moderate to severe primary dysmenorrhea showed the same doses of lemon balm significantly decreased the severity of menstruation-associated fatigue, lethargy, and nervous symptoms during two consecutive menstrual cycles (Mirabi et al., 2018).

Sexual problems: In a 4-week, double-blind RCT in 89 women with hypoactive sexual desire disorder, sexual desire, arousal, lubrication, orgasm, satisfaction, frequency of intercourse, and total Female Sexual Function Index were significantly enhanced by aqueous extract of lemon balm (100 mg twice daily), compared to placebo (Darvish-Mofrad-Kashani et al., 2018).

Preclinical Evidence

IBS: Hydroethanolic extract of lemon balm (100, 200, or 300 mg/kg/day for 3 days; intragastric) could significantly decrease visceral sensitivity and defecation frequency in acetic acid- and restraint stress-induced diarrhea-prominent IBS in rats. The extract could also improve pain thresholds and stool consistency, and reduced TNF-α, MPO, and MDA levels (Dolatabadi et al., 2018).

Peptic ulcer: Pretreatment with lemon balm methanolic extract (150, 300, and 450 mg/kg, orally) significantly decreased ulcer index in indomethacin- or water immersion restraint-induced peptic ulcer in rats in a dose-dependent manner. Moreover, lemon balm improved SOD activity and decreased MDA level which shows the antioxidant properties (Saberi et al., 2016).

Central nervous system problems: Lemon balm essential oil (10%) administered orally with a dose of 100 mg/kg/day for 2 weeks pre- and postischemia could protect two-vessel occlusion-induced transient hippocampal ischemia in rats. The increased levels of caspase-3 like protease activity and the number of TUNEL positive cells hippocampal neuronal cell damage were significantly attenuated. HIF-1α mRNA gene expression and MDA levels were also significantly lowered; while antioxidant capacity in the hippocampus was increased (Bayat et al., 2012). In a model of spinal cord injury, treatment with lemon balm (150 mg/kg, intraperitoneal) in combination with dexamethasone significantly improved motor and sensory functions compared to dexamethasone alone. Moreover, lemon balm alone and in combination with dexamethasone significantly increased recovery from neuronal injury and postinjury cavity formation (Hosseini et al., 2017). Methanolic and aqueous extracts of lemon balm (250, 500 mg/kg) showed potent antiepileptic activity against maximal electroshock- and PTZ-induced epilepsy in mice (Bhat et al., 2012).

Cardiovascular problems: Ethanol extract of lemon balm reduced the occurrence of ventricular premature beats, ventricular fibrillation and ventricular tachycardia following $CaCl_2$-induced arrhythmias in rats (Akhondali et al., 2015). Aqueous extract of lemon balm could prolong QRS, QTc, JT and Tpeak-Tend intervals of ECG in rats possibly via modulating the expression or conductance properties of sodium and potassium channels in the heart (Joukar and Asadipour, 2015). At a dose of 50 mg/kg, it increased the heart resistance in isoproterenol-induced cardiac injury in rats as evidenced by decreased MDA levels of the injured hearts. However, at higher doses (200 mg/kg) the extract worsened the ischemic heart injury (higher serum cardiac troponin I levels) possibly by enhancing cardiac contractility and myocardial oxygen demand (Joukar et al., 2016).

Angiogenesis: Hydroalcoholic extract of lemon balm with a dose of 100 mg/kg/day has been reported to inhibit laser-induced choroidal neovascularization development in a dose-dependent manner in rats through inhibition of VEGF and MMP-9 (Lee et al., 2014). In another experiment, 3-week oral administration of an ethyl acetate fraction from ethanolic extract of lemon balm (100 or 200 mg/kg/day) reduced laser-induced choroidal neovascularization in mice by 44.3% and 68.1%, respectively. The size of the isolectin B4-labeled area also significantly decreased by lemon balm. Fluorescein angiography showed significantly less leakage of fluorescent material in lemon balm-treated mice compared to the control animals. The extract also reduced VEGF-induced human umbilical vein endothelial cell tube formation in a dose-dependent manner. The expression of phosphorylated extracellular signal-regulated kinase 1/2 was also inhibited by the extract (Roh et al., 2016).

ADVERSE REACTIONS

TPM Literature

None.

Current Evidence

Oral (up to 600 mg per day for 8 weeks) and topical (up to 10 days) administration of lemon balm extract are considered relatively safe based on the available clinical trials (Shakeri et al., 2016). Two systematic reviews and meta-analyzes of several RCTs showed no serious side effects related to the oral use of lemon balm (Heshmati et al., 2020; Liao et al., 2021).

Preclinical studies suggest that lemon balm may affect the level of thyroid hormones and inhibit the attachment of TSH to its receptors, but no clinical evidence is available (Gardner and McGuffin, 2013).

CONTRAINDICATIONS

TPM Literature

None.

Current Evidence

None.

PREGNANCY AND LACTATION

TPM Literature

Oral use of high doses should be avoided during pregnancy due to its emmenagogue effects.

Current Evidence

None.

DRUG INTERACTIONS

None.

METHOD OF ADMINISTRATION

TPM Literature

For oral administration, a decoction of the lemon balm leaves can be used. For dental and oral cavity problems, the decoction can be used as a mouthwash. Inhalation of the plant aroma is recommended for mental health. Crushed fresh plant or an infusion of lemon balm powder in oils such as olive and almond oils is administered topically. The decoction can be used as sitz bath for uterine problems (Aghili Khorasani 1771).

Current Evidence

For oral administration, the plant infusion, aqueous extract or dry extract can be used (Blumenthal et al., 2000). An infused oil or essential oil mixed with a proper fix oil is administered topically or as massage oil.

DOSAGE

Fresh plant: 1.5–4.5 g several times daily.
Infusion: 1.5–4.5 g in 150 mL water (Gruenwald et al., 2007).

REFERENCES

Aghili Khorasani MH 1771. *Makhzan-al-Adviah* (*The treasury of drugs*) (rewritten by Shams Ardakani MR, Rahimi R, Farjadmand F, 1st ed). Tehran: Tehran University of Medical Sciences; 2009.

Akhondali Z, Dianat M, Radan M. Negative chronotropic and antidysrhythmic effects of hydroalcoholic extract of lemon balm (*Melissa officinalis* L.) on $CaCl_2$-induced arrhythmias in rats. Electron Physician. 2015;7(1):971–976.

Akhondzadeh S, Noroozian M, Mohammadi M, et al. Melissa officinalis extract in the treatment of patients with mild to moderate Alzheimer's disease: A double blind, randomised, placebo controlled trial. J Neurol Neurosurg Psychiatr. 2003;74(7):863–866.

Avicenna 1025. *Al-Qanoon fi al-Tibb* (*The canon of medicine*) (rewritten by Masoudi A, ed.). Tehran: Almaei; 2015.

Ballard CG, O'Brien JT, Reichelt K, Perry EK. Aromatherapy as a safe and effective treatment for the management of agitation in severe dementia: The results of a double-blind, placebo-controlled trial with Melissa. J Clin Psychiatr. 2002;63(7):553–558.

Bayat M, Azami Tameh A, Hossein Ghahremani M, et al. Neuroprotective properties of *Melissa officinalis* after hypoxic-ischemic injury both in vitro and in vivo. DARU J Pharm Sci. 2012; 20:1–10.

Bhat JU, Nizami Q, Asiaf A, et al. Anticonvulsant activity of methanolic and aqueous extracts of *Melissa parviflora* in experimentally induced Swiss albino mice. EXCLI J. 2012;11:1–6.

Blumenthal M, Goldberg A, Brinckmann J. *Herbal medicine: Expanded Commission E monographs*. Ann Arbor: Integrative Medicine Communications; 2000.

Darvish-Mofrad-Kashani Z, Emaratkar E, Hashem-Dabaghian F, et al. Effect of *Melissa officinalis* (lemon balm) on sexual dysfunction in women: A double-blind, randomized, placebo-controlled study. Iran J Pharm Res. 2018;17(suppl):89–100.

Dastjerdi MN, Darooneh T, Nasiri M, et al. Investigating the effect of *Melissa officinalis* on after-pains: A randomized single-blind clinical trial. J Caring Sci. 2019;8(3):129–138.

Gardner Z, McGuffin M. *Botanical safety handbook*. Boca Raton: Taylor & Francis; 2013.

Ghazizadeh J, Sadigh-Eteghad S, Marx W, et al. The effects of lemon balm (*Melissa officinalis* L.) on depression and anxiety in clinical trials: A systematic review and meta-analysis. Phytother Res. 2021;35(12):6690–6705.

Gruenwald J, Brendler T, Jaenicke C. *PDR for herbal medicines*. Montvale: Thomson Reuters; 2007.

Heshmati J, Morvaridzadeh M, Sepidarkish M, et al. Effects of *Melissa officinalis* (lemon balm) on cardio-metabolic outcomes: A systematic review and meta-analysis. Phytother Res. 2020;34(12):3113–3123.

Hosseini SR, Kaka G, Joghataei MT, et al. Coadministration of dexamethasone and *Melissa officinalis* has neuroprotective effects in rat animal model with spinal cord injury. Cell J (Yakhteh). 2017;19(1):102–116.

Joukar S, Asadipour H. Evaluation of *Melissa officinalis* (lemon balm) effects on heart electrical system. Res Cardiovasc Med. 2015;4(2):e27013.

Joukar S, Asadipour H, Sheibani M, et al. The effects of *Melissa officinalis* (lemon balm) pretreatment on the resistance of the heart to myocardial injury. Pharm Biol. 2016;54(6):1005–1013.

Kennedy DO, Scholey AB, Tildesley NT, et al. Modulation of mood and cognitive performance following acute administration of *Melissa officinalis* (lemon balm). Pharmacol Biochem Behav. 2002;72(4):953–964.

Lee EK, Kim YJ, Kim JY, et al. *Melissa officinalis* extract inhibits laser-induced choroidal neovascularization in a rat model. PLoS One. 2014;9(10):e110109.

Liao D, Liu Y, Ouyang Z, et al. Effects of *Melissa officinalis* L. (lemon balm) extract supplementation on cardiovascular risk factors: A pooled analysis of randomized controlled trials. J Food Nutr Res. 2021;9(7):357–362.

Mirabi P, Alamolhoda SH, Yazdkhasti M, Mojab F. The effects of lemon balm on menstrual bleeding and the systemic manifestation of dysmenorrhea. Iran J Pharm Res. 2018;17(suppl2):214–223.

Mirabi P, Namdari M, Alamolhoda S, Mojab F. The effect of *Melissa officinalis* extract on the severity of primary dysmenorrhea. Iran J Pharm Res. 2017;16(suppl):171–177.

Noguchi-Shinohara M, Hamaguchi T, Sakai K, et al. Effects of *Melissa officinalis* extract containing rosmarinic acid on cognition in older adults without dementia: A randomized controlled trial. J Alzheimer's Dis. 2023;91(2):805–814.

Noguchi-Shinohara M, Ono K, Hamaguchi T, et al. Safety and efficacy of *Melissa officinalis* extract containing rosmarinic acid in the prevention of Alzheimer's disease progression. Sci Rep. 2020;10(1):18627.

Roh YJ, Jee D, Rho CR, et al. Anti-angiogenic effect of ALS-L1023, an extract of *Melissa officinalis* L., on experimental choroidal neovascularization in mice. Clin Exp Ophthalmol. 2016;44(1):43–51.

Saberi A, Abbasloo E, Sepehri G, et al. The effects of methanolic extract of *Melissa officinalis* on experimental gastric ulcers in rats. Iran Red Crescent Med J. 2016;18(7):e24271.

Shakeri A, Sahebkar A, Javadi B. *Melissa officinalis* L.: A review of its traditional uses, phytochemistry and pharmacology. J Ethnopharmacol. 2016; 188:204–228.

b S. British Herbal Pharmacopoeia. Exeter: British Herbal Medicine Association, 1996.

Wölbling RH, Leonhardt K. Local therapy of herpes simplex with dried extract from *Melissa officinalis*. Phytomedicine. 1994;1(1):25–31.

Zeraatpishe A, Oryan S, Bagheri MH, et al. Effects of *Melissa officinalis* L. on oxidative status and DNA damage in subjects exposed to long-term low-dose ionizing radiation. Toxicol Ind Health. 2011;27(3):205–212.

21 *Mentha spicata* L., *Mentha piperita* L.

Sajad Fakhri and Mohammad Hosein Farzaei

Scientific name: *Mentha spicata* L., *Mentha piperita* L.
Family: Lamiaceae
Common names:

- **English:** Mint, mentha, spearmint (*M. spicata*), peppermint (*M. piperita*)
- **Persian:** *na'nā*
- **Arabic:** *na'nā*

Medicinal part(s): Aerial parts (Figure 21.1)
Temperament (nature): Hot and dry in the second degree
Major chemical constituents:

- **Phenolic compounds:** Phenolic acids, flavonoids, lignans, and stilbenes
- **Essential oil:**
  - **Peppermint:** Total of 0.5–4% essential oil: Menthol (30–55%), menthone (14–32%), menthyl acetate (3–5%) as major components, minor constituents including menthofuran, 1,8-cineole, α-pinene, β-pinene, and limonene (WHO, 2002; Gruenwald et al., 2007)
  - **Spearmint:** Total of 0.8–2.5% essential oil: carvone (40–80%), limonene (5–15%) as major ingredients, minor constituents including 1,8-cineole, caryophyllene, trans-sabinene hydrate, and dihydrocarveol (Gruenwald et al., 2007)
- **Fatty acids:** Linoleic, linolenic acid, and palmitic acid
- Triterpenoids and steroids

THERAPEUTIC USE

TPM Literature

Mint is an antidepressant and antiplatelet. It can be used topically for headaches due to cold dystemperament. Chewing fresh mint is recommended for toothache. The decoction is useful for hemorrhage and hemoptysis. The decoction can be used for chest pain, pulmonary disorders, and acts as an expectorant to purge abnormal phlegm of lung and upper respiratory tract. It is also useful for stomachache, as well as heartburn, bloat, dyspepsia, and is suggested as a digestive, antiflatulent, appetizer, spasmolytic, and anthelmintic in GI tract. Mint can tonify cardia sphincter which makes it a treatment choice for GERD. Furthermore, it is a stomach and liver tonic, and is useful for jaundice. Drinking pomegranate juice in which mint aerial parts are macerated, is useful for hiccup, nausea, vomiting, gastroenteritis, and stomachache, as well as heartburn. Topical application of mint as a poultice on abdomen can warm and tonify stomach, and improve appetite. Furthermore, the poultice is useful for hemorrhoid (Aghili Khorasani 1771; Avicenna 1025).

 DOI: 10.1201/b22971-21

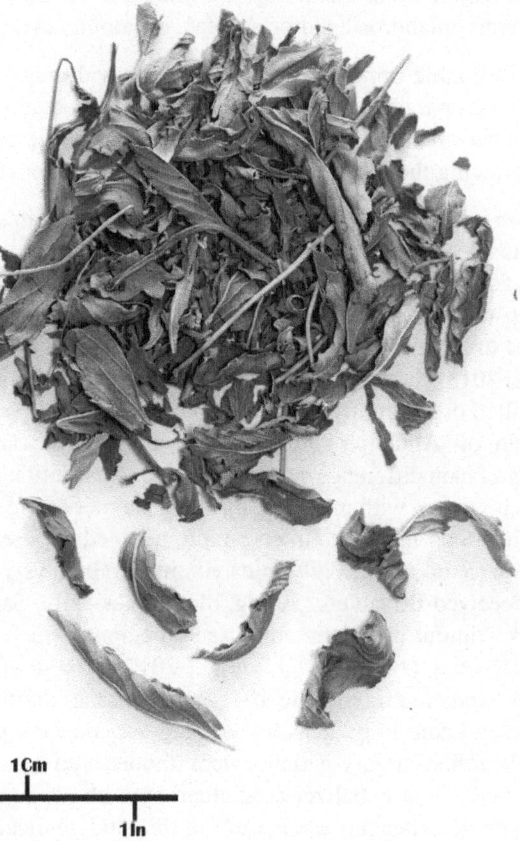

FIGURE 21.1 Peppermint aerial parts.

Current Evidence

Clinical Evidence

Anxiety: In a group of 64 nursing students, the effect of aromatherapy with peppermint oil (one drop on a gauze, inserted in face mask and inhaled for 20 min) was compared with placebo. After 4 days of intervention, peppermint oil could increase accuracy in the students; however, no significant difference was observed in terms of anxiety (Khodadoost et al., 2020). In a placebo-controlled RCT in 80 cardiac patients undergoing intravenous catheterization, aromatherapy via inhalation of peppermint oil (three drops on a cotton ball, inserted to the collar) for 5 min could significantly decrease anxiety in these patients (Akbari et al., 2019). In another RCT in 64 patients diagnosed with acute coronary syndrome in the emergency department, cases underwent aromatherapy with peppermint oil (a cotton ball soaked in the oil and kept 20 cm from nose) or placebo (water) for 1 h. A significant reduction in anxiety was observed in patients treated with peppermint oil (Soleimani et al., 2022). A placebo-controlled RCT in 36 healthy adults showed that consumption of a drink containing 50 μL of peppermint oil for 20 days causes a significant improvement in state and trait anxiety, as well as blood pressure and TAG (Sinclair et al., 2023).

Hirsutism: In an uncontrolled clinical study, 21 female hirsute patients with idiopathic hirsutism and PCOS, received 250 mL of *M. spicata* tea (20 g/L) twice a day for 5 days in the follicular phase of their menstrual cycles. Results indicated a significant increase in LH, FSH, and estradiol. They also found a decrease in free testosterone, but no significant decrease was observed in the levels of total testosterone or dehydroepiandrostenedione sulfate (Akdoğan et al., 2007).

Migraine headache: In a double-blind RCT in 120 patients with migraine, a nasal drop containing 1.5% peppermint oil was compared with placebo and lidocaine in treatment of pain during migraine attack. Accordingly, peppermint oil showed a similar effect to lidocaine and significantly better effect than placebo in reducing the intensity of pain (Rafieian-Kopaei et al., 2019).

Nausea and vomiting: In a double-blind RCT, 50 patients with any cancer diagnosis, received spearmint and peppermint capsules via the oral route (containing two drops of each essential oil every 4 h, filled with sugar, and administered 30 minutes before they received their chemotherapy treatment, again 4 h after first capsule and finally 4 h later in home). The volatile oil from the *M. spicata* and *M. piperita* reduced the intensity and number of emetic events during 24 h postchemotherapy (Tayarani-Najaran et al., 2013). In an RCT in a group of 42 patients with postoperative nausea and vomiting, simple controlled breathing technique was compared with controlled breathing technique while inhaling peppermint oil. Although both treatments could significantly reduce the symptoms of patients, there was no significant difference between the two intervention groups (Sites et al., 2014). In another RCT, 74 pregnant women with moderate morning sickness were divided into two groups (the herbal syrup and vitamin B6 groups). The intervention included the use of pomegranate-spreармint syrup, a TPM formulation (5 mL, thrice daily) plus vitamin B6 in the syrup group; on the other hand, the control group only received B6 tablets (20 mg, three times daily) for 1 week. The subjects were followed up for 1 week without any interventions. Pomegranate-spearmint syrup reduced nausea and vomiting during pregnancy (Abdolhosseini et al., 2017). In a double-blind RCT, use of a soft gel capsule containing *M. spicata* oil (equal to 10–12 mg carvone) during 24 h of postoperative time decreased nausea, bloat, and pain in patients undergoing appendectomy (Shahdadi et al., 2015). In another clinical trial, 60 cardiac surgery patients were divided into control and intervention groups. The intervention group underwent nebulizer aromatherapy with peppermint essential oil before the endotracheal tube was removed after surgery. Results of this study indicated that inhalation of peppermint essential oil reduced nausea and vomiting after open-heart surgery (Maghami et al., 2020).

Dysphagia: In a pilot clinical study in a group of 38 patients with dysphagia and noncardiac chest pain, a lozenge containing 11% peppermint oil was administered as two tablets before meal for dysphagia or as needed for chest pain for a median of 6 months. While 63% of patients reported improvement in their symptoms, it seems that those with distal esophageal spasm or esophagogastric junction outflow obstruction are more responsive to this treatment (Khalaf et al., 2019).

IBS: In a double-blind, placebo-controlled RCT, 72 patients with moderate to severe nonconstipated IBS were randomized to receive peppermint or placebo. Subjects who received a novel formulation of peppermint three times a day for 28 days experienced a statistically significant decrease from baseline in mean Total IBS Symptom Score, a global IBS symptom score, compared with placebo (Cash et al., 2016). A systematic review and meta-analysis on nine RCTs introduced the peppermint oil (as one or two capsules administered three times daily for a minimum of 2 weeks) as an effective treatment for the symptoms of IBS with minor adverse events, e.g., heartburn (Khanna et al., 2014). A more recent meta-analysis of 12 RCTs also confirmed the capability of peppermint oil against the pain and global symptoms in adults with IBS (Alammar et al., 2019).

Abdominal pain and gut microbiome: In a clinical study in 30 children with abdominal pain, three doses of oral peppermint oil (180 mg, once, twice, or thrice daily) were administered for 1 week. Comparison of the microbiome in feces samples after the intervention with the baseline microbiome showed a significant change in *Collinsella* genus, while only the highest dose caused a significant reduction of Firmicutes/Bacteroidetes ratio. Though, studies with a longer follow up period are recommended to confirm the effect of peppermint oil on microbiome modulation (Thapa et al., 2022).

GI imaging: In a prospective RCT, peppermint oil (85 mg), when added to simethicone, N-acetylcysteine, and sodium bicarbonate improved visualization for the lower and upper gastric body in esophagogastroduodenoscopy (Mahawongkajit and Kanlerd, 2021). Another study has reported that coadministration of 40 mL of a peppermint oil solution (16 mL peppermint oil dissolved in water with an emulsifier to make 21 mL of the final solution) and barium suspension reduced the incidence of colonic spasm during the examination in barium enema (Sparks et al., 1995). As evaluated in a double-blind, double-dummy RCT, 40 mL of peppermint oil solution (16 mL of peppermint oil and 2 g of emulsifier dissolved in 1 liter of water) which was sprayed by endoscope around pyloric ring at two phases, reduced gastric spasm during upper GI endoscopy (Hiki et al., 2003). The antispasmodic effects of peppermint oil were also confirmed by a nonrandomized prospective study during esophagogastroduodenoscopy, for elderly patients. Among the elderly patients, those treated with peppermint oil solution (20 mL, 1.6% in water) had similar scores to those in the group received hyoscine butyl bromide, and significantly better scores than those in the group received glucagon (Imagawa et al., 2012). A systematic review and meta-analysis of six RCTs confirmed the antispasmodic effects of peppermint oil in colonoscopy via reduction of spasticity and peristalsis and improvement of adenoma detection rate (Aziz et al., 2020).

Reactive agility: During a double-blind, placebo-controlled RCT, 142 healthy, recreationally active men and women received 900 mg of spearmint aqueous extract or placebo daily for 90 days. Results indicated that spearmint improved specific measures of reactive agility in a young, active population (Falcone et al., 2018).

Lung function: During a quasi-experimental uncontrolled before-and-after study, *M. spicata* oil improved the lung status for the students by increasing FEV-1 and Forced Vital Capacity. Moreover, it made a significant reduction in the means of the running time. The normal spirometry results were 50%; while after inhalation with *M. spicata* oil, the ratio was 60% (Jaradat et al., 2016). In another randomized experiment, 106 healthy participants inhaled nebulized peppermint, eucalyptus, or rosemary essential oil for 15 min or no treatment (control); however, *M. piperita* showed no changes in spirometry of healthy individuals (Köteles et al., 2018).

Memory impairment: In a pilot study, 30-day treatment of spearmint aqueous extract (900 mg daily) improved cognitive function, i.e., planning, attention/concentration, and reasoning, in 11 subjects with self-reported memory impairment (Nieman et al., 2014). In a double-blind, placebo-controlled RCT including 90 cases with age-associated memory impairment, spearmint extract (600 or 900 mg per day) improved working memory during 90 days of supplementation (Herrlinger et al., 2018). In line, in a double-blind, placebo-controlled RCT, 142 healthy, recreationally active men and women received 900 mg of spearmint aqueous extract or placebo daily for 90 days. This study indicated that spearmint extract led to attention-enhancing effects in healthy men and women (Falcone et al., 2019).

Osteoarthritis: In a controlled clinical study, a 16-week daily consumption of high-rosmarinic acid containing spearmint tea (3 g per teabag, two teabags per day) was compared with commercial spearmint tea as control in adults with knee osteoarthritis. Both types of tea could improve physical disability scores and stiffness; while only high-rosmarinic acid spearmint tea could significantly decrease pain (Connelly et al., 2014).

Skin aging: A noncontrolled multicentric clinical trial was done in 121 healthy subjects. The use protocol calls for a session every 2 weeks for a total of four sessions. Subjects were evaluated before each subsequent session at the first and at 2nd–4th–8th weeks after the fourth and last treatment. Results showed that peppermint soft peeling was effective and safe to treat subject with chrono- and photo-aging skin, thereby it can be a potent remedy in the revitalization of dermis and epidermis layers via chemical exfoliation and hydration (Scarano et al., 2019).

Pressure injury: A double-blind RCT was conducted on 150 patients with head trauma admitted to the ICU. The intervention group received peppermint gel three times a day up to 14 days during the skin care as a layer on the skin areas exposed to the risk of pressure injuries. Results showed that in comparison to the placebo gel, peppermint gel was significantly more effective to prevent pressure injuries in these patients (Babamohamadi et al., 2019).

Preclinical Evidence

Colitis: In TNBS-induced IBD in mice, oral consumption of spearmint hydroethanolic extract (15 mg/kg for 4 days) could significantly decrease iNOS expression in the colon tissue, which subsequently improved colon damage by reduction of oxidative stress and inflammation (Direito et al., 2019).

Memory impairment: In APP/PS1 transgenic mice, administration of peppermint oil as inhalation (twice daily, one each time, for 21 days) improved memory via reduction of LPO and Aβ deposition, as well as elevation of GSH and SOD levels in the brain tissue (Lv et al., 2022).

ADVERSE REACTIONS

TPM Literature

Fresh mint leaves may cause flatulence. High doses of mint can induce itching in throat and ingestion with celery can prevent this adverse effect (Aghili Khorasani 1771).

Current Evidence

Peppermint leaf and oil should be used with caution in patients with GERD and hiatal hernia, GI ulcers, and severe GI inflammation (Gardner and McGuffin, 2013).

Some adverse reactions have been reported from peppermint oil including diarrhea, flushing, headache, heartburn, mouth ulcer, bronchospasm (topical), contact dermatitis (topical), laryngospasm, respiratory collapse, skin irritation (Gruenwald et al., 2007; Ulbricht, 2010).

CONTRAINDICATIONS

TPM Literature

None.

Current Evidence

Like most of the essential oils, peppermint oil can be toxic and even lethal at excessive dosages; it has been associated with interstitial nephritis and acute renal failure (Schulz et al., 2001). It may have a choleretic effect and is contraindicated in patients with cholelithiasis or cholecystitis. Peppermint oil is relatively contraindicated in patients with hiatal hernia or significant GERD, because its effect on the lower esophageal sphincter can lead to exacerbation of symptoms (Gruenwald et al., 2007).

Peppermint oil should not be used internally or on or near the face in infants and young children because of its potential to cause bronchospasm, tongue spasms, and, possibly, respiratory arrest (Blumenthal et al., 2000).

PREGNANCY AND LACTATION

TPM Literature

Mint has been emphasized to change the taste of mother's milk to be unpleasant. So, it has been recommended not to be used during breastfeeding (Aghili Khorasani 1771).

Current Evidence

Peppermint oil has been used to trigger menstruation and should be avoided during pregnancy. There is insufficient data to assess its safety during lactation. However, the amount of peppermint in over-the-counter medications, topical preparations, and herbal teas is likely safe in pregnant and lactating women and in young children (Bokelmann, 2021).

DRUG INTERACTIONS

Cyclosporine and Felodipine: Peppermint oil appears to increase cyclosporin and felodipine levels and is recommended to not use pharmaceutical preparations containing peppermint oil with these medications.
Topical preparations: It may also enhance the skin penetration of some topical medicines when applied concomitantly.
Digoxin: Peppermint tea contains digoxin-like constituents and may increase the effects of digoxin theoretically. However, the clinical relevance of this is unclear.
Iron supplements: It may impair iron absorption and should not be used with iron-containing supplements (Williamson et al., 2013).

METHOD OF ADMINISTRATION

TPM Literature

Its fresh aerial part or decoction is administered orally. Rubbing its powder to teeth has been recommended for dental conditions and its poultice has been applied for GI disorders (Aghili Khorasani 1771).

Current Evidence

Peppermint and spearmint are recommended as tea, tincture, or oil. Peppermint oil is also administered topically or via inhalation for aromatherapy.

DOSAGE

Peppermint leaf: 3–6 g per day may be prepared as infusion or tea, 3–4 times daily between meals (Gruenwald et al., 2007).
Peppermint oil: 6–12 drops for inhalation, 3–4 drops in hot water for oral use (for IBS: 0.6 mL as single dose or 0.2 mL as enteric-coated products) (Gruenwald et al., 2007).
Spearmint leaf: RCTs have used a 600–900 mg daily dose of spearmint aqueous extract, or 3 g teabags twice daily.

REFERENCES

Abdolhosseini S, Hashem-Dabaghian F, Mokaberinejad R, et al. Effects of pomegranate and spearmint syrup on nausea and vomiting during pregnancy: A randomized controlled clinical trial. Iran Red Crescent Med J. 2017;19(10):e13542.

Aghili Khorasani MH 1771. *Makhzan-al-Adviah* (*The treasury of drugs*) (rewritten by Shams Ardakani MR, Rahimi R, Farjadmand F, 1st ed.). Tehran: Tehran University of Medical Sciences; 2009.

Akbari F, Rezaei M, Khatony A. Effect of peppermint essence on the pain and anxiety caused by intravenous catheterization in cardiac patients: A randomized controlled trial. J Pain Res. 2019;12:2933–2939.

Akdoğan M, Tamer MN, Cüre E, et al. Effect of spearmint (*Mentha spicata* Labiatae) teas on androgen levels in women with hirsutism. Phytother Res. 2007;21(5):444–447.

Alammar N, Wang L, Saberi B, et al. The impact of peppermint oil on the irritable bowel syndrome: A meta-analysis of the pooled clinical data. BMC Compl Alternative Med. 2019;19(1):21.

Avicenna 1025. *Al-Qanoon fi al-Tibb* (*The canon of medicine*) (rewritten by Masoudi A, ed.). Tehran: Almaei; 2015.

Aziz M, Sharma S, Ghazaleh S, et al. The anti-spasmodic effect of peppermint oil during colonoscopy: A systematic review and meta-analysis. Minerva Gastroenterol Dietol. 2020;66(2):164–171.

Babamohamadi H, Ansari Z, Nobahar M, Mirmohammadkhani M. The effects of peppermint gel on prevention of pressure injury in hospitalized patients with head trauma in neurosurgical ICU: A double-blind randomized controlled trial. Complement Ther Med. 2019; 47:102223.

Blumenthal M, Goldberg A, Brinckmann J. *Herbal medicine: Expanded Commission E monographs*. Ann Arbor: Integrative Medicine Communications; 2000.

Bokelmann JM. *Medicinal herbs in primary care: An evidence-guided reference for healthcare providers*. Philadelphia: Elsevier Health Sciences; 2021.

Cash BD, Epstein MS, Shah SM. A novel delivery system of peppermint oil is an effective therapy for irritable bowel syndrome symptoms. Dig Dis Sci. 2016;61(2):560–571.

Connelly AE, Tucker AJ, Tulk H, et al. High-rosmarinic acid spearmint tea in the management of knee osteoarthritis symptoms. J Med Food. 2014;17(12):1361–1367.

Direito R, Rocha J, Lima A, et al. Reduction of inflammation and colon injury by a spearmint phenolic extract in experimental bowel disease in mice. Medicines. 2019;6(2):65.

Falcone PH, Nieman KM, Tribby AC, et al. The attention-enhancing effects of spearmint extract supplementation in healthy men and women: A randomized, double-blind, placebo-controlled, parallel trial. Nutr Res. 2019;64:24–38.

Falcone PH, Tribby AC, Vogel RM, et al. Efficacy of a nootropic spearmint extract on reactive agility: A randomized, double-blind, placebo-controlled, parallel trial. J Int Soc Sports Nutr. 2018;15(1):58.

Gardner Z, McGuffin M. *Botanical safety handbook*. Boca Raton: Taylor & Francis; 2013.

Gruenwald J, Brendler T, Jaenicke C. *PDR for herbal medicines*. Montvale: Thomson Reuters; 2007.

Herrlinger KA, Nieman KM, Sanoshy KD, et al. Spearmint extract improves working memory in men and women with age-associated memory impairment. J Altern Complement Med. 2018;24(1):37–47.

Hiki N, Kurosaka H, Tatsutomi Y, et al. Peppermint oil reduces gastric spasm during upper endoscopy: A randomized, double-blind, double-dummy controlled trial. Gastrointest Endosc. 2003;57(4):475–482.

Imagawa A, Hata H, Nakatsu M, et al. Peppermint oil solution is useful as an antispasmodic drug for esophagogastroduodenoscopy, especially for elderly patients. Dig Dis Sci. 2012;57(9):2379–2384.

Jaradat NA, Al Zabadi H, Rahhal B, et al. The effect of inhalation of *Citrus sinensis* flowers and *Mentha spicata* leave essential oils on lung function and exercise performance: A quasi-experimental uncontrolled before-and-after study. J Int Soc Sports Nutr. 2016;13(1):36.

Khalaf MH, Chowdhary S, Elmunzer BJ, et al. Impact of peppermint therapy on dysphagia and non-cardiac chest pain: A pilot study. Dig Dis Sci. 2019;64:2214–2218.

Khanna R, MacDonald JK, Levesque BG. Peppermint oil for the treatment of irritable bowel syndrome: A systematic review and meta-analysis. J Clin Gastroenterol. 2014;48(6):505–512.

Khodadoost E, Nakhaei M, Askari A, Nasirizade M. The effect of inhalation of peppermint essential oil on anxiety and accuracy of nursing students in emergency department of Birjand educational hospitals. J Med Plants. 2020;19(75):132–140.

Köteles F, Babulka P, Szemerszky R, et al. Inhaled peppermint, rosemary and eucalyptus essential oils do not change spirometry in healthy individuals. Physiol Behav. 2018;194:319–323.

Lv X, Feng Y, Ma R, et al. Effects of peppermint essential oil on learning and memory ability in APP/PS1 transgenic mice. Molecules. 2022;27(7):2051.

Maghami M, Afazel MR, Azizi-Fini I, Maghami M. The effect of aromatherapy with peppermint essential oil on nausea and vomiting after cardiac surgery: A randomized clinical trial. Complement Ther Clin Pract. 2020;40:101199.

Mahawongkajit P, Kanlerd A. A prospective randomized controlled trial comparing simethicone, N-acetylcysteine, sodium bicarbonate and peppermint for visualization in upper gastrointestinal endoscopy. Surg Endosc. 2021;35(1):303–308.

Nieman K, Herrlinger K, Sanoshy K, et al. Tolerance and cognitive function effects of a proprietary spearmint extract in men and women with self-reported memory impairment: A pilot study (LB402). FASEB J. 2014;28:LB402.

Rafieian-Kopaei M, Hasanpour-Dehkordi A, Lorigooini Z, et al. Comparing the effect of intranasal lidocaine 4% with peppermint essential oil drop 1.5% on migraine attacks: A double-blind clinical trial. Int J Prev Med. 2019;10:121.

Scarano A, Amodeo V, Leonardi V, et al. Evaluation of the effectiveness and safety of peppermint peel (PMP) soft peeling for skin ageing. J Biol Regul Homeost Agents. 2019;33:93–101.

Schulz V, Hänsel R, Tyler VE. *Rational phytotherapy: A physician's guide to herbal medicine*. Heidelberg: Psychology Press; 2001.

Shahdadi H, Balouchi A, Taheri S, Darban F. Study effect of mint essence on pain, bloat and nausea in patients undergoing appendectomy. Pharm Lett. 2015;7(10):193–197.

Sinclair J, Murray H, Smith V, et al. Effects of peppermint oil (*Mentha piperita* L.) on cardiometabolic and other health-related outcomes: A parallel placebo randomized controlled trial. Sport Sci Health. 2023:1–10.

Sites DS, Johnson NT, Miller JA, et al. Controlled breathing with or without peppermint aromatherapy for postoperative nausea and/or vomiting symptom relief: A randomized controlled trial. J Perianesth Nurs. 2014;29(1):12–19.

Soleimani M, Kashfi LS, Ghods AA. The effect of aromatherapy with peppermint essential oil on anxiety of cardiac patients in emergency department: A placebo-controlled study. Complement Ther Clin Pract. 2022;46:101533.

Sparks MJ, O'sullivan P, Herrington AA, Morcos SK. Does peppermint oil relieve spasm during barium enema? Br J Radiol. 1995;68(812):841–843.

Tayarani-Najaran Z, Talasaz-Firoozi E, Nasiri R, Jalali N, Hassanzadeh MK. Antiemetic activity of volatile oil from *Mentha spicata* and *Mentha* × piperita in chemotherapy-induced nausea and vomiting. Ecancermedicalscience. 2013;7:290.

Thapa S, Luna RA, Chumpitazi BP, et al. Peppermint oil effects on the gut microbiome in children with functional abdominal pain. Clin Transl Sci. 2022;15(4):1036–1049.

Ulbricht C, Costa D, M Grimes Serrano J, Guilford J, Isaac R, Seamon E, Varghese M. An evidence-based systematic review of spearmint by the natural standard research collaboration. J Diet Suppl. 2010;7(2):179–215.

WHO. *WHO monographs on selected medicinal plants*, volume 2. Malta: World Health Organization; 2002.

Williamson E, Driver S, Baxter K (eds). *Stockley's herbal medicines interactions*. London: Pharmaceutical Press; 2013.

22 *Myrtus communis* L.

Asie Shojaii

Scientific name: *Myrtus communis* L.
Family: Myrtaceae
Common name:

- **English:** Myrtle, common myrtle
- **Persian:** *mūrd*
- **Arabic:** *'ās*

Medicinal parts: Leaves, fruits (berries), fresh flowering branches (Figure 22.1)
Temperament (nature): Cold in the first degree and dry in the second degree
Major chemical constituents:

- **Leaves:**
  - **Essential oil:** Major components include 1,8-cineole (9.9–20.3%), α-pinene (3.8–23.0%), myrtenyl acetate, limonene (5.5–17.8%), linalool (12.3–17.6%), α-terpinyl acetate (1.8–7.0%), geraniol, geranyl acetate (1.2–3.1%)
  - **Phenolic compounds:** Tannins, flavonoids such as quercetin, catechin, and myricetin derivatives, phenolic acid such as caffeic acid, gallic acid, and ellagic acids, coumarins, myrtucommulone A and B, semimyrtucommulone, galloyl-glucosides, ellagitannins, galloyl-quinic acids (Alipour et al., 2014)

- **Berries:**
  - **Essential oil:** The major components include α-pinene (28.6%), 1,8-cineole (26.7%), limonene (18.0%), α-terpinyl acetate (5.4%), linalyl acetate (3.4%), and linalool (2.3%)
  - **Phenolic compounds:** Tannins, flavonoids such as kaempferol, quercetin, myricetin derivatives, and anthocyanins
  - **Fatty acids:** Linoleic acid, palmitic acid, oleic acid, and stearic acids

- **Other components:** Resins, citric acid, malic acid, caffeic acid, and arabinosides (Alipour et al., 2014; Pezhmanmehr et al., 2009)

THERAPEUTIC USE

TPM LITERATURE

Myrtle is a brain tonic in oral use and as inhalation. It is useful for headache, especially those secondary to GI problems (gastrointestinal headaches), vertigo, and dizziness. It improves eyesight, relieves conjunctivitis as eye drop and earache as ear drop. It is also helpful in toothache, dental abscess, and aphthous stomatitis as mouthwash. Myrtle can be used to treat swellings and to stop hemorrhage from any organs, either in external or internal use. It is also a potent wound healing agent. Topical application of fresh myrtle leaves poultice on the forehead, either alone or mixed with vinegar, is helpful to stop nosebleed.

DOI: 10.1201/b22971-22

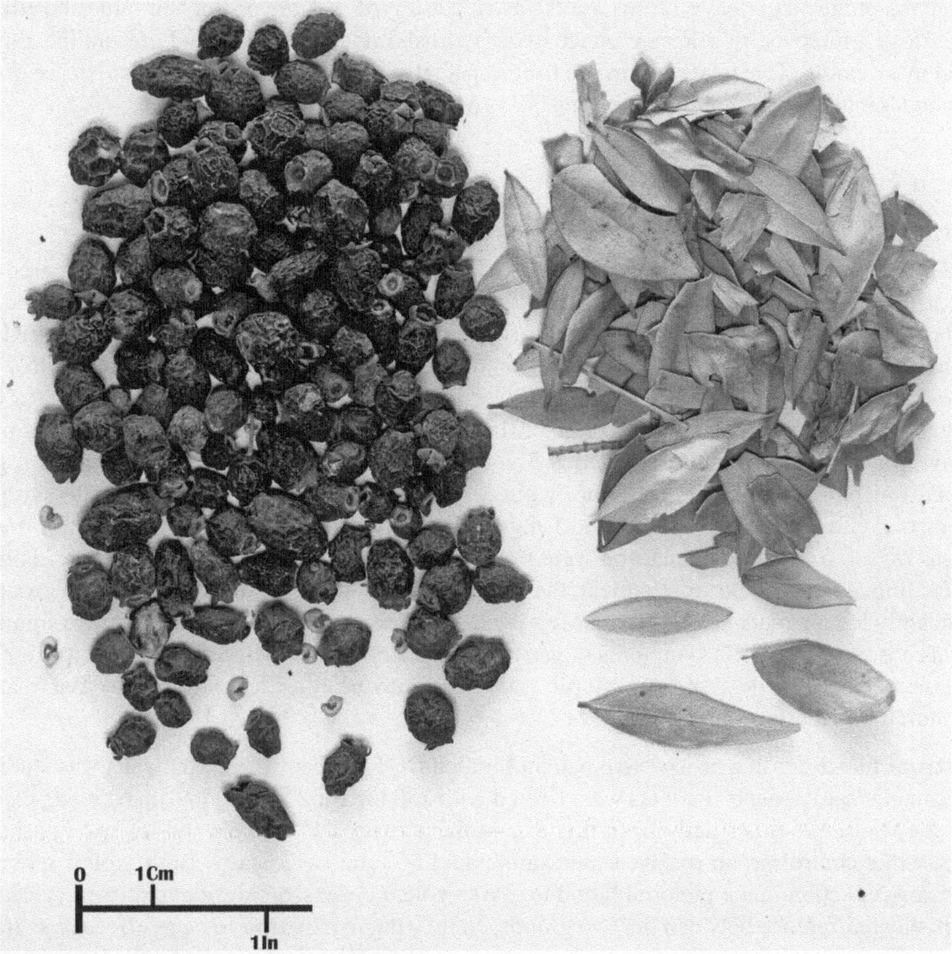

FIGURE 22.1 Myrtle fruits (left) and leaves (right).

This plant acts as a cardiotonic and can show its effects via inhalation of its aroma, or oral intake of ripe fruits and fruit preparations, e.g., syrup and concentrated juice. Myrtle fruit syrup is suggested for palpitation, as well as cough due to catarrh.

Myrtle fruit is a tonic for stomach and visceral organs, especially in the form of concentrated juice or powder, and is recommended for the treatment of GERD and chronic diarrhea. Also, topical application of myrtle leaves poultice at the bottom of the navel is useful in some types of diarrheas.

Myrtle has diuretic effect and can be used in dysuria, bladder ulcers, and kidney weakness. It is highly recommended for the treatment of hemorrhoids, both in the oral and topical applications. It can also be used to stop abnormal menstrual bleeding and vaginal discharge.

Topical use of myrtle leaves and oil is recommended for urticaria, fire burns, wound healing of palms and soles, and erythema. Myrtle oil can be used in conditions like paronychia. Also, decoction of myrtle leaves can be used topically for joint pain and accelerate the conjunction of bone fracture. It is helpful in improvement of weakness of limbs and nerves, and in joint lassitude. Topical usage of leaves can be effective in abrasion of foot heel. Myrtle fruits can be used topically in skin hyperpigmentation such as freckles, lentigo, and skin dark spots.

All parts of the plant (leaves, fruits, roots), as well as myrtle oil, are potent hair tonic and effective for hair loss. Moreover, myrtle can reduce hyperhydrosis, smelly armpits, and prevent the abrasion caused by sweating. Topical use of myrtle fruit, especially with wine, may be helpful in case of scorpion and tarantula bites (Aghili Khorasani 1771; Avicenna 1025).

Current Evidence

Clinical Evidence

GERD: Efficacy of myrtle berries freeze-dried aqueous extract in GERD was compared with omeprazole in a double-blind three-arm RCT for 6 weeks. Forty-five patients were treated with 1,000 mg per day of myrtle, 20 mg per day of omeprazole, or both. In all groups, both GERD and dyspeptic scores significantly decreased in comparison with the respective baselines. Also, there were no differences in the postintervention measures between groups, showing myrtle to be as effective as omeprazole (Zohalinejad et al., 2016). In another double-blind RCT, efficacy of myrtle fruit syrup was studied in children aged 1–7 years old, diagnosed with GERD. The control group received omeprazole and placebo syrup, while the intervention group received myrtle syrup and omeprazole. Omeprazole was prescribed 1 mg/kg/day in two divided doses, 15 min before feeding whereas myrtle fruit syrup or placebo were prescribed 0.21 mL/kg per dose, three times daily and after feeding. After 8 weeks of treatment, the symptom "refusal to eat" in the intervention group was significantly less than in placebo group. Moreover, 4 weeks after cessation of treatment, a significant rise was observed in GERD symptoms of patients in placebo group; while no such rise was reported for those received myrtle syrup. So, myrtle fruit syrup may be considered as an effective treatment for children GERD (Paknejad et al., 2021).

Menstrual bleeding: In a prospective patient blinded RCT, efficacy of myrtle fruits was studied in menorrhagia in 40 patients. Patients were treated with 750 mg (one 500 mg and one 250 mg capsule) of myrtle fruit three times daily from first day of menstruation for 5 days and for two consecutive cycles, while control group received tranexamic acid 500 mg twice daily. Both groups reported a significant reduction in the pictorial blood loss assessment chart score during treatment cycles with no statistical difference between the two groups, suggesting myrtle fruit to be as effective as tranexamic acid for the management of heavy menstrual bleeding (Umarami et al., 2020). In another pilot RCT, efficacy of myrtle syrup (5 mL three times a day) was compared with placebo in 30 women with abnormal uterine bleeding (menometrorrhagia). The treatments were administered for 7 days, starting from the onset of bleeding and for three consecutive menstrual cycles. Results showed that mean number of bleeding days significantly declined after 3 months treatment with the syrup and consequently, the participants in the intervention group used fewer pads after 3 months compared with the number of pads used at the beginning of the treatment (Qarraaty et al., 2014).

Hemorrhoid: In a triple-blind RCT, efficacy of myrtle ointment (5% myrtle essential oil in ointment base) and anti-hemorrhoid ointment (containing lidocaine, hydrocortisone acetate, aluminum subacetate, and bicarbonate oxide) were evaluated in 134 postpartum women with grade I and II hemorrhoid. The ointments were used twice a day with an applicator containing 3–4 g of the drug through the rectum for a duration of 4 weeks. Findings showed that myrtle ointment was able to reduce the symptoms of hemorrhoid and improve the quality of life with a similar efficacy to the anti-hemorrhoid group; however, the participants in the myrtle ointment group had a significantly lower anal itching and were more satisfied with their drug use (Malekuti et al., 2019).

Vaginitis: Masoudi et al. studied the effect of a vaginal gel containing metronidazole 0.75% and myrtle 2% ethanolic extract vs. metronidazole 0.75% vaginal gel alone in the treatment of recurrent bacterial vaginosis in 80 married women of 18–40 years old for five consecutive nights. Findings suggested that combination of myrtle extract with metronidazole increases the efficiency of bacterial vaginosis treatment, Also, the patients received combination therapy did not experience a recurrent infection; whereas 30% of those treated with metronidazole alone had a recurrent bacterial vaginosis after 3 weeks (Masoudi et al., 2017).

HPV infection: In a double-blind, placebo-controlled RCT on 60 women, 18–50 years old, with cervicovaginal HPV infection, vaginal suppositories contained 10% of myrtle aqueous extract and 0.5% of myrtle essential oil or placebo were prescribed for 3 months (20 suppositories at each menstrual cycle). At the end of the study, the HPV test was negative in 92.6% of patients in the intervention group which was a statistically higher response vs. placebo (62.6%). Also, based on colposcopic findings, the improvement in cervical lesion size was 71.4% in patients used myrtle suppository, while it was 30.4% in the placebo group. It seems that herbal suppository can speed up virus clearance and can be effective in treating HPV infection (Nikakhtar et al., 2018).

Wart: In a pilot RCT in 100 patients with total number of warts ≤20 and diameter ≤1 cm, the effect of salving leaves of myrtle, processed by 1× leaves of myrtle and 2× water (twice daily) was compared with 16.5% salicylic acid (once daily). The interventions were topically applied on each wart for 40 days. The number of warts decreased in the myrtle group faster than salicylic acid and the maximum reduction in the number of warts was seen in myrtle group on day 40. Also, reduction of the size of warts in myrtle group was more than the other group on days 20, 40, and 90 (Ghadami Yazdi et al., 2014).

Dandruff: Effect of topical myrtle solution, prepared as a combination of myrtle aqueous extract and vinegar, in the treatment of 90 cases with dandruff was compared with ketoconazole shampoo in a double-blind RCT. Results showed that myrtle solution was effective in the treatment of dandruff with a powerful and rapid effect on scaly scalps. Myrtle solution had a similar efficacy to the standard control without any serious adverse effect (Chaijan et al., 2018).

Aphthous stomatitis: According to an RCT on 45 patients with recurrent aphthous stomatitis, application of an oral paste containing 5% myrtle leaf aqueous extract, four times a day for 6 days, caused a significant reduction in ulcer size, pain, erythema, and exudate vs. placebo paste. The paste could improve oral health impact profile and patient overall assessment of their treatment (Babaee et al., 2010).

Wound healing: In a placebo-controlled RCT, the effect of myrtle cream (10% leaf ethanolic extract) on wound healing and severity of episiotomy pain was studied on 100 nulliparous women. Myrtle cream or placebo were topically applied twice a day for 10 days. According to the REEDA scale for episiotomy healing assessment, myrtle cream could accelerate the healing of episiotomy wound and decrease the pain severity in comparison to the placebo cream (Mirzaee et al., 2019).

Acne vulgaris: A comparative split-face study on 55 patients with mild to moderate acne vulgaris, evaluated the efficacy of topical myrtle leaf ethanolic extract and clindamycin 1% solution. The patients received topical myrtle solution to the right side of the face and clindamycin solution to the left side twice daily for 12 weeks, followed by 4 weeks of drug-free period for follow up. Considering treatment outcomes, such as number of comedones, inflammatory lesion, sebum percentage change, and acne severity index, myrtle lotion demonstrated a similar or better efficacy vs. clindamycin (Salmanian et al., 2020).

Preclinical Evidence

Heart failure: Myrtle is considered as a cardiotonic plant in TPM. Protective effect of myrtle fruit and leaf hydroalcoholic extracts (300, 700 mg/kg) was evaluated on isoproterenol-induced heart failure in rats. Results showed that administration of myrtle for 4 weeks, significantly reduced the MDA and increased SOD and GSH levels in the group treated with myrtle (Aboutaleb et al., 2021).

Hypnotic effect: Efficacy of ethanolic extract of myrtle leaves on sleep and anxiety were evaluated in rats using open field, grip strength, and righting reflex models. The extract showed a muscle relaxant and anxiolytic activity with a 200 mg/kg dose. It also exhibited a significant hypnotic effect with the same dose which was accompanied with a reduction of REM sleep, as well as an increase in total and non-REM sleep time (Hajiaghaee et al., 2016).

Anti-inflammatory and analgesic effect: Several studies have indicated the anti-inflammatory and analgesic properties of the essential oil and extracts of myrtle in animal models. The ethanolic (0.05 g/kg) and aqueous extracts (0.005, 0.015, and 0.03 g/kg) of myrtle demonstrated anti-inflammatory effects in cotton pellet test and xylene-induced ear edema. Additionally, both extracts showed central and peripheral antinociceptive effects in hot plate and acetic acid-induced writhing test, possibly via opioid receptors (Hosseinzadeh et al., 2011). In another study, topical anti-inflammatory activity of myrtle essential oil was studied in croton oil-induced ear edema and cotton pellet test in mice. Results showed a significant reduction of MPO, TNF-α, IL-6, and leukocyte migration to the damaged tissue (Maxia et al., 2011). In another study in a rat model of cerulean-induced acute pancreatitis, protective effects of myrtle leaf ethanolic extract was assessed, which was administered by oral gavage (100 mg/kg/day) for 14 days. Results showed that administration of myrtle extract could inhibit the development of acute pancreatitis via reduction of IL-1β, IL-6, and MDA, as well restoration of IL-10 and GSH (Ozbeyli et al., 2020).

Diarrhea: Oral administration of myrtle berries aqueous extract (25, 50 and 100 mg/kg) in castor oil-induced acute diarrhea in rats caused a significant and dose-dependent delay of the diarrhea onset and decrease in the stooling frequency, weight of wet stools, and the diarrhea score. Though, the standard antidiarrheal drug, loperamide (20 mg/kg), produced a more potent inhibitory effect on all diarrhea parameters compared to the highest dose of myrtle extract (Jabri et al., 2016a). In another study in mice, antidiarrheal effect of 80% methanol extract and solvent fractions of myrtle leaves were evaluated using a similar animal model. Results revealed that the extract, at all doses (100, 200 and 400 mg/kg), as well as the chloroform fraction and methanol fraction at 300 and 400 mg/kg, respectively, produced a significant antimotility effect and decline in the weight and volume of intestinal contents (Sisay et al., 2017).

Effect on gastrointestinal disorders: Myrtle berries showed protective effects on gastric ulcers induced by ethanol, indomethacin, and pyloric ligation models in rats. Aqueous (105 and 175 mg/kg) and methanolic (93 and 154 mg/kg) extracts of myrtle berry significantly reduced the ulcer index, gastric juice volume and acidity, and increased gastric pH and gastric wall mucus content compared with omeprazole in the ethanol-induced ulcer (Sumbul et al., 2010). Also, the protective effect of the myrtle berries aqueous extract (25, 50 and 100 mg/kg, orally) against esophageal reflux-induced damage in esophagus mucosa in rats was evaluated. Findings suggest that various doses of myrtle extract significantly reduced the severity of esophageal lesions in a dose-dependent manner and exerted potential protective effect against esophageal reflux-induced damage in rat esophagus, at least in part, due to its antioxidant properties (Jabri et al., 2016b).

Wound: In a study in 76 cows and calves between 1 and 5 years of age with clinical sing of foot and mouth disease, myrtle essential oil (5% concentration) has been demonstrated to be effective in treatment of wounds in foot and mouth ulcers as it causes faster improvement of mouth ulcers and reduces purulent discharge (Najafi et al., 2011). In another study, application of a topical gel containing 6% aqueous extract of myrtle berries for 3 weeks on wound healing in STZ-induced diabetic rats showed a significant improvement in wound healing by accelerating epidermal and dermal maturation (Khodaei et al., 2021). In a study in third-degree burn wound in rats, protective role of oral (100 mg/kg/day) or topical (5% ointment) myrtle ethanolic extract was investigated. Myrtle extract was applied for 2 days either orally or topically. The findings showed that both oral and topical treatments could decrease burn-induced oxidative injury and skin damage. However, oral administration of myrtle extract was found to be more effective than the topical administration in terms of increased GSH and NO levels, increased SOD activities (Ozkan et al., 2019).

ADVERSE REACTIONS

TPM Literature

It is harmful for headaches caused by hot dystemperament and coryza. Smelling of myrtle for long time may cause insomnia; thus, because of these adverse effects, it is better to be taken with violet fresh flower or lily (Aghili Khorasani 1771).

Current Evidence

No health hazards or side effects are reported as a result of the proper administration of designated therapeutic dosages. Systemic administration of myrtle essential oil as a drug may lead to nausea, vomiting and diarrhea in rare cases (Gruenwald et al., 2007).

Overdoses of myrtle essential oil (more than 10 g) can cause life-threatening poisoning, due to the high amount of cineole. Symptoms include drop in blood pressure, circulatory disorders, collapse, and respiratory failure. Vomiting should not be induced in case of poisoning, due to the danger of aspiration. Management of toxicity includes administration of activated charcoal, treating spasms with diazepam (intravenous), treating colic with atropine, and providing electrolyte substitution. Possible cases of acidosis can be managed with sodium bicarbonate infusions. Intubation and oxygen respiration may also be necessary (Alipour et al., 2014; Gruenwald et al., 2007).

CONTRAINDICATIONS

TPM Literature

None.

Current Evidence

The medicine should not be administered in case of inflammatory illnesses of the GI tract or of the biliary ducts, or in the case of severe liver diseases (Gruenwald et al., 2007).

Because of the possibility of triggering glottal spasm, asthma like attacks or even respiratory failure, preparations containing myrtle essential oil should not be administered to infants or young children (Alipour et al., 2014; Gruenwald et al., 2007).

PREGNANCY AND LACTATION

TPM Literature

None.

Current Evidence

None.

DRUG INTERACTIONS

None.

METHOD OF ADMINISTRATION

TPM Literature

For oral administration, decoction of fruits, ripe fruits, leaf or fruit juice, fruit syrup, fruit concentrated juice are used.

For topical administration, myrtle oil (myrtle leaves boiled in water and filtered, the filtrate is then boiled with olive or sesame oil until the water is completely evaporated; the remaining oil is myrtle oil) and ointment from myrtle oil are used.

Myrtle leaves are used in the forms of poultice (mixing leaves powder with water, wine, or olive oil to form a paste), some kinds of ointment prepared by mixing wax in oil and herbal medicine, liniment, plaster, nasal or ear drop, mouth wash, decoction, pulverized dry leaves sprinkled on or rubbed on an infected area, ash of leaves, irrigation solution of leave decoction.

Myrtle fruits are used as decoction, mouth wash, fruit juice, ointment, decoction with wine (in joint weakness). Smelling of fresh leaves is also recommended (Aghili Khorasani 1771)

Current Evidence

Myrtle leaves infusion is given by mixing 15–30 g of the drug with 1 L water for 15 minutes as a solution for wash.

Myrtle oil is recommended up to 0.2 mg per day for internal use (Gruenwald et al., 2007).

DOSAGE

Leaves: The average daily dosage of powder from the leaves is 5 g taken in divided doses before meals. Three cups of an infusion may be taken each day. Washes may be used several times daily (Gruenwald et al., 2007).

REFERENCES

Aboutaleb N, Hashem-Dabaghian F, Elahian-Boroujeni A, Shojaii A. Protective effects of *Myrtus communis* Linn fruit and leaf extracts on isoproterenol-induced heart failure in rat. Trad Integr Med. 2021;6(2):138–151.

Aghili Khorasani MH 1771. *Makhzan-al-Adviah* (*The treasury of drugs*) (rewritten by Shams Ardakani MR, Rahimi R, Farjadmand F, 1st ed.). Tehran: Tehran University of Medical Sciences; 2009.

Alipour G, Dashti S, Hosseinzadeh H. Review of pharmacological effects of *Myrtus communis* L. and its active constituents. Phytother Res. 2014;28(8):1125–1136.

Askari SF, Jahromi BN, Dehghanian A, et al. Effect of a novel herbal vaginal suppository containing myrtle and oak gall in the treatment of vaginitis: A randomized clinical trial. Daru. 2020; 28(2):603–614.

Avicenna 1025. *Al-Qanoon fi al-Tibb* (*The canon of medicine*) (rewritten by Masoudi A, ed.). Tehran: Almaei; 2015.

Babaee N, Mansourian A, Momen-Heravi F, et al. The efficacy of a paste containing *Myrtus communis* (Myrtle) in the management of recurrent aphthous stomatitis: A randomized controlled trial. Clin Oral Invest. 2010;14:65–70.

Bureau J, Ginouves P, Guilbaud J, Roux M. Essential oils and low-intensity electromagnetic pulses in the treatment of androgen-dependent alopecia. Adv Ther. 2003;20:220–229.

Chaijan MR, Handjani F, Zarshenas M, et al. The *Myrtus communis* L. solution versus ketoconazole shampoo in treatment of dandruff: A double blinded randomized clinical trial. J Pak Med Assoc. 2018;68(5):715–720.

Ghadami Yazdi E, Minaei MB, Hashem Dabaghian F, et al. Efficacy of *Myrtus communis* L. and *Descurainia sophia* L. versus salicylic acid for wart treatment. Iran Red Cresc Med J. 2014;16(10):e16386.

Gruenwald J, Brendler T, Jaenicke C. *PDR for herbal medicines*. Montvale: Thomson Reuters; 2007.

Hajiaghaee R, Faizi M, Shahmohammadi Z, et al. Hydroalcoholic extract of *Myrtus communis* can alter anxiety and sleep parameters: A behavioral and EEG sleep pattern study in mice and rats. Pharm Biol. 2016;54:2141–2148.

Hosseinzadeh H, Khoshdel M, Ghorbani M. Antinociceptive, anti-inflammatory effects and acute toxicity of aqueous and ethanolic extracts of *Myrtus communis* L. aerial parts in mice. J Acupunct Merid Stud. 2011;4:242–247.

Jabri MA, Rtibi K, Ben-Said A, et al. Antidiarrhoeal, antimicrobial and antioxidant effects of myrtle berries (*Myrtus communis* L.) seeds extract. J Pharm Pharmacol. 2016a;68(2):264–274.

Jabri MA, Tounsi H, Rtibi K, et al. Ameliorative and antioxidant effects of myrtle berry seed (*Myrtus communis*) extract during reflux-induced esophagitis in rats. Pharma Biol. 2016b;54(9):1575–1585.

Karimlar S, Naderi A, Mohammadi SF, et al. Hypoglycemic and hypolipidemic effects of *Myrtus communis*, *Trachyspermum copticum* and *Ferula gummosa* essential oils on streptozotocin induced diabetic rats. Nutr Food Sci Res. 2019;6(1):1–8.

Khodaie SA, Emadi F, Naseri M, et al. The effect of *Myrtus communis* aqueous extract-containing gel on wound healing in streptozotocin-induced diabetic rats. Curr Drug Discov Technol. 2021;18(4):542–547.

Malekuti J, Mirghafourvand M, Samadi K, et al. Comparison of the effect of *Myrtus communis* herbal and anti-hemorrhoid ointments on the hemorrhoid symptoms and quality of life in postpartum women with grade I and II internal hemorrhoid: A triple-blinded randomized controlled clinical trial. J Integr Complement Med. 2019;0180147.

Masoudi M, Rafieian Kopaei M, Miraj S. A comparison of the efficacy of metronidazole vaginal gel and myrtus (*Myrtus communis*) extract combination and metronidazole vaginal gel alone in the treatment of recurrent bacterial vaginosis. Avicenna J Phytomed. 2017;7(2):129–136.

Maxia A, Frau M, Falconieri D, et al. Essential oil of *Myrtus communis* inhibits inflammation in rats by reducing serum IL-6 and TNF-alpha. Nat Prod Commun. 2011;6:1545–1548.

Mirzaee F, Jannesari S, Kariman N, et al. The effect of *Myrtus communis* cream on wound healing and severity of episiotomy pain: Double-blind clinical trial. Iran J Obstetr Gynec Infert. 2019;22(8):52–61.

Najafi MR, Torabi Goudarzi M, Bahonar A, et al. Clinical evaluation of the effect of Myrtus oil on the oral lesions of FMD in cattle. J Med Plants. 2011;10:135–141.

Nikakhtar Z, Hasanzadeh M, Hamedi SS, et al. The efficacy of vaginal suppository based on myrtle in patients with cervicovaginal human papillomavirus infection: A randomized, double-blind, placebo trial. Phytother Res. 2018;32(10):2002–2008.

Ozbeyli D, Sen A, Cilingir Kaya OT, et al. *Myrtus communis* leaf extract protects against cerulein-induced acute pancreatitis in rats. J Food Biochem. 2020;44(2):e13130.

Ozcan O, Ipekci H, Alev B, et al. Protective effect of Myrtle (*Myrtus communis*) on burn induced skin injury. Burns. 2019;45(8):1856–1863.

Paknejad MS, Eftekhari K, Rahimi R, et al. Myrtle (*Myrtus communis* L.) fruit syrup for gastroesophageal reflux disease in children: A double-blind randomized clinical trial. Phytother Res. 2021;35(11):6369–6376.

Pezhmanmehr M, Dastan D, Nejad Ebrahimi S, Hadian J. Essential oil constituents of leaves and fruits of *Myrtus communis* L. from Iran. J Essent Oil-Bear Plants. 2009;75(9):1–7.

Qaraaty M, Kamali SH, Dabaghian FH, et al. Effect of myrtle fruit syrup on abnormal uterine bleeding: A randomized double-blind, placebo-controlled pilot study. Daru. 2014;22(45):1–7.

Salmanian M, Shirbeigi L, Hashem-Dabaghian F, et al. The effects of Myrtle (*Myrtus communis*) and clindamycin topical solution in the treatment of mild to moderate acne vulgaris: A comparative split-face study. J Pharmacopuncture. 2020;23(4):220–229.

Sepici-Dincel A, Açıkgöz Ş, Çevik C, et al. Effects of in vivo antioxidant enzyme activities of myrtle oil in normoglycaemic and alloxan diabetic rabbits. J Ethnopharmacol. 2007;110(3):498–503.

Sisay M, Engidawork E, Shibeshi W. Evaluation of the antidiarrheal activity of the leaf extracts of *Myrtus communis* Linn (Myrtaceae) in mice model. BMC Complement Altern Med. 2017;17(1):103.

Sumbul S, Ahmad MA, Asif M, et al. Evaluation of *Myrtus communis* Linn. berries (common myrtle) in experimental ulcer models in rats. Hum Exp Toxicol. 2010;29(11):935–944.

Umarami RB, Roqaiya M, Quadri MA. Efficacy of Habbul aas (fruits of *Myrtus communis*) in menorrhagia: A single blinded randomized standard control study. J Complement Integr Med. 2020;18(1):123–130.

Yılmaz H, Ekinci, N, Ömerli A, et al. The protective effect of *Myrtus communis* L. against experimental kidney stone in rats. Adv Trad Med. 2022;23(1):241–249.

Zohalinezhad ME, Hosseini-Asl MK, Akrami R, et al. *Myrtus communis* L. freeze-dried aqueous extract versus omeprazol in gastrointestinal reflux disease: A double-blind randomized controlled clinical trial. J Evid-Based Complementary Altern Med. 2016;21(1):23–29.

23 *Nardostachys jatamansi* (D.Don) DC.

Zahra Memariani

Scientific name: *Nardostachys jatamansi* (D.Don) DC.
Family: Caprifoliaceae
Common names:

- **English:** Jatamansi, Indian nard, Indian spikenard, spikenard, nard
- **Persian:** *sonbol-e ṭīb*, *nārdīn*
- **Arabic:** *sumbul hindī*

Medicinal part(s): Rhizome, root (Figure 23.1)
Temperament (nature): Hot and dry in the second degree
Major chemical constituents

- **Volatile oil (0.3–0.4%):** Sesquiterpenoids (jatamansone, calarene, aristolone, β-maaliene, nardol, valerenal), monoterpenoids (α-thujene, α-pinene, β-pinene, linalool) (Cornara et al., 2020; Xue et al., 2023)
- **Phenolic compounds:** pyranocoumarins: jatamansin, jatamansinol, jatamansinone; furanocumarins: angelicin, oroselol, flavonoids: catechin, epicatechin, rutin (Razack et al., 2015; Chatterjee et al., 2005)
- **Others:** Steroids, carbohydrates, fatty acids (Gruenwald, 2007; Wang, et al., 2021)

THERAPEUTIC USE

TPM Literature

Jatamansi has been introduced in TPM as a tonic for the brain, stomach and liver, and an enhancer of their functionality. In topical use on the eyes, it reduces eye redness and abnormal secretions, improves eyesight, and eyelash growth. It can also improve the delivery of other medicines to different layers of the eye. In the respiratory system, it is useful for asthma and productive coughs. It has also been recommended for flatulence, jaundice, cold-tempered liver (fatty liver), spleen pain, internal swellings or inflammations, diarrhea, hemorrhoid, and kidney stones. Its consumption with cold water is beneficial for nausea, stomach bloating, and heart palpitations. As a vaginal suppository, it is recommended to reduce abnormal uterine bleeding and secretions. To relieve inflammation of the uterus and its pains and to induce menstruation, jatamansi decoction is recommended to be used as sitz bath, or as a warm compress on the uterus area. Topical application of jatamansi on the stomach is recommended as a tonic for cardia sphincter and reduces its inflammation. In topical use, it acts as an antiperspirant and deodorant. Also, jatamansi powder has wound healing properties in topical application (Aghili Khorasani 1771; Avicenna 1025).

DOI: 10.1201/b22971-23

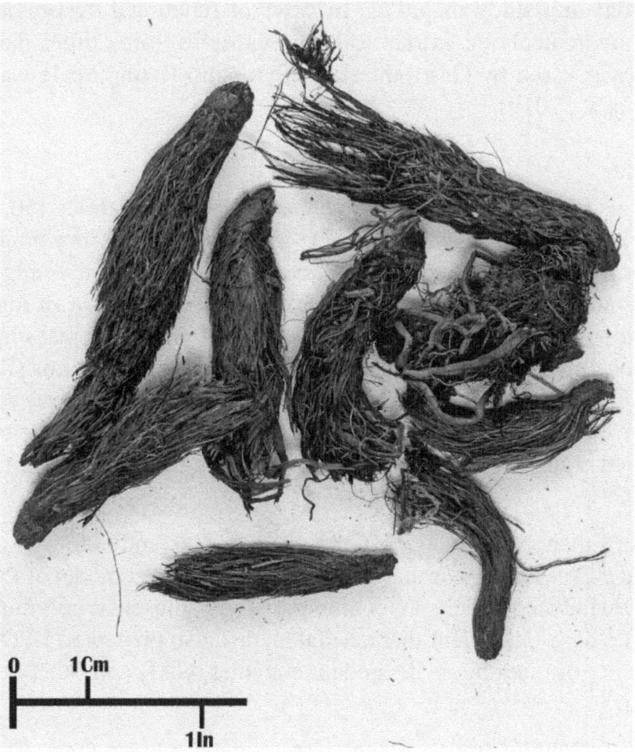

FIGURE 23.1 Jatamansi rhizomes and roots.

Current Evidence

Clinical Evidence

Hypertension: A single-blind placebo-controlled RCT on 40 adult patients with stage 1 hypertension showed that using jatamansi powder (3 g per day) for 4 weeks, significantly reduced average SBP and DBP (Bhat and Malik, 2020). It has also been reported in an open-labeled study that using jatamansi liquid (10 mL twice daily for 15 days: containing 500 mg of extract equivalent to 2.5 g herb) by 10 patients with type 2 diabetes and hypertension led to a decrease in SBP and DBP, as well as a reduction in random blood sugar, hs-CRP, and IL-6. It also showed antioxidant activity via improving GSH and reducing MDA (Rajyalakshmi et al., 2018).

Insomnia: An open-labeled comparative study has shown that administration of jatamansi or *Valeriana wallichii* DC. powder (4 g thrice daily with milk) for 1 month in patients with primary insomnia both resulted in significant improvement in sleep initiation and duration, disturbed sleep, and disruption in routine works (Toolika et al., 2015).

PMS: In a single-blind RCT, the effect of jatamansi (4 g three times daily) on PMS symptoms was studied in 60 healthy women. After two consecutive menstrual cycles, a significant decrease in average scores of questionnaires PMTS-O and PMTS-SR was observed vs. placebo. Also, jatamansi group showed a significant decrease in all VAS domains comparing the before and after treatment scores except in swelling of extremities; while no significant decrease in VAS scores was reported in placebo (Malik et al., 2018).

Functional dyspepsia: In a study including 16 cases of functional dyspepsia, 1-month administration of jatamansi hydroalcoholic extract (500 mg capsules, three times daily), the mean score of symptoms severity assessed by Gastrointestinal Symptom Rating Scale was improved in these subjects (Mirzapour et al., 2019).

Preclinical Evidence

Alzheimer's disease: Three oral doses of jatamansi ethanolic extract (50, 100, and 200 mg/kg) were evaluated in diazepam and scopolamine-induced amnesia in young and aged mice for 8 days and the highest dose could significantly reverse the amnesia in young mice. Furthermore, it improved learning and memory and reversed aging-induced amnesia in mice (Joshi and Parle, 2006). Jatamansi extract (200 mg/kg) was also shown to protect against chronic stress-induced impairments in hippocampus-dependent spatial learning and memory in rats (Karkada et al., 2012). Methanolic extract of jatamansi (200 and 400 mg/kg orally for 14 days) was studied to evaluate its effect on sleep deprived amnesic mice. Compared to piracetam (200 mg/kg orally), in behavioral tests, jatamansi caused a significant improvement in learning and cognition factors (Rahman and Muralidharan, 2010).

Parkinson's disease: Ethanolic extract of jatamansi (200, 400, and 600 mg/kg orally for 3 weeks) as pretreatment could decrease the neuronal damage in 6-OHDA-rat model of Parkinson's disease. It could restore 6-OHDA-induced deficits in locomotor activity, muscular coordination, and decreased level of dopamine in a dose-dependent manner. Jatamansi also prevented LPO and GSH depletion and restored the activity of glutathione dependent enzymes, CAT, and SOD in the substantia nigra (Ahmad et al., 2006).

Anxiety and sedation: Administration of jatamansi powder with a dose of 270 mg/kg in Swiss albino mice showed significant decrease in the horizontal activity in open field test. It also reduced the latency of onset of sleep, and prolonged the total duration of sleep in pentobarbital-induced sleep test without any influence on gross behavior and muscle coordination in rotarod test (Panara et al., 2020).

In an animal model of chronic fatigue syndrome, oral administration of jatamansi extract (200 and 500 mg/kg) was shown to significantly reverse the locomotor activity and the anxiety state of stressed rats (Lyle et al., 2009). More, oral administration of its hydroethanolic extract in the same doses in rats exposed to cold restraint stress led to improvement in central monoaminergic and oxidative changes (Lyle et al., 2012).

Also, oral administration of jatamansi extract in mice (250 mg/kg) showed anxiolytic effects in several behavioral examinations. Treatment with the extract for 7 days revealed significant anxiolytic effects and elevated the content of brain monoamine and GABA neurotransmitter (Razack et al., 2018).

Depression: Antidepressant effect of the total methanolic extract of jatamansi (58, 116, and 255 mg/kg orally for 7 days), and one of its water-soluble fractions (36, 73, and 160 g/kg) with serotonin transporter (SERT) enhancing constituents has been shown in mice via tail suspension test and open-field test behavioral models (Li et al., 2021). Also, jatamansi ethanolic extract was evaluated with a dose of 200 mg/kg for its antidepressant effect in a radiation-induced depression in mice which could successfully induce a significant decrease in the duration of immobility in behavioral tests compared to control (Deepa et al., 2013). Another study indicated the antidepressant effect of ethanolic extract (100, 200, and 400 mg/kg orally for 14 days) of jatamansi in both tail suspension and forced swim tests in young albino mice. The antidepressant effect was comparable to imipramine and sertraline, probably via interaction with $GABA_B$ receptors (Dhingra and Goyal, 2008).

Convulsion: In maximal electroshock-induced seizure in rats, jatamansi ethanolic extract with 125–500 mg/kg doses was able to increase the seizure threshold and reduce extension/flexion ratio upon 15 days of administration. Pretreatment of rats with phenytoin (12.5, 25, 50, and 75 mg/kg) in combination with jatamansi (50 mg/kg) led to a significant increase in the protective index of phenytoin, suggesting the synergistic effect of the two drugs without any sign of neurotoxicity. Nevertheless, the extract was not effective in PTZ-induced seizure (Rao et al., 2005).

Peptic ulcer: The gastroprotective effect of jatamansi hydroethanolic extract has been shown in an ethanol-induced gastric ulcer model in rats. Oral pretreatment with 20 mg/kg of the extract significantly reduced ulcer index, increased GSH, CAT and HO-1 compared with control group (Memariani et al., 2017). Also, pretreatment with hydroethanolic extract (200 and 500 mg/kg orally) in stress-induced ulcer animal model resulted in significant antioxidant activity, inhibition of the gastric ulceration occurrence, and reversed alterations in biochemical markers (Lyle et al., 2009).

Hepatotoxicity: Pretreatment with ethanolic extract of jatamansi (800 mg/kg orally) in rats significantly decreased the thioacetamide-induced elevated levels of AST, ALT, and ALP (Ali et al., 2000).

Cardiotoxicity: Jatamansi ethanolic extract with an oral dose of 500 mg/kg for 7 days could decrease doxorubicin-induced myocardial mitochondrial/lysosomal damage in rats (Subashini et al., 2007).

ADVERSE REACTIONS

TPM LITERATURE

It may be harmful to kidneys and to prevent the possible side effects, it is recommended to be taken with tragacanth (Aghili Khorsaani 1771).

CURRENT EVIDENCE

No health hazards have been reported relevant to the proper administration of therapeutic doses (Gruenwald et al., 2007). It has potential emmenagogue and diuretic effects (Gardner and McGuffin, 2013).

CONTRAINDICATIONS

TPM LITERATURE

None.

CURRENT EVIDENCE

None.

PREGNANCY AND LACTATION

TPM LITERATURE

Due to emmenagogue properties, it is contraindicated in pregnancy (Aghili Khorasani 1771).

CURRENT EVIDENCE

It is contraindicated in pregnancy except under the supervision of a qualified healthcare practitioner. Although there are not any reported concerns for use while breastfeeding, safety has not been conclusively proven.

DRUG INTERACTIONS

None.

METHOD OF ADMINISTRATION

TPM Literature

Jatamansi root can be used as infusion, decoction, syrup, and dry powder for oral intake. For topical use, the decoction may be applied as a warm compress for eyes and the dry powder can be used for skin problems. For intrauterine use, it is recommended as sitz bath (Aghili Khorasani 1771).

Current Evidence

Its rhizome is used in forms of a whole, cut, or powdered drug for internal and topical use. There are also preparations including capsules and compound preparations, infusion, and tinctures.

DOSAGE

Plant powder: 0.6 to 1.3 for single dose administration.
Pure drug with a cup of water: 5 g of the drug, three times daily (Gruenwald et al., 2007).

REFERENCES

Aghili Khorasani MH 1771. *Makhzan-al-Adviah* (*The treasury of drugs*) (rewritten by Shams Ardakani MR, Rahimi R, Farjadmand F, 1st ed.). Tehran: Tehran University of Medical Sciences; 2009.

Ahmad M, Yousuf S, Khan MB, et al. Attenuation by *Nardostachys jatamansi* of 6-hydroxydopamine-induced parkinsonism in rats: Behavioral, neurochemical, and immunohistochemical studies. Pharmacol Biochem Behav. 2006;83(1):150–160.

Ali S, Ansari KA, Jafry MA, et al. *Nardostachys jatamansi* protects against liver damage induced by thioacetamide in rats. J Ethnopharmacol. 2000;71(3):359–363.

Avicenna 1025. *Al-Qanoon fi al-Tibb* (*The canon of medicine*) (rewritten by Masoudi A, ed.). Tehran: Almaei; 2015.

Bhat MD, Malik SA. Efficacy of *Nardostachys jatamansi* (D. Don) DC in essential hypertension: A randomized controlled study. Complement Ther Med. 2020;53:102532.

Chatterjee A, Basak B, Datta U, et al. Studies on the chemical constituents *of Nardostachys jatamansi* DC (Valerianaceae). Indian J Chem. 2005;44(B):430–433.

Cornara L, Ambu G, Trombetta D, et al. Comparative and functional screening of three species traditionally used as antidepressants: *Valeriana officinalis* L., *Valeriana jatamansi* jones ex roxb. and *Nardostachys jatamansi* (D. Don) DC. Plants. 2020;9(8):994.

Deepa B, Suchetha K, Rao S. Antidepressant activity of *Nardostachys jatamansi* in electron beam irradiated mice. Int J Res Ayurveda Pharm. 2013;4(1):101–103.

Dhingra D, Goyal PK. Inhibition of MAO and GABA: Probable mechanisms for antidepressant-like activity of *Nardostachys jatamansi* DC. in mice. Indian J Exp Biol. 2008:46(4):212–218.

Gardner Z, McGuffin M. *Botanical safety handbook*. Boca Raton: Taylor & Francis; 2013.

Gruenwald J, Brendler T, Jaenicke C. *PDR for herbal medicines*. Montvale: Thomson Reuters; 2007.

Joshi H, Parle M. *Nardostachys jatamansi* improves learning and memory in mice. J Med Food. 2006;9(1):113–118.

Karkada G, Shenoy KB, Halahalli H, Karanth K. *Nardostachys jatamansi* extract prevents chronic restraint stress-induced learning and memory deficits in a radial arm maze task. J Nat Sci Biol Med. 2012;3(2):125–132.

Li R, Wang ZM, Wang Y, et al. Antidepressant activities and regulative effects on serotonin transporter of *Nardostachys jatamansi* DC. J Ethnopharmacol. 2021;268:113601.

Lyle N, Bhattacharyya D, Sur TK, et al. Stress modulating antioxidant effect of *Nardostachys jatamansi*. Indian J Biochem Biophys. 2009;46(1):93–98.

Lyle N, Chakrabarti S, Sur T, et al. *Nardostachys jatamansi* protects against cold restraint stress induced central monoaminergic and oxidative changes in rats. Neurochem Res. 2012;37(12):2748–2757.

Lyle N, Gomes A, Sur T, et al. The role of antioxidant properties of *Nardostachys jatamansi* in alleviation of the symptoms of the chronic fatigue syndrome. Behav Brain Res. 2009;202(2):285–290.

Malik R, Firdose KF, Bhat MD. Efficacy of *Nardostachys jatamansi* DC. in the management of premenstrual syndrome: A randomized controlled study. J Herb Med. 2018;14:17–21.

Memariani Z, Hajimahmoodi M, Minaee B, et al. Protective effect of a polyherbal traditional formula consisting of *Rosa damascena* Mill., *Glycyrrhiza glabra* L. and *Nardostachys jatamansi* DC., against ethanol-induced gastric ulcer. Iran. J Pharm Res. 2017;16(2):694–707.

Mirzapour M, Mojahedi M, Shokri J, et al. Treatment of patients with refractory functional dyspepsia using *Nardostachys jatamansi* (D. Don) DC. hydroalcoholic extract: A case series. Tradit Integr Med. 2019;4(4):191–199.

Panara K, Nariya M, Karra N. Central nervous system depressant activity of Jatamansi (*Nardostachys jatamansi* DC.) rhizome. AYU. 2020;41(4):250–254.

Rahman H, Muralidharan P. *Nardostacys Jatamansi* DC protects from the loss of memory and cognition deficits in sleep deprived Alzheimer's disease (AD) mice model. Int J Pharm Sci Rev Res. 2010;5(3):160–167.

Rajyalakshmi I, Rao VA, Potti RB. Effects of *Nardostachys jatamansi* extract on inflammatory and oxidative stress markers in hypertensive, hyperglycaemic patients: An open-label, prospective study. Int J Res Pharm Sci. 2018;9(4):1096–1098.

Rao VS, Rao A, Karanth KS. Anticonvulsant and neurotoxicity profile of *Nardostachys jatamansi* in rats. J Ethnopharmacol. 2005;102(3):351–356.

Razack S, Hemanth Kumar K, Nallamuthu I, et al. Antioxidant, biomolecule oxidation protective activities of *Nardostachys jatamansi* DC and its phytochemical analysis by RP-HPLC and GC-MS. Antioxidants. 2015;4(1):185–203.

Razack S, Kandikattu HK, Venuprasad MP, et al. Anxiolytic actions of *Nardostachys jatamansi* via GABA benzodiazepine channel complex mechanism and its biodistribution studies. Metab Brain Dis. 2018;33(5):1533–1549.

Subashini R, Gnanapragasam A, Senthilkumar S, et al. Protective efficacy of *Nardostachys jatamansi* (rhizomes) on mitochondrial respiration and lysosomal hydrolases during doxorubicin induced myocardial injury in rats. J Health Sci. 2007;53(1):67–76.

Toolika E, Bhat NP, Shetty SK. A comparative clinical study on the effect of Tagara (*Valeriana wallichii* DC.) and Jatamansi (*Nardostachys jatamansi* DC.) in the management of Anidra (primary insomnia). AYU. 2015;36(1):46–49.

Wang M, Yang TT, Rao Y, et al. A review on traditional uses, phytochemistry, pharmacology, toxicology and the analytical methods of the genus Nardostachys. J Ethnopharmacol. 2021;280:114446.

Xue BX, Liu SX, Oduro PK, et al. Vasodilatory constituents of essential oil from *Nardostachys jatamansi* DC.: Virtual screening, experimental validation and the potential molecular mechanisms. Arab J Chem. 2023;16(8):104911.

24 *Nigella sativa* L.

Ayeh Naghizadeh

Scientific name: *Nigella sativa* L.
Family: Ranunculaceae
Common names:

- **English:** Black cumin, black seed, black caraway, Roman coriander, kalonji
- **Persian:** *sīyāhdāneh*, šonīz
- **Arabic:** *ḥabbat al-saudā'*

Medicinal part(s): Seed (Figure 24.1)
Temperament (nature): Hot and dry in the third degree
Major chemical constituents:

- **Volatile oil:** Trans-anethole, *p*-cymene, limonene, thymoquinone, α-thujene, carvone, carvacrol, thymol, sabinene, and β-pinene
- **Fatty acids:** Linoleic acid, oleic acid, and palmitic acid (Nickavar et al., 2003; Kesen et al., 2018).

THERAPEUTIC USE

TPM Literature

Black seed is a frequently used medicinal herb in TPM. Aromatherapy or nasal administration of preparations of this seed is considered an efficient treatment for specific types of chronic headaches, tremors, and also chronic sinusitis. Regarding ophthalmic disorders, topical use of black seed preparations can prevent progression of cataract if administered in early stages. As mouthwash, black seed boiled in vinegar has been recommended for toothaches. Respiratory disorders including productive coughs, and orthopnea can also be ameliorated with topical or oral use. It is considered an antidote of toxins, and used to manage rabid dog and tarantula bites. Black cumin can help ameliorate a number of gastrointestinal symptoms including nausea, jaundice, and some types of colicky pains, and is also beneficial in hemorrhoids. It is also used in infections, including chronic fevers, common cold, sinusitis, and infections caused by intestinal helminths. Topical use with vinegar is used in dermatologic diseases such as warts, while the oil can act as a facial skin abstergent. Oral administration and also topical use of black cumin as oil or in hot packs is an efficient remedy for relieving both musculoskeletal and neurological pains.

Furthermore, due to antilithiasis activities, this seed is used in formulations to treat kidney and bladder stones.

Being an emmenagogue, persistent use of this plant helps treat oligomenorrhea and amenorrhea. It is also used to reduce uterine pain in the puerperal period, and has dual benefits in this period as it has galactagogue activity and can help increase breast milk supply. This herb is also used in formulations to treat reduced sex drive. Moreover, topical use of black cumin oil

DOI: 10.1201/b22971-24

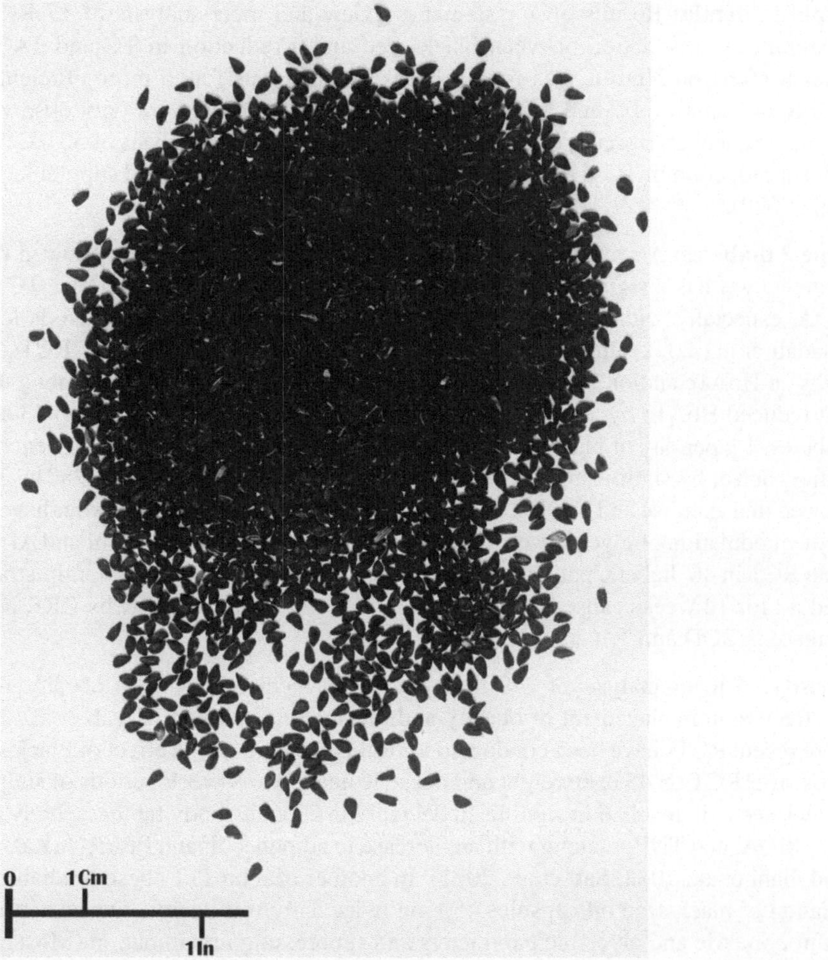

FIGURE 24.1 Black seed.

on lumbar and genital areas can help ameliorate erectile dysfunction (Aghili Khorasani 1771; Avicenna 1025).

Current Evidence

Clinical Evidence

Hypertension: In a meta-analysis of 11 RCTs on hypertensive and normotensive individuals, it was demonstrated that short-term administration of black seed powder (mean of 8.3 weeks duration) reduces both SBP and DBP significantly. A –3.26 mmHg and –2.80 mmHg reduction was observed in SBP and DBP compared to control/standard groups, respectively. Oil preparations were less efficient (Sahebkar, et al., 2016). In an RCT on 76 elderly patients, administration of 300 mg black seed extract, twice daily for 4 weeks, resulted in a slight nonsignificant reduction of blood pressure (Rizka et al., 2017). Results of a more recent trial on 26 hypertensive individuals, showed that administration of 2.5 mL of black seed oil resulted in significant reduction of both SBP and DBP compared to placebo (Shoaei-Hagh et al., 2021).

Hyperlipidemia: Results of a systematic review and meta-analysis of 17 RCTs were indicative of significant association between black seed and a reduction in TC and TAG, although no significant effect on HDL-C was found. Black seed oil was found more efficient than seed powder on improvement of TC and LDL-C, while increased HDL-C were only observed with black seed powder (Sahebkar, Beccuti, et al., 2016). A more recent meta-analysis of 50 RCTs demonstrated significant reduction in TC, TAG, LDL-C and VLDL-C with black seed supplementation (Hallajzadeh et al., 2020).

Type 2 diabetes: A systematic review and meta-analysis of 11 RCTs showed that black seed supplementation has a significant effect on the improvement of FBS, HbA1c, TC, LDL-C, CRP, and MDA, especially with doses larger than 1 g per day and treatment periods longer than 8 weeks (Saadati et al., 2022). In a review that investigated 25 meta-analyses of RCTs on effectiveness of herbs on HbA1c and/or FBS in type 2 diabetic patients, black seed was among the medicinal plants that reduced HbA1c by at least 0.5% (Willcox et al., 2021). In an RCT on 43 subjects with type 2 diabetes, 1 g per day of black seed oil in soft gel capsules for 8 weeks had beneficial effects on glycemic control by significantly decreasing FBS and HbA1c (Hadi et al., 2021). Two clinical studies showed that exercise and black seed intake in the form of tea or seed powder have a synergistic effect on the modulation of glycemic profile in type 2 diabetic patients (Alyami and Al-Hariri, 2023). Also, in an RCT in 46 diabetic patients undergoing hemodialysis, daily oral administration of 2 g of black seed oil for 12 weeks caused a significant reduction in FBS, HbA1c, hs-CRP, MDA, along with an increase in SOD and TAC (Rahmani et al., 2022).

Obesity: A meta-analysis of 279 trials on herbal medicines used in obesity, found black seed to be effective in management of obesity and metabolic syndrome (Payab et al., 2020). Additionally, more recent RCTs have been conducted to further investigate the effect of black seed on obesity. In a cross-over RCT on 45 overweight and obese women, two 8-week periods of supplementation with 2 g black seed oil, resulted in significant decrease in appetite, body fat mass, body fat percentage, BW, WC, MDA, and TNF-α, along with an increase in adiponectin and PPAR-γ (Razmpoosh et al., 2022; Abdollahi et al., 2022; Safi et al., 2021). In another trial on 117 obese prediabetic subjects, administration of black seed oil capsules 450 mg twice daily was as effective as metformin in improving anthropometric and glycemic parameters and suppressing inflammation (Mostafa et al., 2021).

Liver and kidney parameters/diseases: Based on findings of a meta-analysis of 19 trials ($n = 1,295$ subjects), a daily dose of 1,100–1,500 mg black seed significantly reduced ALP and BUN. Moreover, interventions of longer than 12 weeks decreased AST. However, doses higher than 2 g per day significantly increased BUN (Razmpoosh et al., 2020). Similarly, the results of a more recent meta-analysis indicated significant reduction of AST by black seed (Azizi et al., 2021). A recent meta-analysis assessing six RCTs (n=358) on the effect of black seed on NAFLD demonstrated the plant to significantly improve the grade and severity of this disease; though, the optimum dose and treatment duration should be further clarified (Tang et al., 2021).

Inflammation/oxidative stress: Black seed has beneficial effects on inflammation and oxidative stress. A recent systematic review and meta-analysis assessed the effects of black seed and seed oil consumption on oxidative stress and inflammation markers in ten RCTs. Results indicated that it significantly reduced hs-CRP, TNF-α, and MDA, and increased SOD and TAC (Montazeri et al., 2021). However, another meta-analysis performed in the same year did not report significant difference in hs-CRP, IL-6, and MDA; while other results conformed with the former study (Malekian et al., 2021). An earlier meta-analysis of five RCTs indicated that a reduction in CRP was only significant in participants with BMI ≥ 30 (Tavakoly et al., 2019).

Hashimoto's thyroiditis: An RCT in 40 cases with Hashimoto's thyroiditis has shown that daily oral administration of 2 g black seed powder for 8 weeks can significantly improve lipid profile, atherogenic index, and anthropometric parameters in these patients (Farhangi et al., 2018). Significant reductions in TSH, anti-TPO antibodies, MDA, VCAM-1, VEGF, and IL-23, as well as an increase in T3, TAC, and SOD were also reported (Farhangi et al., 2016; Tajmiri et al., 2016; Farhangi and Tajmiri, 2020).

Respiratory diseases: A meta-analysis of four RCTs on asthmatic patients has demonstrated that black seed as 1 g per day of the powdered seeds, 15–30 mg/kg of the oil, or 15 mL/kg of 0.1% boiled seeds, administered for 1–3 months, can significantly increase Asthma Control Test scores, and FEV1 in asthmatic individuals, but has no obvious impact on peak expiratory flow, IL-4, or IFN-γ (He and Xu, 2020). Also, one clinical report on the oral use of black seed oil (40–80 mg/kg) in patients with a series of allergies, including allergic rhinitis and bronchial asthma, confirmed the efficacy of this product in the reduction of subjective allergic symptoms in these patients (Kalus et al., 2003). An open-label RCT on 173 patients with mild COVID-19 showed that administration of 500 mg black seed oil twice daily for 10 days resulted in faster recovery of symptoms compared with routine treatment (Koshak et al., 2021).

Functional dyspepsia: Results of an RCT on oral administration of a traditional honey-based black seed formula (equal to 5 mL per day of the oil) for 8 weeks demonstrated significant symptomatic improvement in mean Hong Kong index of dyspepsia severity and also *H. pylori* infection based on urease test (Mohtashami et al., 2015). Another RCT also confirmed the beneficial effect of black seed powder, 2 g per day added to quadruple therapy for 8 weeks in patients with *H. pylori* infection (Alizadeh-naini et al., 2020).

Rheumatoid arthritis: Two RCTs assessed the effect of 1 g per day of oral black seed oil vs. placebo on 40 and 42 females for 4 and 8 weeks, respectively. The disease activity score, the number of swollen joints, and the duration of morning stiffness improved significantly following black seed oil use (Gheita and Kenawy, 2012). Also, a significant elevation of IL-10, and a reduction in MDA and NO were reported (Hadi et al., 2016).

Osteopenia: A triple-blind RCT on postmenopausal women with low bone mass density demonstrated an increase in expression level of miRNA-21 upon 6-month daily oral intake of 1 g black seed oil (Farshbaf-Khalili et al., 2021).

Vitiligo: Twice daily topical application of black seed oil for 6 months in 52 patients with vitiligo was found to be more effective than fish oil in deceasing VASI (Ghorbanibirgani et al., 2014).

Radiation-induced dermatitis: An RCT on 62 breast cancer subjects demonstrated that 5% black seed gel can significantly reduce the severity and incidence of acute radiation dermatitis. Moreover, moist desquamation was delayed in intervention group compared with placebo (Rafati et al., 2019).

Acne vulgaris: An RCT assessed the effect of a black seed hydrogel applied twice daily for 2 months on 60 patients with acne vulgaris. Results were indicative of significant decrease in Investigator's Global Assessment grading score for acne severity and Acne Disability Index, as well as the number of comedones, papules, and pustules (Soleymani et al., 2020).

Memory and cognition: A research on the effects of black seed powder supplementation (500 mg twice daily for 9 weeks) on memory, attention, and cognition in 40 healthy elderly volunteers, showed significant improvement in tasks including logical memory test, total score of digit span, 30 min delayed recall, percent score in Rey-Osterrieth complex figure test, time to complete letter cancellation test, and time taken in trail-making test (Bin Sayeed et al., 2013).

Infertility: Results of an RCT on infertile men demonstrated significant improvement in sperm count, motility, and morphology as well as semen volume, pH, and round cells following 2-month administration of daily 5 mL black seed oil (Kolahdooz et al., 2014).

Preclinical Evidence

Tissue protection from injury: Black seed extract and oil have been investigated in several studies regarding protective effects on tissues. Research has revealed that via antioxidative, anti-inflammatory, and antiapoptotic properties, black seed can reverse injuries or protect tissues from deleterious effects of toxins. These preventive and therapeutic effects have been demonstrated in various organs including the brain (Madkour et al., 2021), heart (Bocsan et al., 2021), liver (Adam et al., 2016; Alam et al., 2021), lungs (Tayman et al., 2013), kidneys (Alkis et al., 2021; Cascella et al., 2017; Hannan et al., 2021), thyroid (Mohebbati et al., 2017), stomach (Kanter et al., 2006), and testes (Uchendu and Okoroiwu, 2021). Radioprotective effects of black seed have also been revealed in a few studies (Çanakci et al., 2018; Rastogi et al., 2010).

Thyroid disorders: Oral administration of black seed (200 mg/kg/day) to rats has been shown to modulate thyroid hormones in both hyper- and hypothyroidism (Avci et al., 2021). In a study on hypothyroid rats, 4-week administration of black seed oil increased thyroid hormones; while decreased TSH and parotid weight (El-Din and Fattah, 2020). Hypothyroidism-associated liver dysfunction (Hosseini et al., 2020) and learning and memory impairment (Beheshti et al., 2017) have also been shown to ameliorate with black seed.

Neurologic disorders: An animal study has shown anti-epileptogenic properties of oral black seed oil (12 mL/kg) in PTZ-induced seizure in mice (Ilhan et al., 2005). The seed ethanolic extract (400 mg/kg) could also provide some protection against cognitive impairment resulting from seizure (Tahmasebi et al., 2020). Moreover, administration of black seed oil (0.2 mL per rat) for 6 weeks significantly ameliorated haloperidol-induced extrapyramidal syndrome-like behaviors and oral dyskinesia, and also decrease astrogliosis in caudate and accumbens nuclei (Malik et al., 2016).

Immunity and infections: The immunomodulatory effects of black seed and its compounds have been revealed in several studies (Khazdair, Gholamnezhad, et al., 2021; Kulyar et al., 2021). This seed has shown antibacterial (Lorina Badger et al., 2015; Mahmoudvand et al., 2014), antiviral (Khazdair, Ghafari, et al., 2021; Ulasli et al., 2014), antiparasitic (Ayaz et al., 2007), antimalarial (Okeola et al., 2011; Udu et al., 2021), and antifungal activities (Khan et al., 2003; Rusda et al., 2020) in several animal and *in vitro* studies.

Infertility: In a study on obese male rats, concurrent administration of metformin and black seed (200–400 mg/kg/day) for 8 weeks significantly improved weight and testosterone compared with control group. The group that received 400 mg/kg/day black seed experienced an improved sperm concentration, but reduced sperm viability (Leisegang et al., 2021).

PCOS: Black seed hydroethanolic extract (50, 100 and 200 mg/kg) improved histopathological changes and increased serum levels of LH, testosterone, FBS, insulin resistance, MDA, insulin, and estrogen in PCOS rats in a dose-dependent manner (Khani et al., 2021).

ADVERSE REACTIONS

TPM Literature

Excessive oral use of black seed can cause dizziness and also pharyngeal swelling with possible difficulty in breathing and swallowing in hot-tempered individuals. It is also mentioned to be harmful to the kidneys and is thus advised to be used with tragacanth as the corrigent (Aghili Khorasani 1771).

Current Evidence

Black seed is generally safe when taken in food amounts. Safety assessments of black seed essential and fixed oils have also proved it safe for human use (Sultan et al., 2009). An animal study on black seed fixed oil indicated that chronic administration (2 mg/kg for 12 weeks) is associated with an increase in hemoglobin and reduction of leukocyte and platelet count (Zaoui et al., 2002). Both of the abovementioned studies found anorexic effects for black seed.

Topical use of black seed may cause skin irritation. There are reports of gastrointestinal side effects including dyspepsia, nausea, and constipation in a clinical trial on elderly patients (Rizka et al., 2017).

CONTRAINDICATIONS

TPM Literature

None.

Current Evidence

Black seed should be avoided in individuals with known allergy or sensitivity. Additionally, caution should be taken when administered to individuals with immune disorders (Ulbricht, 2010).

PREGNANCY AND LACTATION

TPM Literature

Black seed is an emmenagogue and used for induction of abortion and removal of retained products of conception. Hence its use is contraindicated in pregnancy (Aghili Khorasani 1771).

Current Evidence

According to current evidence, black seed should be avoided in women who are pregnant or trying to conceive, as it may inhibit uterine contractions and conception. Also, it should be used cautiously in patients under treatment for fertility or labor induction. Lactating women should also avoid black seed (Ulbricht, 2010).

DRUG INTERACTIONS

Black seed may increase the effects of some drugs with antibiotic, antiparasitic, antioxidant, and anti-inflammatory activities. Caution should be taken in concurrent use of this plant with drugs and supplements used for management of asthma, hyperlipidemia, cancer, and immune disorders and also drugs cleared through CYP450 2D6-catalyzed metabolism (Ulbricht, 2010; Bin Jardan et al., 2021).

METHOD OF ADMINISTRATION

TPM Literature

Black seed is mainly used orally. However, topical application on the skin in poultices or hot packs or oil preparations is also common. Black cumin preparations can be delivered via otic, nasal, and ophthalmic routes. Other methods of administration include inhalation of vapors, mouthwash, and vaginal use (Aghili Khorasani 1771).

Current Evidence

Black seed powder or oil is administered orally for various conditions. Topical use of oil on the scalp and skin and also otic administration for earache have also been suggested. The vapor may be inhaled to relieve sinusitis and respiratory symptoms.

DOSAGE

Adults (18 years and older): Doses of 40–80 mg/kg have been used for treatment of allergies. Usual doses of black seed oil in clinical trials are 900–2,000 mg per day.
Children (younger than 18 years): There is no proven safe or effective dose in children, and therefore use is not recommended in this age group (Ulbricht, 2010).

REFERENCES

Abdollahi N, Nadjarzadeh A, Salehi-Abargouei A, et al. The effect of *Nigella sativa* on TAC and MDA in obese and overweight women: Secondary analysis of a crossover, double blind, randomized clinical trial. J Diabetes Metab Disord. 2022;21(1):171–179.

Adam GO, Rahman MM, Lee SJ, et al. Hepatoprotective effects of *Nigella sativa* seed extract against acetaminophen-induced oxidative stress. Asian Pac J Trop Med. 2016;9(3):221–227.

Aghili Khorasani MH 1771. *Makhzan-al-Adviah* (*The treasury of drugs*) (rewritten by Shams Ardakani MR, Rahimi R, Farjadmand F, 1st ed.). Tehran: Tehran University of Medical Sciences; 2009.

Alam T, Rizwan S, Farooqui Z, et al. Oral *Nigella sativa* oil administration alleviates arsenic-induced redox imbalance, DNA damage, and metabolic and histological alterations in rat liver. Environ Sci Pollut Res Int. 2021;28(30):41464–41478.

Alizadeh-naini M, Yousefnejad H, Hejazi N. The beneficial health effects of *Nigella sativa* on *Helicobacter pylori* eradication, dyspepsia symptoms, and quality of life in infected patients: A pilot study. Phytother Res. 2020;34(6):1367–1376.

Alkis H, Demir E, Taysi MR, et al. Effects of *Nigella sativa* oil and thymoquinone on radiation-induced oxidative stress in kidney tissue of rats. Biomed Pharmacother. 2021;139:111540.

Alyami HH, Al-Hariri MT. Synergistic effects of *Nigella sativa* and exercise on diabetic profiles: A systematic review. Diabetes Ther. 2023;14:467–478.

Avci G, Ulutas E, Ozdemir V, et al. The positive effect of black seed (*Nigella sativa* L.) essential oil on thyroid hormones in rats with hypothyroidism and hyperthyroidism. J Food Biochem. 2022;46(4):e13801.

Avicenna 1025. *Al-Qanoon fi al-Tibb* (*The canon of medicine*) (rewritten by Masoudi A, ed.). Tehran: Almaei; 2015.

Ayaz E, Yilmaz H, Ozbek H, et al. The effect of *Nigella sativa* oil against *Aspiculuris tetraptera* and *Hymenolepis nana* in naturally infected mice. Saudi Med J. 2007;28(11):1654–1657.

Azizi N, Amini MR, Djafarian K, Shab-Bidar S. The effects of *Nigella sativa* supplementation on liver enzymes levels: A systematic review and meta-analysis of randomized controlled trials. Clin Nutr Res. 2021;10(1):72–78.

Beheshti F, Hosseini M, Shafei MN, et al. The effects of *Nigella sativa* extract on hypothyroidism-associated learning and memory impairment during neonatal and juvenile growth in rats. Nutr Neurosci. 2017;20(1):49–59.

Bin Jardan YA, Ahad A, Raish M, et al. Effects of garden cress, fenugreek and black seed on the pharmacodynamics of metoprolol: An herb-drug interaction study in rats with hypertension. Pharm Biol. 2021;59(1):1086–1095.

Bin Sayeed MS, Asaduzzaman M, Morshed H, et al. The effect of *Nigella sativa* Linn. seed on memory, attention and cognition in healthy human volunteers. J Ethnopharmacol. 2013;148(3):780–786.

Bocsan IC, Pop RM, Sabin O, et al. Comparative protective effect of *Nigella sativa* oil and *Vitis vinifera* seed oil in an experimental model of isoproterenol-induced acute myocardial ischemia in rats. Molecules. 2021;26(11):3221.

Çanakci H, Yilmaz AA, Canpolat MS, et al. Evaluation of the effect of topical application of *Nigella sativa* on acute radiation-induced nasal mucositis. J Craniofac Surg. 2018;29(3):e279–282.

Cascella M, Palma G, Barbieri A, et al. Role of *Nigella sativa* and its constituent thymoquinone on chemotherapy-induced nephrotoxicity: evidences from experimental animal studies. Nutrients. 2017;9(6):625.

El-Din WA, Fattah IO. Histopathological and biochemical alterations of the parotid gland induced by experimental hypothyroidism in adult male rats and the possible therapeutic effect of *Nigella sativa* oil. Tissue Cell. 2020;65:101366.

Farhangi MA, Dehghan P, Tajmiri S. Powdered black cumin seeds strongly improves serum lipids, atherogenic index of plasma and modulates anthropometric features in patients with Hashimoto's thyroiditis. Lipids Health Dis. 2018;17:59.

Farhangi MA, Dehghan P, Tajmiri S, Abbasi MM. The effects of *Nigella sativa* on thyroid function, serum vascular endothelial growth factor (VEGF)-1, Nesfatin-1 and anthropometric features in patients with Hashimoto's thyroiditis: A randomized controlled trial. BMC Complement Altern Med. 2016;16:1–9.

Farhangi MA, Tajmiri S. The effects of powdered black cumin seeds on markers of oxidative stress, intracellular adhesion molecule (ICAM)-1 and vascular cell adhesion molecule (VCAM)-1 in patients with Hashimoto's thyroiditis. Clin Nutr ESPEN. 2020;37:207–212.

Farshbaf-Khalili A, Farajnia S, Pourzeinali S, et al. The effect of nanomicelle curcumin supplementation and *Nigella sativa* oil on the expression level of miRNA-21, miRNA-422a, and miRNA-503 gene in postmenopausal women with low bone mass density: A randomized, triple-blind, placebo-controlled clinical trial with factorial design. Phytother Res. 2021;35(11):6216–6227.

Gheita TA, Kenawy SA. Effectiveness of *Nigella sativa* oil in the management of rheumatoid arthritis patients: A placebo controlled study. Phytother Res. 2012;26(8):1246–1248.

Ghorbanibirgani A, Khalili A, Rokhafrooz D. Comparing *Nigella sativa* oil and fish oil in treatment of vitiligo. Iran Red Crescent Med J. 2014;16(6):e4515.

Hadi MY, Mohammed GJ, Hameed IH. Analysis of bioactive chemical compounds of *Nigella sativa* using gas chromatography-mass spectrometry. J Pharmacognosy Phytother. 2016;8(2):8–24.

Hadi S, Daryabeygi-Khotbehsara R, Mirmiran P, et al. Effect of *Nigella sativa* oil extract on cardiometabolic risk factors in type 2 diabetes: A randomized, double-blind, placebo-controlled clinical trial. Phytother Res. 2021;35(7):3747–3755.

Hadi V, Kheirouri S, Alizadeh M, et al. Effects of *Nigella sativa* oil extract on inflammatory cytokine response and oxidative stress status in patients with rheumatoid arthritis: A randomized, double-blind, placebo-controlled clinical trial. Avicenna J Phytomed. 2016;6(1):34.

Hallajzadeh J, Milajerdi A, Mobini M, et al. Effects of *Nigella sativa* on glycemic control, lipid profiles, and biomarkers of inflammatory and oxidative stress: A systematic review and meta-analysis of randomized controlled clinical trials. Phytother Res. 2020;34(10):2586–2608.

Hannan MA, Zahan MS, Sarker PP, et al. Protective effects of black cumin (*Nigella sativa*) and its bioactive constituent, thymoquinone against kidney injury: An aspect on pharmacological insights. Int J Mol Sci. 2021;22(16):9078.

He T, Xu X. The influence of Nigella sativa for asthma control: A meta-analysis. Am J Emerg Med. 2020;38(3):589–593.

Hosseini M, Ghasemi S, Hadjzadeh MA, et al. Administration of *Nigella sativa* during neonatal and juvenile growth period improved liver function of propylthiouracil-induced hypothyroid rats. J Matern Fetal Neonatal Med. 2020;33(5):718–725.

Ilhan A, Gurel A, Armutcu F, et al. Antiepileptogenic and antioxidant effects of *Nigella sativa* oil against pentylenetetrazol-induced kindling in mice. Neuropharmacology. 2005;49(4):456–464.

Kalus U, Pruss A, Bystron J, et al. Effect of *Nigella sativa* (black seed) on subjective feeling in patients with allergic diseases. Phytother Res. 2003;17(10):1209–1214.

Kanter M, Coskun O, Uysal H. The antioxidative and antihistaminic effect of *Nigella sativa* and its major constituent, thymoquinone on ethanol-induced gastric mucosal damage. Arch Toxicol. 2006;80(4):217–224.

Kesen S, Amanpour A, Tsouli Sarhir S, et al. Characterization of aroma-active compounds in seed extract of black cumin (*Nigella sativa* L.) by aroma extract dilution analysis. Foods. 2018;7(7):98.

Khan MA, Ashfaq MK, Zuberi HS, et al. The in vivo antifungal activity of the aqueous extract from *Nigella sativa* seeds. Phytother Res. 2003;17(2):183–186.

Khani S, Abdollahi M, Khalaj A, et al. The effect of hydroalcoholic extract of *Nigella sativa* seed on dehydroepiandrosterone-induced polycystic ovarian syndrome in rats: An experimental study. Int J Reprod Biomed. 2021;19(3):271–282.

Khazdair MR, Ghafari S, Sadeghi M. Possible therapeutic effects of *Nigella sativa* and its thymoquinone on COVID-19. Pharm Biol. 2021;59(1):694–701.

Khazdair MR, Gholamnezhad Z, Rezaee R, Boskabady MH. A qualitative and quantitative comparison of *Crocus sativus* and *Nigella sativa* immunomodulatory effects. Biomed Pharmacother. 2021;140:111774.

Kolahdooz M, Nasri S, Modarres SZ, et al. Effects of Nigella sativa L. seed oil on abnormal semen quality in infertile men: a randomized, double-blind, placebo-controlled clinical trial. Phytomedicine. 2014;21(6):901–905.

Koshak AE, Koshak EA, Mobeireek AF, et al. *Nigella sativa* for the treatment of COVID-19: An open-label randomized controlled clinical trial. Complement Ther Med. 2021;61:102769.

Kulyar MF, Li R, Mehmood K, et al. Potential influence of *Nagella sativa* (black cumin) in reinforcing immune system: A hope to decelerate the COVID-19 pandemic. Phytomedicine. 2021;85:153277.

Leisegang K, Almaghrawi W, Henkel R. The effect of *Nigella sativa* oil and metformin on male seminal parameters and testosterone in Wistar rats exposed to an obesogenic diet. Biomed Pharmacother. 2021;133:111085.

Lorina Badger E, Promise Madu E, Tahir Mehmood K. Antimicrobial activity of *Nigella sativa* L. seed oil against multi-drug resistant *Staphylococcus aureus* isolated from diabetic wounds. Pak J Pharm Sci. 2015;28(6):1985–1990.

Madkour DA, Ahmed MM, Orabi SH, et al. *Nigella sativa* oil protects against emamectin benzoate-induced neurotoxicity in rats. Environ Toxicol. 2021;36(8):1521–1535.

Mahmoudvand H, Sepahvand A, Jahanbakhsh S, et al. Evaluation of antifungal activities of the essential oil and various extracts of *Nigella sativa* and its main component, thymoquinone against pathogenic dermatophyte strains. J Mycol Med. 2014;24(4):e155–161.

Malekian S, Ghassab-Abdollahi N, Mirghafourvand M, Farshbaf-Khalili A. The effect of *Nigella sativa* on oxidative stress and inflammatory biomarkers: A systematic review and meta-analysis. J Complement Integr Med. 2021;18(2):235–259.

Malik T, Hasan S, Pervez S, et al. *Nigella sativa* oil reduces extrapyramidal symptoms (EPS)-like behavior in haloperidol-treated rats. Neurochem Res. 2016;41:3386–3398.

Mohebbati R, Hosseini MA, Haghshenas M, et al. The effects of *Nigella sativa* extract on renal tissue oxidative damage during neonatal and juvenile growth in propylthiouracil-induced hypothyroid rats. Endocr Regul. 2017;51(2):105–113.

Mohtashami R, Huseini HF, Heydari M, et al. Efficacy and safety of honey based formulation of *Nigella sativa* seed oil in functional dyspepsia: A double blind randomized controlled clinical trial. J Ethnopharmacol. 2015;175:147–152.

Montazeri RS, Fatahi S, Sohouli MH, et al. The effect of *Nigella sativa* on biomarkers of inflammation and oxidative stress: A systematic review and meta-analysis of randomized controlled trials. J Food Biochem. 2021;45(4):e13625.

Mostafa TM, Hegazy SK, Elnaidany SS, et al. *Nigella sativa* as a promising intervention for metabolic and inflammatory disorders in obese prediabetic subjects: A comparative study of *Nigella sativa* versus both lifestyle modification and metformin. J Diabetes Complications. 2021;35(7):107947.

Nickavar B, Mojab F, Javidnia K, Amoli MA. Chemical composition of the fixed and volatile oils of *Nigella sativa* L. from Iran. Z Naturforsch C J Biosci. 2003;58(9–10):629–631.

Okeola VO, Adaramoye OA, Nneji CM, et al. Antimalarial and antioxidant activities of methanolic extract of *Nigella sativa* seeds (black cumin) in mice infected with *Plasmodium yoelli nigeriensis*. Parasitol Res. 2011;108:1507–1512.

Payab M, Hasani-Ranjbar S, Shahbal N, et al. Effect of the herbal medicines in obesity and metabolic syndrome: A systematic review and meta-analysis of clinical trials. Phytother Res. 2020;34(3):526–545.

Rafati M, Ghasemi A, Saeedi M, et al. *Nigella sativa* L. for prevention of acute radiation dermatitis in breast cancer: A randomized, double-blind, placebo-controlled, clinical trial. Complement Ther Med. 2019;47:102205.

Rahmani A, Niknafs B, Naseri M, et al. Effect of *Nigella sativa* oil on oxidative stress, inflammatory, and glycemic control indices in diabetic hemodialysis patients: A randomized double-blind, controlled trial. Evid-Based Complement Altern Med. 2022;2022:2753294.

Rastogi L, Feroz S, Pandey BN, et al. Protection against radiation-induced oxidative damage by an ethanolic extract of *Nigella sativa* L. Int J Radiat Biol. 2010;86(9):719–731.

Razmpoosh E, Safi S, Abdollahi N, et al. The effect of *Nigella sativa* on the measures of liver and kidney parameters: A systematic review and meta-analysis of randomized-controlled trials. Pharmacol Res. 2020;156:104767.

Razmpoosh E, Safi S, Nadjarzadeh A, et al. Effects of *Nigella sativa* supplementation on blood concentration and mRNA expression of TNF-α, PPAR-γ and adiponectin, as major adipogenesis-related markers, in obese and overweight women: A crossover, randomised-controlled trial. Br J Nutr. 2022;129(4),627–636.

Rizka A, Setiati S, Lydia A, Dewiasty E. Effect of *Nigella sativa* seed extract for hypertension in elderly: A double-blind, randomized controlled trial. Acta Med Indones. 2017;49(4):307–313.

Rusda M, Ganis Siregar MF, Lelo A, et al. A therapeutic effect of *Nigella sativa* extract on female Wistar rats vulvovaginal candidiasis model. Med Glas (Zenica). 2020;17(2):472–476.

Saadati S, Naseri K, Asbaghi O, et al. *Nigella sativa* supplementation improves cardiometabolic indicators in population with prediabetes and type 2 diabetes mellitus: A systematic review and meta-analysis of randomized controlled trials. Front Nutr. 2022;9:977756.

Safi S, Razmpoosh E, Fallahzadeh H, et al. The effect of *Nigella sativa* on appetite, anthropometric and body composition indices among overweight and obese women: A crossover, double-blind, placebo-controlled, randomized clinical trial. Complement Ther Med. 2021;57:102653.

Sahebkar A, Beccuti G, Simental-Mendia LE, et al. *Nigella sativa* (black seed) effects on plasma lipid concentrations in humans: A systematic review and meta-analysis of randomized placebo-controlled trials. Pharmacol Res. 2016;106:37–50.

Sahebkar A, Soranna D, Liu X, et al. A systematic review and meta-analysis of randomized controlled trials investigating the effects of supplementation with *Nigella sativa* (black seed) on blood pressure. J Hypertens. 2016;34(11):2127–2135.

Shoaei-Hagh P, Kamelan Kafi F, Najafi S, et al. A randomized, double-blind, placebo-controlled, clinical trial to evaluate the benefits of *Nigella sativa* seeds oil in reducing cardiovascular risks in hypertensive patients. Phytother Res. 2021;35(8):4388–4400.

Soleymani S, Zargaran A, Farzaei MH, et al. The effect of a hydrogel made by *Nigella sativa* L. on acne vulgaris: A randomized double-blind clinical trial. Phytother Res. 2020;34(11):3052–3062.

Sultan MT, Butt MS, Anjum FM. Safety assessment of black cumin fixed and essential oil in normal Sprague Dawley rats: Serological and hematological indices. Food Chem Toxicol. 2009;47(11):2768–2775.

Tahmasebi S, Oryan S, Mohajerani HR, et al. Probiotics and *Nigella sativa* extract supplementation improved behavioral and electrophysiological effects of PTZ-induced chemical kindling in rats. Epilepsy Behav. 2020;104:106897.

Tajmiri S, Farhangi MA, Dehghan P. *Nigella Sativa* treatment and serum concentrations of thyroid hormones, transforming growth factor β (TGF-β) and interleukin 23 (IL-23) in patients with Hashimoto's thyroiditis. Eur J Integr Med. 2016;8(4):576–580.

Tang G, Zhang L, Tao J, Wei Z. Effect of *Nigella sativa* in the treatment of nonalcoholic fatty liver disease: A systematic review and meta-analysis of randomized controlled trials. Phytother Res. 2021;35(8):4183–4193.

Tavakoly R, Arab A, Vallianou N, et al. The effect of *Nigella sativa* L. supplementation on serum C-reactive protein: A systematic review and meta-analysis of randomized controlled trials. Complement Ther Med. 2019;45:149–155.

Tayman C, Cekmez F, Kafa IM, et al. Protective effects of *Nigella sativa* oil in hyperoxia-induced lung injury. Arch Bronconeumol. 2013;49(1):15–21.

Tiruppur Venkatachallam SK, Pattekhan H, Divakar S, Kadimi US. Chemical composition of *Nigella sativa* L. seed extracts obtained by supercritical carbon dioxide. J Food Sci Technol. 2010;47:598–605.

Uchendu IK, Okoroiwu HU. Evaluation of blood oxidant/antioxidant changes and testicular toxicity after sub-acute exposure to cadmium in albino rats: Therapeutic effect of *Nigella sativa* seed extracts. Comb Chem High Throughput Screen. 2021;24(1):79–87.

Udu R, Oyweri J, Gathirwa J. Antimalarial activity of *Nigella sativa* L. seed extracts and selection of resistance in *Plasmodium berghei* ANKA in a mouse model. J Pathog. 2021;2021:1–10.

Ulasli M, Gurses SA, Bayraktar R, et al. The effects of *Nigella sativa* (Ns), *Anthemis hyalina* (Ah) and *Citrus sinensis* (Cs) extracts on the replication of coronavirus and the expression of TRP genes family. Mol Biol Rep. 2014;41(3):1703–1711.

Ulbricht CE. *Mosby's natural standard herb & supplement guide*. St. Luis: Elsevier; 2010.

Willcox ML, Elugbaju C, Al-Anbaki M, et al. Effectiveness of medicinal plants for glycaemic control in type 2 diabetes: An overview of meta-analyses of clinical trials. Front Pharmacol. 2021:3402.

Zaoui A, Cherrah Y, Mahassini N, et al. Acute and chronic toxicity of *Nigella sativa* fixed oil. Phytomedicine. 2002;9(1):69–74.

25 *Phyllanthus emblica* L.

Ayeh Naghizadeh and Raefeh Mardi

Scientific name: *Phyllanthus emblica* L. (syn. *Emblica officinalis* Gaertn.)
Family: Phyllanthaceae
Common names:

- **English:** Amla, aonla, Indian gooseberry, amlika, emblic, emblic myrobalan, myrobalan, Malacca tree
- **Persian:** *'āmeleh*
- **Arabic:** *'āmlağ*

Medicinal part(s): Fruit (Figure 25.1)
Temperament (nature): Cold in the second degree and dry in the third degree
Major chemical constituents:

- **Phenolic compounds:** Gallic acid (5%), methyl gallate, ellagic acid, trigallayl glucose
- **Hydrolysable tannins:** Emblicanin B, emblicanin A, punigluconin, pedunculagin, chebulinic acid, chebulagic acid, corilagin, geraniin
- **Alkaloids:** Phyllantine, phyllantidine
- **Flavonoids:** Quercetin, kaempferol
- **Amino acids:** Glutamic acid, proline, aspartic acid, alanine, lysine, cystine
- **Vitamins:** Vitamin C (193–720 mg/100 g) (Gul et al., 2022; Saini et al., 2022)

THERAPEUTIC USE

TPM Literature

Amla fruit has considerable effects on the brain and nervous system and combined with honey or its jam made with honey is recommended in palsy, paresis, tremor, memory impairments, and psychological disorders such as depression and melancholy. Regarding ophthalmologic conditions, oral formulations are suggested for improving eyesight; while topical use is recommended for some diseases including cataracts. Amla is known in TPM for special significant beneficial effects on the heart. Dietary use is recommended as cardiotonic, as well as strengthening other organs; though, due to its cold nature, cold-tempered individuals are better to take it with honey, cinnamon, or mastic. Amla is an astringent and therefore, a good tonic of the gastrointestinal tract. It can be used as an appetizer and for excessive salivation. This fruit can help management of chronic diarrhea, dysuria, and anal burning or irritation. Moreover, it is recommended for management of bleeding disorders and intestinal ulcers. Topical compresses are used to prevent hemorrhage due to hemorrhoids. Likewise, compresses of amla powder mixed with water on the forehead can stop nosebleed. This plant enhances sexual function. It is also beneficial in nocturia. Amla oil can hasten hair growth and retain hair color (Aghili Khorasani 1771; Avicenna 1025).

 DOI: 10.1201/b22971-25

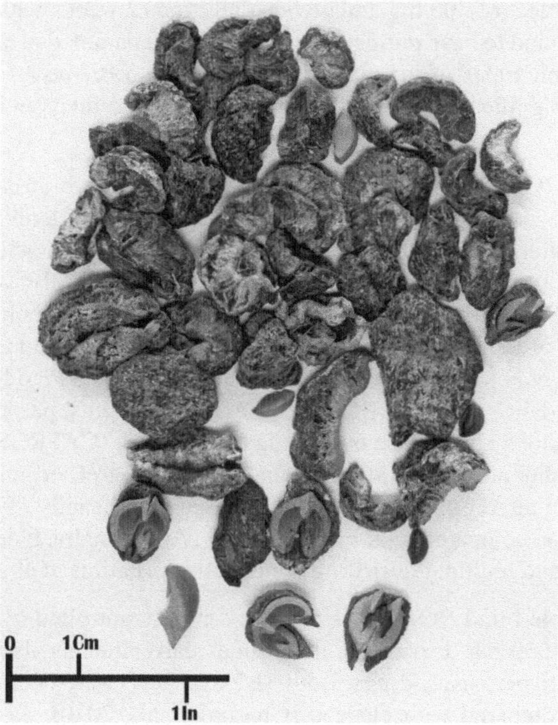

FIGURE 25.1 Amla fruits.

Current Evidence

Clinical Evidence

Systemic inflammation and oxidative stress: In a clinical trial on overweight (class-1 obese) adults, 500 mg of a standardized extract of amla (CAPROS®) was administered twice a week for 12 weeks. Results showed a considerable reduction in LDL-C and TC/HDL-C at the end of intervention. Circulatory hs-CRP notably reduced. Moreover, amla extract significantly ameliorated ADP- and collagen-induced platelet aggregation. Therefore, results of this study demonstrated advantageous effects on CVD risk factors in overweight individuals (Khanna et al., 2015).

Fifteen healthy volunteers were investigated in a double-blind, crossover RCT. They were treated with either 500 mg amla capsules or placebo once a day for 4 weeks. Considerable enhancement was seen in amla group in terms of blood fluidity, endothelial function, and lipid profile. Also, 8-OHdG and vWF were significantly decreased; while no sign of hepatic, hematologic, or renal toxicity was observed (Kapoor et al., 2020).

Hyperlipidemia: In a pilot clinical study, a purified, standardized, dried extract of amla was administered in two doses of 500 and 1,000 mg per day. This extract was found to have positive effects on TC, LDL-C, CRP, and HDL-C after 3 and 6 months of intervention (Antony et al., 2008). An RCT on 60 individuals with hyperlipidemia, indicated significant reduction of BP, as well as TC, TAG, LDL-C, and VLDL-C, along with a raise in HDL-C compared with baseline values which was similar to the control drug simvastatin (Gopa et al., 2012). In a double-blind RCT, amla aqueous extract was given to 65 individuals with metabolic syndrome in two doses of 250 and 500 mg twice daily. After 12 weeks of treatment, significant reductions of LDL-C, TC, TAG, MDA, and hs-CRP, as well as elevation of GSH, HDL-C, and NO were observed in amla-treated patients in a dose-dependent manner (Usharani et al., 2019). Another double-blind RCT on 98 dyslipidemic patients compared the effect of 500 mg amla twice daily for 12 weeks with placebo. At the end of intervention amla was found to have mitigating effects on lipid parameter such as TAG, TC, LDL-C, VLDL-C, and atherogenic index of the plasma. Moreover, Apo B/Apo A1 ratio was lowered after amla use, although no significant difference was found between intervention and placebo groups (Upadya et al., 2019).

Diabetes: A four-arm RCT was designed to examine the effects of an aqueous extract of amla (highly standardized to contain low-molecular-weight hydrolyzable tannins) on endothelial dysfunction and oxidative stress in 80 diabetic patients. For 12 weeks, participants received either amla extract as 250 mg or 500 mg twice daily, placebo, or atorvastatin. All groups except the placebo group showed significant improvements in HbA1c, lipid profile, endothelial function, biomarkers of oxidative stress, and systemic inflammation, including MDA, NO, and GSH, hs-CRP compared with baseline (Usharani et al., 2013). Amla has also been demonstrated to have antiplatelet activity in diabetics. In an open-label crossover RCT on 10 diabetic patients, participants were divided by washout periods, including a single dose of 500 mg amla extract (CAPROS®), 75 mg clopidogrel, 75 mg ecosprin, or 10-day administration of amla and clopidogrel, or amla and ecosprin. At the end of the study, platelet aggregation factor had decreased significantly after both single-dose and 10-day drug consumption compared with baseline levels. Additionally, bleeding and clotting times prolonged after single- and multiple-dose drug combinations (Fatima et al., 2014).

Hypertension: In a triple-blind RCT on 81 patients with uncontrolled hypertension, participants were treated with amla 500 mg or placebo, three times daily after meals for 8 weeks in combination with standard antihypertensive drugs. Both SBP and DBP were decreased more significantly in intervention group compared with placebo (Ghaffari et al., 2020). Another RCT investigated the effect of amla aqueous extract on 150 patients with essential hypertension. Participants were given 500 mg amla capsules or placebo twice daily for 12 weeks as an add on to the conventional antihypertensive medication. However, this trial did not find any significant reduction in SBP, DBP, or arterial stiffness parameters with amla use (Shanmugarajan et al., 2021).

GERD: An RCT was performed on 68 individuals with a minimum 3-month history of GERD. Patients were treated with either 500 mg amla or placebo tablets twice a day for 28 days. Based on the frequency and severity scale for the symptoms of nonerosive reflux disease, a significant reduction in frequency and intensity of heartburn and regurgitation was observed in the intervention group (Varnosfaderani et al., 2018).

COVID-19: In a double-blind RCT performed on 61 COVID-19 patients, 31 patients were given amla tea (2 g fruit powder in 100 mL hot water) as an adjunct therapy and compared with a placebo for 10 days. RT-PCR test, hospitalization period, extent of pulmonary involvement, clinical symptoms (fever, cough severity, shortness of breath, myalgia, severity of chills, sore throat, weakness) and laboratory factors were evaluated during the study. Although amla did not have a significant effect on RT-PCR, it was able to reduce the intensity of symptoms and shorten hospitalization period. Also, three paraclinical variables, including the mean SpO_2, mean percentage of lung involvement on CT, and CRP levels showed significant improvement in the intervention group (Varnasseri et al., 2022).

Oral hygiene: In an examiner-blinded crossover RCT on 20 healthy individuals, the efficacy of a sugar-free chewing gum containing amla fruit extract in changing the oral microbiome was compared with placebo. Saliva samples were collected at intervals up to 80 min after each intervention. Salivary flow rate and pH levels were significantly higher after 0–2, 2–5, and 5–10 min in the amla gum group. Moreover, total bacteria, *Streptococcus mutans*, *Porphyromonas gingivalis*, and volatile sulfur compound concentrations showed significant difference between the two groups at 75–80 min (Gao et al., 2018).

Periodontitis: Forty-six subjects participated in an RCT to investigate the effect of a 10% amla sustained-release gel in chronic periodontitis. Patients received scaling and root planing as routine care and either amla sustained-release gel or placebo as an adjunct therapy. Significantly better periodontal variables including plaque index, gingival index, probing pocket depth, clinical attachment level, and modified sulcus bleeding index were demonstrated in the intervention group, confirming anti-inflammatory effect of amla sustained-release gel (Grover et al., 2016).

Preclinical Evidence

Memory and cognition: In an animal model of epilepsy, hydroalcoholic extract of amla (500 and 700 mg/kg) delayed kainic acid-induced seizure onset, inhibited lipid peroxidation, and restored GSH. Also, the higher dose prominently ameliorated cognitive damage (Golechha et al., 2011). Another study assessed the effect of 60-day administration of amla aqueous extract (250 mg/kg/day) to rats with alcohol-induced brain mitochondrial dysfunction. A significant reduction of NO, protein carbonyls, and LPO, as well as enhanced SDH, NADH dehydrogenase, and cytochrome c oxidase, thereby protecting the brain against mitochondrial dysfunction was reported (Reddy et al., 2011). In a study on scopolamine-induced amnesia and oxidative stress in mice, the effect of a hydroalcoholic extract of amla fruit was examined in memory impairment. Four doses of the extract (150, 300, 450 and 600 mg/kg, i.e.) were administered for 7 consecutive days which caused a significant AChE activity (Golechha et al., 2012). Another study reported that oral administration of 100 mg per day of amla powder to fluoride-induced memory impairment can significantly increase protein content and AChE activity in the brain, thereby ameliorating neuronal fluoride toxicity (Shalini and Sharma, 2015). In another animal study, ripe and unripe amla ethanolic extracts were orally administered to evaluate its effects on cognitive functions, brain antioxidant enzymes, and AChE activity. Results indicated amla fruit, especially the ripe fruit, improved memory function, as well as brain content of SOD, CAT, GSH, and Gpx, along with a decrease in AChE activity and MDA level (Uddin et al., 2016).

Depression: Oral administration of an aqueous extract of amla with a dose range of 200 and 400 mg/kg for 14 days to mice demonstrated antidepressant effect based on the behavioral evaluations, along with reduced brain MAO-A levels (Dhingra et al., 2012).

Cardiac damage: To investigate the effect of amla on myocardial ischemia-reperfusion injury, 100 mg/kg of an aqueous extract was administered orally to rats for 30 days. Accordingly, amla could upregulate the PI3K/Akt/GSK3β/β-catenin cardioprotective pathway and thus, protected cardiac tissue from injury. Moreover, a raise in the ejection fraction, and reduction in left ventricular internal diameter and fibrosis percentage were observed (Thirunavukkarasu et al., 2015). Another study on rats demonstrated that 30-day oral administration of fresh fruit homogenate of amla in three different doses (250, 500 and 750 mg/kg) causes myocardial adaptation via increasing endogenous antioxidants and protecting rat hearts from ischemia/reperfusion-induced injury (Rajak et al., 2004).

Diarrhea: Animal studies indicate that amla possesses antidiarrheal and spasmolytic activities. A study performed on Wistar rats, demonstrated the inhibitory effect of the methanol extract of amla on diarrhea induced by castor oil and magnesium sulfate in rats. Significant reduction in GI motility, and inhibition of enteropooling were also observed (Perianayagam et al., 2005). Likewise, in doses of 500–700 mg/kg, amla extract could prevent castor oil-induced diarrhea and intestinal fluid accumulation in mice (Mehmood et al., 2011).

ADVERSE REACTIONS

TPM Literature

Amla may be harmful for the spleen and is thus advised to be used with honey or spikenard, as corrigents. Additionally, it may lead to intestinal colic and is thus used with sweet almond oil to minimize this risk (Aghili Khorasani 1771).

Current Evidence

Amla is used in food, and no specific adverse effects have been reported in current literature. Four-week daily intake of 500 mg amla extract in healthy individuals caused no sign of nephrotoxicity, hepatotoxicity, hematological toxicity, or adverse effects (Kapoor et al., 2020). However, another clinical study in type 2 diabetic patients suggests that 10-day intake of amla extract with a dose of 500 mg per day significantly decreases platelet aggregation and increases clotting and bleeding time (Fatima et al., 2014).

CONTRAINDICATIONS

TPM Literature

None.

Current Evidence

Since amla consumption is associated with bleeding and bruising in some individuals, it should be used with caution in bleeding disorders. Also, due to an increased risk of bleeding, amla intake should be discontinued 2 weeks prior to surgery (WebMD, January 2024).

PREGNANCY AND LACTATION

TPM Literature

None.

Current Evidence

None

DRUG INTERACTIONS

Anticoagulant sand antiplatelets: Since amla intake may delay the blood-clotting process, caution should be taken in concurrent administration with anticoagulant and antiplatelet agents like aspirin or clopidogrel (Fatima et al., 2014).

Antidiabetics: simultaneous consumption of amla and other antidiabetic drugs may cause hypoglycemic effects (Fatima et al., 2014).

METHOD OF ADMINISTRATION

TPM Literature

Most commonly, amla (water or dried powder) is used orally. It may be prepared as decoction, jam, electuary (mixture of the fruit with honey), or syrup. Topical application in the form of poultices or oil (fruit extracted and boiled in olive oil base) products is also used. Moreover, ophthalmic drops or compress have been suggested for eye problems (Aghili Khorasani 1771).

Current Evidence

Amla can be taken orally in powder, extract, tablet, capsule, or tea forms. Also, it can be used in eye drop preparations, toothpaste combinations, and mouthwash formulas. Topical amla gel is used for skin disorders.

DOSAGE

Suggested oral dose for adults is 500–1,000 mg amla extract daily for 1–3 months (WebMD, January 2024). Doses of up to 1,500 mg per day of the fruit powder have been used in RCTs (Ghaffari et al., 2020).

REFERENCES

Aghili Khorasani MH 1771. *Makhzan-al-Adviah* (*The treasury of drugs*) (rewritten by Shams Ardakani MR, Rahimi R, Farjadmand F, 1st ed.). Tehran: Tehran University of Medical Sciences; 2009.

Antony B, Benny M, Kaimal TN. A pilot clinical study to evaluate the effect *of Emblica officinalis* extract (Amlamax™) on markers of systemic inflammation and dyslipidemia. Indian J Clin Biochem. 2008;23(4):378–381.

Avicenna 1025. *Al-Qanoon fi al-Tibb* (*The canon of medicine*) (rewritten by Masoudi A, ed.). Tehran: Almaei; 2015.

Chaikul P, Kanlayavattanakul M, Somkumnerd J, Lourith N. *Phyllanthus emblica* L. (amla) branch: A safe and effective ingredient against skin aging. J Tradit Complement Med. 2021;11(5):390–399.

Dhingra D, Joshi P, Gupta A, Chhillar R. Possible involvement of monoaminergic neurotransmission in antidepressant-like activity of *Emblica officinalis* fruits in mice. CNS Neurosci Ther. 2012;18(5):419–425.

Fatima N, Pingali U, Muralidhar N. Study of pharmacodynamic interaction of *Phyllanthus emblica* extract with clopidogrel and ecosprin in patients with type II diabetes mellitus. Phytomedicine. 2014;21(5):579–585.

Gao Q, Li X, Huang H, et al. The efficacy of a chewing gum containing *Phyllanthus emblica* fruit extract in improving oral health. Curr Microbiol. 2018;75(5):604–610.

Ghaffari S, Navabzadeh M, Ziaee M, et al. A randomized, triple-blind, placebo-controlled, add-on clinical trial to evaluate the efficacy of *Emblica officinalis* in uncontrolled hypertension. Evid-Based Complement Alternat Med. 2020;2020:8592869.

Golechha M, Bhatia J, Arya DS. Studies on effects of *Emblica officinalis* (amla) on oxidative stress and cholinergic function in scopolamine induced amnesia in mice. J Environ Biol. 2012;33(1):95.

Golechha M, Bhatia J, Ojha S, Arya DS. Hydroalcoholic extract of *Emblica officinalis* protects against kainic acid-induced status epilepticus in rats: Evidence for an antioxidant, anti-inflammatory, and neuroprotective intervention. Pharm Biol. 2011;49(11):1128–1136.

Gopa B, Bhatt J, Hemavathi KG. A comparative clinical study of hypolipidemic efficacy of amla (*Emblica officinalis*) with 3-hydroxy-3-methylglutaryl-coenzyme-A reductase inhibitor simvastatin. Indian J Pharmacol. 2012;44(2):238.

Grover S, Tewari S, Sharma RK, et al. Effect of subgingivally delivered 10% *Emblica officinalis* gel as an adjunct to scaling and root planing in the treatment of Chronic periodontitis: A randomized placebo-controlled clinical trial. Phytother Res. 2016;30(6):956–962.

Gul M, Liu ZW, Rabail R, et al. Functional and nutraceutical significance of amla (*Phyllanthus emblica* L.): A review. Antioxidants. 2022;11(5):816.

Huang CZ, Tung YT, Hsia SM, et al. The hepatoprotective effect of *Phyllanthus emblica* L. fruit on high fat diet-induced non-alcoholic fatty liver disease (NAFLD) in SD rats. Food Funct. 2017;8(2):842–850.

Kapoor MP, Suzuki K, Derek T, et al. Clinical evaluation of Emblica Officinalis Gatertn (amla) in healthy human subjects: Health benefits and safety results from a randomized, double-blind, crossover placebo-controlled study. Contemp Clin Trials Commun. 2020;17:100499.

Khanna S, Das A, Spieldenner J, et al. Supplementation of a standardized extract from *Phyllanthus emblica* improves cardiovascular risk factors and platelet aggregation in overweight/class-1 obese adults. J Med Food. 2015;18(4):415–420.

Mehmood MH, Siddiqi HS, Gilani AH. The antidiarrheal and spasmolytic activities of Phyllanthus emblica are mediated through dual blockade of muscarinic receptors and Ca2+ channels. J Ethnopharmacol. 2011;133(2):856–865.

Perianayagam JB, Narayanan S, Gnanasekar G, Pandurangan A, Raja S, Rajagopal K, Rajesh R, Vijayarajkumar P, Vijayakumar SG. Evaluation of Antidiarrheal Potential of Emblica officinalis. Pharm Biol. 2005;43(4):373–377.

Rajak S, Banerjee SK, Sood S, et al. Emblica officinalis causes myocardial adaptation and protects against oxidative stress in ischemic-reperfusion injury in rats. Phytother Res. 2004;18(1):54–60.

Reddy VD, Padmavathi P, Kavitha G, et al. *Emblica officinalis* ameliorates alcohol-induced brain mitochondrial dysfunction in rats. J Med Food. 2011;14(1–2):62–68.

Reddy VD, Padmavathi P, Varadacharyulu NC. *Emblica officinalis* protects against alcohol-induced liver mitochondrial dysfunction in rats. J Med Food. 2009;12(2):327–333.

Saini R, Sharma N, Oladeji OS, et al. Traditional uses, bioactive composition, pharmacology, and toxicology of Phyllanthus emblica fruits: A comprehensive review. J Ethnopharmacol. 2022;282:114570.

Shalini B, Sharma JD. Beneficial effects of *Emblica officinalis* on fluoride-induced toxicity on brain biochemical indexes and learning-memory in rats. Toxicol Int. 2015;22(1):35.

Shanmugarajan D, Girish C, Harivenkatesh N, et al. Antihypertensive and pleiotropic effects of *Phyllanthus emblica* extract as an add-on therapy in patients with essential hypertension: A randomized double-blind placebo-controlled trial. Phytother Res. 2021;35(6):3275–3285.

Thilakchand KR, Mathai RT, Simon P, et al. Hepatoprotective properties of the Indian gooseberry (*Emblica officinalis* Gaertn): A review. Food Funct. 2013;4(10):1431–1441.

Thirunavukkarasu M, Selvaraju V, Tapias L, et al. Protective effects of *Phyllanthus emblica* against myocardial ischemia-reperfusion injury: the role of PI3-kinase/glycogen synthase kinase 3β/β-catenin pathway. J Physiol Biochem. 2015;71:623–633.

Uddin MS, Al Mamun A, Hossain MS, et al. Exploring the effect of *Phyllanthus emblica* L. on cognitive performance, brain antioxidant markers and acetylcholinesterase activity in rats: Promising natural gift for the mitigation of Alzheimer's disease. Ann Neurosci. 2016;23(4):218–229.

Upadya H, Prabhu S, Prasad A, et al. A randomized, double blind, placebo controlled, multicenter clinical trial to assess the efficacy and safety of *Emblica officinalis* extract in patients with dyslipidemia. BMC Complement Altern Med. 2019;19:1–4.

Usharani P, Fatima N, Muralidhar N. Effects of *Phyllanthus emblica* extract on endothelial dysfunction and biomarkers of oxidative stress in patients with type 2 diabetes mellitus: A randomized, double-blind, controlled study. Diabetes Metab Syndr Obes. 2013;26:275–284.

Usharani P, Merugu PL, Nutalapati C. Evaluation of the effects of a standardized aqueous extract of *Phyllanthus emblica* fruits on endothelial dysfunction, oxidative stress, systemic inflammation and lipid profile in subjects with metabolic syndrome: A randomised, double blind, placebo controlled clinical study. BMC Complement Altern Med. 2019;19:1–8.

Varnasseri M, Siahpoosh A, Hoseinynejad K, et al. The effects of add-on therapy of *Phyllanthus emblica* (amla) on laboratory confirmed COVID-19 cases: A randomized, double-blind, controlled trial. Complement Ther Med. 2022;65:102808.

Varnosfaderani SK, Hashem-Dabaghian F, Amin G, et al. Efficacy and safety of amla (*Phyllanthus emblica* L.) in non-erosive reflux disease: A double-blind, randomized, placebo-controlled clinical trial. J Integr Med. 2018;16(2):126–131.

WebMD. Indian gooseberry: Uses, side effects, and more. January 2024; www.webmd.com/vitamins/ai/ingredientmono-784/indian-gooseberry

26 *Pimpinella anisum* L.

Roja Rahimi

Scientific name: *Pimpinella anisum* L.
Family: Apiaceae
Common names:

- **English:** Anise, aniseed
- **Persian:** *'anīsūn, bādīyān-e rūmī, zīre-ye rūmī*
- **Arabic:** *kamūn al-ḥulw, rāziyānağ al-šāmī, rāziyānağ al-rūmī*

Medicinal part(s): Fruit (Figure 26.1)
Temperament (nature): Hot in the second degree and dry in the third degree
Major chemical constituents:

- **Volatile oil (2–6%):** Trans-anethole (80–95%), chavicol methyl ether (estragole, 2%), anisaldehyde (1.4%)
- **Caffeic acid derivatives:** Chlorogenic acid, other caffeoyl quinic acids
- **Flavonoids:** Apigenin-7-O-glucoside, isoorientin, isovitexin, luteolin-7-O-glucoside
- **Coumarins:** Scopoletin, umbelliferone, umbelliprenine, bergapten
- Fatty oil (30%) (Gruenwald et al., 2007; Williamson et al., 2013)

THERAPEUTIC USE

TPM Literature

Aniseed is an analgesic and can be used orally as decoction or topically as oil. It is recommended to be used as a spice in the diet of patients with neurological disorders including palsy, epilepsy, and facial palsy. It is suggested that patients with palsy just drink decoction of aniseed in the first week of beginning of disease. Its smoke and inhalation are recommended for headache, migraine, dizziness, catarrh, as well as ear pain due to cold dystemperament. Smelling aniseed which is macerated in vinegar and then dried and roasted is useful for catarrh and rhinorrhea due to cold dystemperament. Aniseed as powder or decoction is beneficial for hypochondriasis. Rubbing aniseed powder to teeth is recommended for teeth whitening as well as halitosis.

Chewing aniseed and its decoction sweetened with honey is useful for respiratory tract disorders including reproductive cough, pneumonia, and asthma. Moreover, its decoction is recommended for liver disease, even those with fibrotic features. Also, the decoction and powder of aniseed can relief flatulence and dyspepsia and act as a digestive aid.

The decoction of aniseed is emmenagogue and galactagogue and can eliminate leucorrhea. Furthermore, it can tonify kidney and is diuretic and useful for urolithiasis (Aghili Khorasani 1771; Avicenna 1025).

DOI: 10.1201/b22971-26

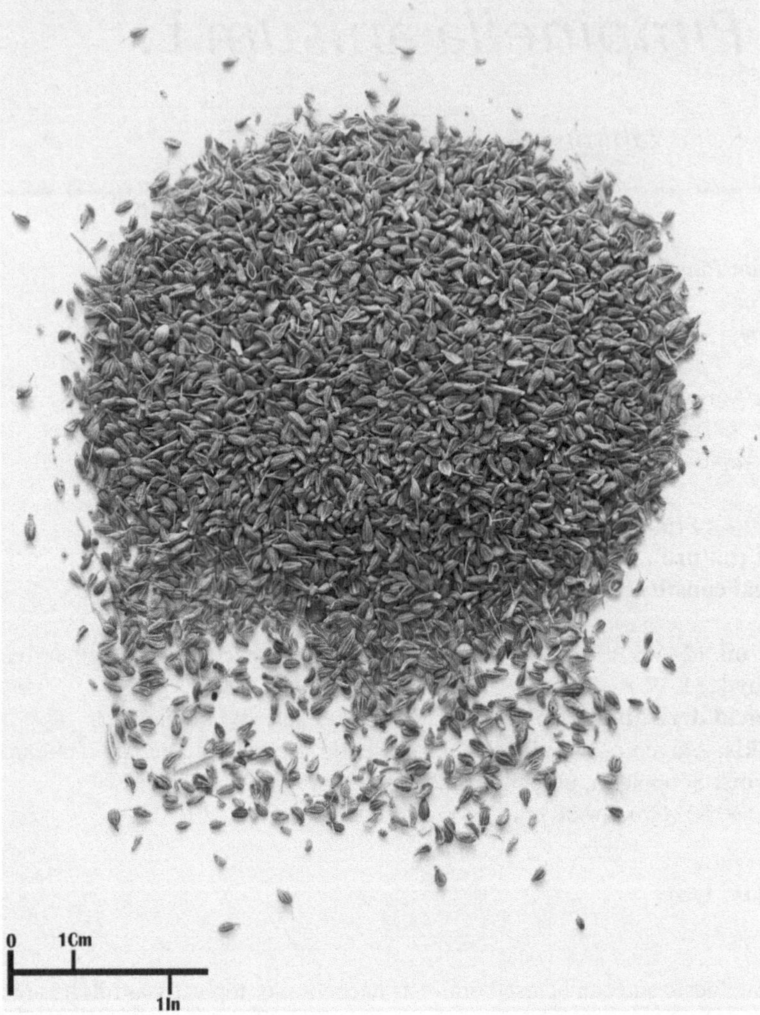

FIGURE 26.1 Anise fruits.

Current Evidence

Clinical Evidence

Migraine headache: In an RCT, a cream containing 7% aniseed essential oil (2 mL of cream on the temporal and forehead zones at the onset of migraine attacks) was administered to patients with migraine headache for 6 weeks. Headache Impact Test (HIT-6) score, the frequency of migraine attacks, the mean duration of migraine attacks, the mean number of analgesic consumptions per week, as well as severity of headache significantly decreased in the anise oil group compared to placebo group (Mosavat et al., 2019).

Rhinosinusitis: In a single-blind RCT including 48 patients with chronic rhinosinusitis without polyps, aniseed oil prepared according to TPM instructions (aqueous extract of aniseed concentrated in almond oil) was compared with fluticasone nasal spray. Patients received two drops of oil in each nostril every 12 hours, while those in the second group received two puffs of fluticasone nasal spray in each nostril every 12 h for 4 weeks. Symptoms were reduced according to 22-item Sino-Nasal

Outcome Test (SNOT-22) by both interventions; however, traditional aniseed oil showed significantly better results than fluticasone. Mean changes in CT scan scoring markedly decreased in both groups. Significant improvement in postnasal drip and nasal obstruction was reported in aniseed oil group compared to fluticasone group (Vazifehkah et al., 2016).

Functional dyspepsia: In a double-blind RCT, patients with postprandial distress syndrome were randomized to receive either aniseed powder 3 g after each meal three times a day (n = 47) or placebo (n = 60) for 4 weeks. The severity of functional dyspepsia symptoms markedly decreased after 2, 4, and 12 weeks in aniseed group compared to placebo (Ghosegir et al., 2015). Moreover, the quality of life significantly increased in aniseed group compared to placebo (Ghosegir et al., 2014).

IBS: In a double-blind RCT, 120 patients with IBS were divided into three groups: enteric coated capsules containing 200 mg essential oil of aniseed (n = 40), placebo (n = 40) and enteric coated capsules containing 187 mg essential oil of peppermint as active control (n = 40). Patients in each group received three similar capsules per day for 4 weeks. Seventy-five percent of patients in the treatment group, 35% in the placebo group and 52.5% in active control group were free from IBS symptoms. The effectiveness of enteric coated capsules of anise oil in improving IBS symptoms (abdominal discomfort or pain, bloating, diarrhea, constipation severity, difficulty in defecation, gastroesophageal reflux, headache, tiredness, overall satisfaction and quality of life) was significantly better than placebo or enteric coated capsules of peppermint oil after the 4-week treatment period and the 2-week follow-up period (Mosaffa-Jahromi et al., 2016). Moreover, aniseed oil capsule markedly improved the total score of Beck Depression Inventory-II in mild to moderate depression in patients suffering from IBS in comparison to peppermint oil and placebo (Mosaffa-Jahromi et al., 2017).

Hot flashes: In a placebo-controlled RCT, post-menopausal women with hot flashes complaint received capsules containing 330 mg dried ethanolic extract of aniseed (n = 36) or placebo capsules (n = 36) three times daily for 4 weeks. The frequency and severity of hot flashes significantly decreased in aniseed group compared to placebo (Nahidi et al., 2012).

PMS: In a double-blind RCT, administration of capsules containing 110 mg dried hydroethanolic extract of aniseed three times daily 7 days before the start of the menstruation and continued until 3 days after, which was a total of 10 days during two consecutive menstruation cycles to women suffering from PMS (n = 37) significantly reduced the intensity of the symptoms of PMS in comparison with placebo (n = 32) (Farahmand et al., 2020).

Preclinical Evidence

Convulsion and neurotoxicity: Intraperitoneal administration of aniseed oil (1–3 mL/kg) to rats significantly prolonged the latency of seizure attacks and reduced the amplitude and duration of epileptiform burst discharges induced by injection of intraperitoneal PTZ. In addition, anise oil significantly inhibited production of dark neurons in different regions of the brain in epileptic rats. Anise oil also significantly enhanced the duration of the appearance of anoxic terminal negativity induced by oxygen withdrawal and inhibited induction of long-term potentiation in hippocampal slices (Karimzadeh et al., 2012).

NAFLD: Hydroethanolic extract (25–200 mg/kg) and essential oil (0.125–0.5 mg/kg) of aniseed significantly reversed increase in the plasma levels of TC, LDL-C, and TAG and decrease in HDL-C level in experimental model of NAFLD. Serum levels of AST and ALT were also significantly reduced by treatment with these interventions. Histological assessments also confirmed the effectiveness of treatments by reduced macrovesicular steatohepatitis (Asadollahpoor et al., 2017).

Milk production: The aqueous extract (1 g/kg) and ethanolic extract (1 g/kg) of aniseed significantly increased the milk production in rats with about 68.1% and 81% more milk being produced, respectively, than in the control group (Hosseinzadeh et al., 2014).

ADVERSE REACTIONS

TPM Literature

It is harmful for intestine and fennel can ameliorate its damage. It can cause headache and ingestion with oxymel can prevent this adverse event (Aghili Khorasani 1771).

Current Evidence

Tongue angioedema was reported in a 58-year-old man after drinking aniseed liqueur (Gázquez García et al., 2007).

Six-week topical administration of a cream containing 7% aniseed essential oil did not show any systemic or dermal side effects (Mosavat et al., 2019).

Nasal administration of traditional aniseed oil was well tolerated by patients with rhinosinusitis (n = 26) and no serious adverse effect was reported. The most common problems reported were increased discharge (n = 7), nausea (n = 3), and headache (n = 1) (Vazifehkah et al., 2016).

Enteric coated capsules containing 200 mg aniseed oil was well tolerated, with no adverse events during the 4-week treatment period and the 2-week follow-up period (Mosaffa-Jahromi et al., 2016).

CONTRAINDICATIONS

TPM Literature

None.

Current Evidence

It is contraindicated in patients allergic to aniseed and anethole (Gruenwald et al., 2007). Because of estrogenic effects, women with hormone-sensitive conditions should avoid using aniseed. Some of these conditions include breast cancer, uterine cancer, ovarian cancer, endometriosis, and uterine fibroids (Pharmacist's Letter, 2013).

PREGNANCY AND LACTATION

TPM Literature

As it is emmenagogue, it may induce bleeding during pregnancy and should be avoided during this period. As it is galactagogue, it can be used during lactation in the form of powder or decoction (Aghili Khorasani 1771).

Current Evidence

Its essential oil and alcoholic preparations are contraindicated during pregnancy and lactation. Mild estrogenic effect and anti-fertility activity of anethole (the major constituent of essential oil) have been demonstrated in rats (ESCOP, 2003).

DRUG INTERACTIONS

Selective estrogen receptor modulators: Because of its estrogenic effect, aniseed should not be used in patients receiving selective estrogen receptor modulators including tamoxifen and raloxifene (Pharmacist's Letter, 2013).

Coumarin anticoagulants: Aniseed contains natural coumarins, but the quantity of these constituents is not established. So, it may have potential to interact with coumarin anticoagulants (Williamson et al., 2013).

METHOD OF ADMINISTRATION

TPM Literature

Aniseed crushed fruits or decoction is administered orally. Rubbing its powder to teeth has been recommended for dental conditions, and its smoke and inhalation has been applied for respiratory tract disorders (Aghili Khorasani 1771).

Current Evidence

It may be recommended as powder, infusion, or decoction for oral administration.

DOSAGE

Adult average daily dose: 3 g of crushed fruits as an infusion or similar preparation.
Children average daily dose: 1–4 years: 1g; 4–10 years: 2 g; ≥10 years: as adult dose (ESCOP, 2003).

REFERENCES

Aghili Khorasani MH 1771. *Makhzan-al-Advíah* (*The treasury of drugs*) (rewritten by Shams Ardakani MR, Rahimi R, Farjadmand F, 1st ed.). Tehran: Tehran University of Medical Sciences; 2009.

Asadollahpoor A, Abdollahi M, Rahimi R. *Pimpinella anisum* L. fruit: Chemical composition and effect on rat model of nonalcoholic fatty liver disease. J Res Med Sci. 2017;22:37.

Avicenna 1025. *Al-Qanoon fi al-Tibb* (*The canon of medicine*) (rewritten by Masoudi A, ed.). Tehran: Almaei; 2015.

ESCOP. *The scientific foundation of herbal medicinal products*. Stuttgart: European Scientific Cooperative on Phytotherapy; 2003.

Farahmand M, Khalili D, Ramezani Tehrani F, et al. Could anise decrease the intensity of premenstrual syndrome symptoms in comparison to placebo? A double-blind randomized clinical trial. J Complement Integr Med. 2020;17(4):20190077.

Gázquez García V, Gaig Jané P, Bartolomé Zavala B. Aniseed-induced nocturnal tongue angioedema. J Investig Allergol Clin Immunol. 2007;17(6):406–408.

Ghoshegir SA, Mazaheri M, Ghannadi A, et al. *Pimpinella anisum* in modifying the quality of life in patients with functional dyspepsia: A double-blind randomized clinical trial. J Res Med Sci. 2014;19:1118–1123.

Ghoshegir SA, Mazaheri M, Ghannadi A, et al. *Pimpinella anisum* in the treatment of functional dyspepsia: A double-blind, randomized clinical trial. J Res Med Sci. 2015;20(1):13–21.

Gruenwald J, Brendler T, Jaenicke C. *PDR for herbal medicines*. Montvale: Thomson Reuters; 2007.

Hosseinzadeh H, Tafaghodi M, Abedzadeh S, Taghiabadi E. Effect of aqueous and ethanolic extracts of *Pimpinella anisum* L. seeds on milk production in rats. J Acupunct Meridian Stud. 2014;7(4):211–216.

Karimzadeh F, Hosseini M, Mangeng D, et al. Anticonvulsant and neuroprotective effects of *Pimpinella anisum* in rat brain. BMC Complement Altern Med. 2012;12:76.

Mosaffa-Jahromi M, Lankarani KB, Pasalar M, et al. Efficacy and safety of enteric coated capsules of anise oil to treat irritable bowel syndrome. J Ethnopharmacol. 2016;194:937–946.

Mosaffa-Jahromi M, Tamaddon AM, Afsharypuor S, et al. Effectiveness of anise oil for treatment of mild to moderate depression in patients with irritable bowel syndrome: A randomized active and placebo-controlled clinical trial. J Evid-Based Complementary Altern Med. 2017; 22:41–46.
Mosavat SH, Jaberi AR, Sobhani Z, et al. Efficacy of anise (*Pimpinella anisum* L.) oil for migraine headache: A pilot randomized placebo-controlled clinical trial. J Ethnopharmacol. 2019;236:155–160.
Nahidi F, Kariman N, Simbar M, Mojab F. The study on the effects of *Pimpinella anisum* on relief and recurrence of menopausal hot flashes. Iran J Pharm Res. 2012;11(4):1079–1085.
Pharmacist's Letter. Natural Medicines Comprehensive Database. Stockton: Therapeutic Research Faculty, 2013.Vazifehkah S, Shams-Ardekani MR, Kamalinejad M, et al. Evaluation of a novel natural drop for treatment of chronic rhinosinusitis without nasal polyps: A single blind randomized trial. Int Forum Allergy Rhinol. 2016;6(9):943–949.
Williamson E, Driver S, Baxter K (eds.). *Stockley's herbal medicines interactions*. London: Pharmaceutical Press; 2013.

27 *Piper nigrum* L.

Azadeh Zarei and Mehrdad Karimi

Scientific name: *Piper nigrum* L.
Family: Piperaceae
Common names:

- **English:** Black pepper
- **Persian:** *polpol, felfel, felfel-e-siyāh*
- **Arabic:** *fulful*

Medicinal part(s): Fruit (Figure 27.1)
Temperament (nature): Hot and dry in the third to fourth degree
Major chemical constituents:

- **Volatile oil (1.2–2.6%):** Bisabolene, sabinene (15–25%), limonene (15–20%), caryophyllene (10–15%), β-pinene (10–12%), α-pinene (8–12%), 3-carene (5%)
- **Alkaloids:** Piperine, piperolein A and B, piperidine, piperlongumine, pipernonaline
- Polysaccharides (45%)
- Fatty oil (10%) (Gruenwald et al., 2007; Williamson et al., 2013)

THERAPEUTIC USE

TPM Literature

Black pepper is a memory enhancer and recommended to be used for patients with neurological disorders such as palsy in the form of oil. Topical application of black pepper powder is recommended to reduce toothache. Its decoction is used to relieve reproductive cough, dyspnea, and reduces chest pain caused by respiratory problems. It is a digestive, GI tonic, and appetizer and is beneficial for cold and wet dystemperament of GI tract. Topical use of black pepper with vinegar can reduce splenomegaly. It is diuretic and emmenagogue and its vaginal application after intercourse acts as a contraceptive. Drinking black pepper with milk and sugar can increase libido. It is the most potent heater of nerve and muscle from the view of TPM. Drinking decoction of crushed fruit until vomiting is recommended as an antidote (Aghili Khorasani 1771; Avicenna 1025).

Current Evidence

Clinical Evidence

Desire for nicotine use: In a comparative study with pre- and posttest criteria, which was performed on 20 volunteers who consumed nicotine daily, the tendency to use nicotine in these individuals was evaluated by aromatherapy intervention with black pepper. In this intervention, the participant inhaled the black pepper essential oil for two minutes as soon as the participant felt the desire to use nicotine. Before and after inhalation, the level of nicotine cravings was assessed on a scale of 0–10.

DOI: 10.1201/b22971-27

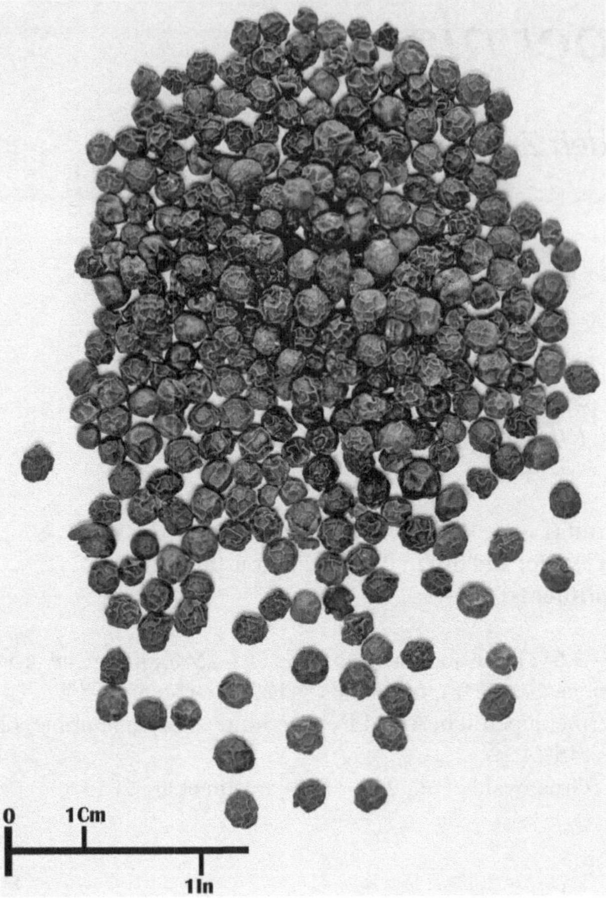

FIGURE 27.1 Black pepper fruits.

The study has shown that black pepper aromatherapy significantly reduces nicotine cravings and can be effective in quitting nicotine (Cordell and Buckle, 2013).

Appetite-suppressing effects: Sixteen healthy participants were examined in a crossover RCT. A black pepper-based beverage containing 20 mg equivalent of gallic acid was prescribed for these people. The results showed that consumption of a black pepper drink before meals can reduce appetite without changing glucose metabolism and the amount of gut or thyroid hormones (Zanzer et al., 2018).

Vein visibility: In a controlled RCT of hospitalized patients, 120 patients who required inferior vena cava placement but did not have visible and palpable vessels for venipuncture were examined. In this study, 20% black pepper essential oil in *Aloe vera* gel was topically applied. Patients were then reexamined for arteries before and after topical application of the gel. Intervention with black pepper compared to routine nursing procedures resulted in a higher percentage of patients obtaining the desired intravenous score (vein score = 2). The number of patients who did not have visible vessels after the intervention was halved, and the effort to catheterize was also halved ($p < 0.05$). This study showed that topical application of black pepper can increase the sight and touch of the vein and improve catheterization (Kristiniak et al., 2012). Another study on 60 patients also demonstrated the same results upon topical application of pepper essential oil which caused a significant improvement in period of appropriate vein selection and successful catheter insertion, as well as satisfaction in both nurses and patients (Handan et al., 2022).

Swallowing dysfunction: In a clinical study performed on patients with poststroke disorders, the rate of swallowing reflex delay and the number of swallowing movements after inhalation of volatile black pepper oil were investigated. Inhalation of the oil for one minute in these patients compared to the control group who were stimulated by smell with distilled water and lavender oil caused a delay in swallowing ($p < 0.03$). It also increased the number of swallowing movements compared to the control group ($p < 0.01$). Inhalation of black pepper oil appears to be beneficial for patients with poststroke dysphagia, at any level of consciousness or physical or mental state (Ebihara et al., 2006).

Preclinical Evidence

Seizure: The anticonvulsant effect of black pepper ethanolic and *n*-hexane extract was evaluated in a rat model of convulsion. *Piper nigrum* at a dose of 500 mg/kg reduced all stages of seizures and the extensor phase ($p < 0.001$) (Belemkar et al., 2013).

Alzheimer's disease: In a rat model of Alzheimer's disease, methanolic extract of black pepper fruits (50 and 100 mg/kg orally for 21 days) significantly improved memory function by increasing working memory and reducing memory errors via reduction in oxidative stress in the rat hippocampus (Hritcu et al., 2014).

Obesity: In a high-fat diet-induced model of obesity in rats, oral treatment with 200 mg/kg of black pepper extracts (obtained with solvents with different polarities) for 42 days, could significantly reduce BW, fat percentage, as well as FBS, insulin resistance, leptin, LPO, and lipid profile parameters. Also, an increase was reported in adiponectin and antioxidant enzymes. Aqueous and ethyl acetate extract of black pepper showed the best pharmacological activities (Parim et al., 2015). Another study in the same animal model also demonstrated antioxidant activity of black pepper via elevation of SOD, CAT, GSH, Gpx, and reduction of LPO (Vijayakumar et al., 2013).

ADVERSE REACTIONS

TPM Literature

It can cause headaches in people with hot temperaments. It is harmful to the lungs and throat. It is also not recommended for people with anemia. It can reduce the volume of semen. It is also harmful to GI ulcers, as well as urinary tract pains. The use with cold-tempered oils in patients with hot temperament and its application with honey in patients with cold temperament can be effective in reducing adverse events (Aghili Khorasani 1771).

Current Evidence

No adverse effects are known with the proper administration of designated therapeutic dosages (Gruenwald et al., 2007).

Large doses of black pepper may irritate the urinary tract. Overdoses of black pepper may cause abdominal heat and burning, thirst, vomiting, fever, and sometimes convulsion and urticaria (Gardner and MacGuffin, 2013).

CONTRAINDICATIONS

TPM Literature

None

Current Evidence

None.

PREGNANCY AND LACTATION

TPM Literature

Since it can provoke menstrual bleeding in women, it is better to use it with caution in pregnancy (Aghili Khorasani 1771).

Current Evidence

Oral administration of 50 mg of black pepper extract to rats for 25 days increased fetal resorption (Gardner and MacGuffin, 2013).

The spasmolytic effect of an aqueous extract of black pepper was observed in uteruses excised from pregnant and nonpregnant rats. At concentrations of 0.125–2 mg/mL, the black pepper extract dose-dependently reduced uterine contractions (Gharib and Yahyavi, 2007).

DRUG INTERACTIONS

No interaction has been reported for black pepper during clinical studies. However, the experimental investigations have demonstrated its interactions with some drugs. Piperine as a major chemical compound of black pepper increases the levels of phenytoin, propranolol, and theophylline. Interactions with amoxicillin, barbiturates, NSAIDs, and oxytetracycline have also been reported in various animal studies and in increasing the amount of these drugs in the body. The antithyroid effect of piperine has also been found in animal studies (Williamson et al., 2013).

METHOD OF ADMINISTRATION

TPM Literature

Its decoction is used orally. It is also used in oral diseases in the form of gargling and in toothpowder. Its poultice is used with suitable herbs for skin, hair, and gum problems. Its oil is used for topical applications. It is also applied as a form of vaginal suppository to prevent pregnancy (Aghili Khorasani 1771).

Current Evidence

It may be recommended as powder, decoction, or administered in the form of oil or ointment.

DOSAGE

Single doses range from 0.3 to 0.6 g. The daily dosage is 1.5 g (Gruenwald et al., 2007).

REFERENCES

Aghili Khorasani MH 1771. *Makhzan-al-Adviah* (*The treasury of drugs*) (rewritten by Shams Ardakani MR, Rahimi R, Farjadmand F, 1st ed.). Tehran: Tehran University of Medical Sciences; 2009.

Avicenna 1025. *Al-Qanoon fi al-Tibb* (*The canon of medicine*) (rewritten by Masoudi A, ed.). Tehran: Almaei; 2015.

Belemkar S, Kumar A, Pata MK. Pharmacological screening of herbal extract of *Piper nigrum* (maricha) and *Cinnamomum zeylanicum* (dalchini) for anticonvulsant activity. Ethnopharmacology. 2013;2(2):1–5.

Cordell B, Buckle J. The effects of aromatherapy on nicotine craving on a US campus: A small comparison study. J Altern Complement Med. 2013;19(8):709–713.

Ebihara T, Ebihara S, Maruyama M, et al. A randomized trial of olfactory stimulation using black pepper oil in older people with swallowing dysfunction. J Am Geriatr Soc. 2006;54(9):1401–1406.

Gardner Z, McGuffin M (eds.). *American Herbal Products Association's botanical safety handbook*. Boca Raton: CRC Press; 2013.

Gharib NM, Yahyavi H. Spasmolytic activity of piper nigrum fruit aqueous extract on rat non-pregnant uterus. Iran J Pharmacol Ther. 2007;6(1):35–40.

Gruenwald J, Brendler T, Jaenicke C. *PDR for herbal medicines*. Montvale: Thomson Reuters; 2007.

Handan ER, Turkmen AS, Aslan A. Effect of topical application of black pepper essential oil on peripheral intravenous catheter insertion: A randomized controlled study. Explore. 2022;18(4):457–462.

Hritcu L, Noumedem JA, Cioanca O, et al. Methanolic extract of *Piper nigrum* fruits improves memory impairment by decreasing brain oxidative stress in amyloid beta (1–42) rat model of Alzheimer's disease. Cell Mol Neurobiol. 2014;34:437–449.

Kristiniak S, Harpel J, Breckenridge DM, Buckle J. Black pepper essential oil to enhance intravenous catheter insertion in patients with poor vein visibility: A controlled study. J Altern Complement Med. 2012;18(11):1003–1007.

Parim B, Harishankar N, Balaji M, et al. Effects of *Piper nigrum* extracts: Restorative perspectives of high-fat diet-induced changes on lipid profile, body composition, and hormones in Sprague–Dawley rats. Pharm Biol. 2015;53(9):1318–1328.

Vijayakumar R, Surya D, Nalini N. Antioxidant efficacy of black pepper (*Piper nigrum* L.) and piperine in rats with high fat diet induced oxidative stress. Redox Report. 2004;9(2):105–110.

Williamson E, Driver S, Baxter K (eds.). *Stockley's herbal medicines interactions*. London: Pharmaceutical Press; 2013.

Zanzer YC, Plaza M, Dougkas A, et al. Black pepper-based beverage induced appetite-suppressing effects without altering postprandial glycaemia, gut and thyroid hormones or gastrointestinal well-being: A randomized crossover study in healthy subjects. Food Funct. 2018;9(5):2774–2786.

28 *Pistacia lentiscus* L.

Seyedeh Mahnaz Karimi

Scientific name: *Pistacia lentiscus* L.
Family: Anacardiaceae
Common names:

- **English:** Mastic gum, lentisk, chios mastic, mastiha
- **Persian:** *maṣṭakī, maṣṭakā*
- **Arabic:** *'ilk al-rūm*

Medicinal part(s): Oleo-gum resin (Figure 28.1)
Temperament (nature): Hot and dry in the second degree
Major chemical constituents:

- **Essential oil (1–3%):** α-pinene (40%), β-pinene (1.5%), β-myrcene (9%), limonene (1.0%), β-caryophyllene (5%) (Koutsoudaki et al., 2005)
- **Resin (90%):** Triterpenes, oleanolic acid, isomastic acid, mastic acid, tirucallol (Gruenwald et al., 2007)

THERAPEUTIC USE

TPM Literature

Mastic is an astringent and general tonic. Chewing mastic strengthens teeth and gums, relieves toothache, and absorbs phlegm humor from head and tongue. Putting a cloth soaked in mastic extract on the eyes is useful for eye pain and dripping mastic oil is useful for ear pain. In oral intake, it is useful for cold-tempered headaches, purifying the lungs, and reducing cough. It is also a tonic for the stomach, intestines, liver, and kidneys. It is recommended to be taken orally for dyspepsia, bloating, hiccups, GERD, and cramps. Mastic is an appetizer, mouth freshener, stomach tonic, and carminative. It is recommended to take it with warm water for mild laxative effects. Its decoction is experienced for diarrhea, fatty liver, nausea, intestinal ulcers, dyspepsia, hemoptysis, umbilical hernia, and uterine bulge. It is also used topically to strengthen the stomach, uterus, kidneys, and bladder. The use of mastic gum orally or topically, by suppressing inflammation and relieving pain, is useful in bone fractures, muscle cramps, and injuries caused by trauma. It can be used in skin care and brightening the facial skin (Aghili Khorasani 1771; Avicenna 1025).

Current Evidence

Clinical Evidence

IBD: In a double-blind RCT, 60 IBD patients were treated with either mastic (four tablets containing 2.8 g per day), placebo, or standard treatment (mesalamine, azathioprine, and corticosteroids) for 3 months. Mastic could decrease IBD symptoms by acting as a prebiotic which was evident from increased iron and decreased fecal lysozyme (Papada et al., 2019). A significant decrease was

 DOI: 10.1201/b22971-28

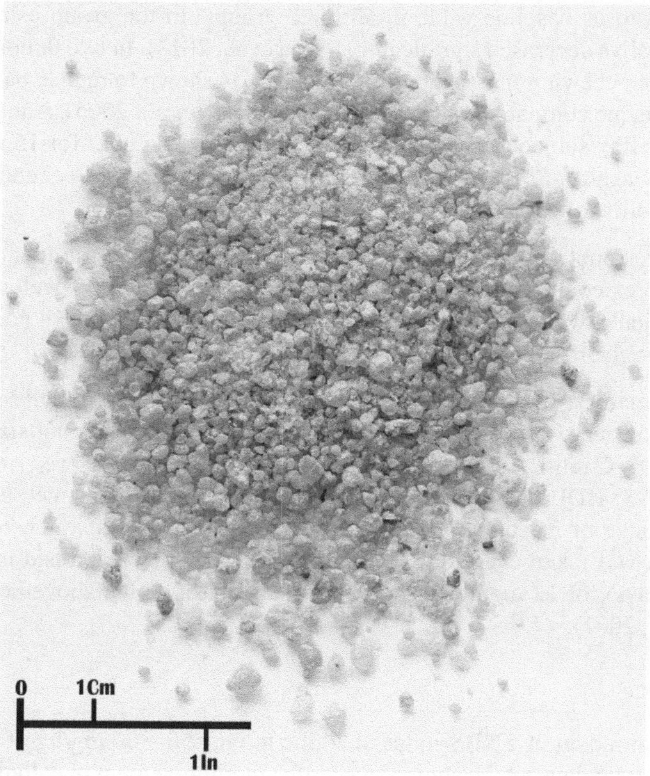

FIGURE 28.1 Mastic gum.

observed in ox-LDL-C, ox-LDL-C/HDL-C, and ox-LDL-C/LDL-C. Change in amino acid profile is an early prognostic marker of IBD and according to the results, alanine, valine, proline, glutamine, fecal calprotectin, and fecal lactoferrin increased only in placebo group (Papada et al., 2018; Papada et al., 2019). In a pilot study in ten patients with mild to moderately active Crohn's disease and eight healthy volunteers as control, a 4-week treatment with mastic (2.22 g daily) could significantly decrease disease activity index and the plasma levels of IL-6 and CRP in these patients (Kaliora et al., 2007).

Functional dyspepsia: In a placebo-controlled RCT on 148 patients with functional dyspepsia, 3-week supplementation with mastic gum (350 mg three times daily) could reduce stomach pain in general, stomach pain when anxious, dull ache in the upper abdomen, and heartburn vs. placebo (Dabos et al., 2010).

***Helicobacter pylori* infection:** A four-arm pilot RCT on 52 patients with *H. pylori* infection assessed the effect of 350 mg mastic three times daily, 1.05 g mastic three times daily, 20 mg pantoprazole twice a day plus 350 mg mastic three times a day for 14 days, or and pantoprazole 20 mg twice daily plus amoxicillin 1g twice daily plus clarithromycin 500 mg twice daily for 10 days. In the two first groups, mastic gum could eradicate *H. pylori* in 4/13 and 5/13 of patients, respectively, compared with 10/13 in the antibiotic therapy and none (no case of negative *H. pylori*) in mastic plus pantoprazole-treated group (Dabos et al., 2010).

Dental problems: In a single-blind RCT, 42 students randomly received pure mastic gum, xylitol mastic gum, or probiotic mastic gum for 3 weeks. Mutans streptococci count showed a significant reduction compared to its baseline value in all three groups. In the group using probiotic mastic gum, the pH of the saliva decreased significantly (Biria et al., 2014). In two double-blinded RCTs on 20 healthy volunteers, chewing mastic gum for 4 hours was shown to reduce bacterial colonization and reduce dental plaque compared to the placebo (Takahashi et al., 2003). Another clinical trial on 25 periodontally healthy subjects showed that chewing the mastic gum for 15 min had significant antibacterial activity against *Streptococcus mutans* and mutans streptococci and it may be a useful adjunct in the prevention of caries (Aksoy et al., 2006; 2007).

Hypertension: In a double-blind, controlled crossover study, daily administration of 2,800 mg mastic gum for 1 week could improve both aortic and peripheral SBP, as well as pulse pressure in 13 hypertensive patients; while no hemodynamic change was observed in 14 normotensive cases in control group (Kontogiannis et al., 2019).

Lipid profile parameters: In a group of 48 subjects over 50 years old, daily administration of 5 g of chios mastic powder (*Pistacia lentiscus* var. *chia*) for 18 months could significantly decrease TC, LDL-C, TC/HDL-C ratio, ApoA1, ApoB, AST, ALT, and GGT; however, no significant change was observed in FBS, HDL-C, and TAG. Another assessment in the same study showed that in 85 subjects, oral intake of mastic solution (5 g of mastic mixed with water, remained overnight, and the supernatant was taken every day, while the mastic powder remained in the glass and was refreshed every 7 days) for 12 months has no significant effect on the abovementioned parameters (Triantafyllou et al., 2007).

Preclinical Evidence

Colitis: In an animal model of TNBS-induced colitis in rats, 50–300 mg/kg of mastic powder was orally administered for 6 days which showed a significant improvement in colonic indices and tissue damage, as well as a significant reduction of MDA, IL-6, IL-8, TNF-α, and ICAM-1 (Gioxari et al., 2011). Also, in acetic acid-induced colitis in rats, 400 mg/kg of mastic (dissolved in sesame oil as oral or intracolonic administration) could significantly decrease MPO, TNF-α, and tissue damage (Ostovan et al., 2020).

Colon cancer: Oral administration of mastic essential oil with a dose of 0.58 mg/kg (diluted in corn oil) for 13 days showed a significant inhibition of tumor growth in mice with colon carcinoma; while α-pinene and myrcene as the major components of the essential oil did not show such an antineoplastic activity neither *in vitro*, nor *in vivo* (Spyridopoulou et al., 2017).

Dermatitis: The effect of topical treatment with 3% or 30% mastic cream were evaluated in toluene-2,4-diisocyanate-induced allergic contact dermatitis in mice which resulted in significant attenuation of the skin thickness, atopic dermatitis score, transepidermal water loss, and itch behavior due to anti-inflammatory activities (Kishimoto et al., 2021).

NASH: In a rat model of high-fat and high-carbohydrate-induced NASH, mastic gum incorporated in food pellets (0.2% w/w) was orally administered for 8 weeks which caused a significant decrease in ALT, improvement of hepatic steatosis and collagen content, and a reduction in NAFLD activity score. Furthermore, it resulted in a partial but significant recovery of gut microbiota diversity and changes in identity and abundance of specific taxa (Kannt et al., 2019).

ADVERSE REACTIONS

TPM Literature

It is harmful to the bladder and should be soaked in grape vinegar overnight, dried before use, and then taken individually or together with tragacanth. Taken together with sugar, gum Arabic, walnuts, and coriander can also ameliorate its side effects (Aghili Khorasani 1771).

Current Evidence

In general, mastic was well tolerated when taken orally in short term. Long-term use of mastic is not recommended. Mastic can decrease blood pressure (Ulbricht, 2010).

CONTRAINDICATIONS

TPM Literature

None.

Current Evidence

Oral use in children and adolescents under 18 years and topical use in children under 12 years have not been recommended due to lack of adequate data (Committee on Herbal Medicinal Products, 2016).

Avoid in people with a known allergy or hypersensitivity to mastic, or members of the Anacardiaceae family such as pistachio, terebinth, Chinese pistache, and *Schinus terebinthifolius* (Brazilian pepper) (Ulbricht, 2010).

PREGNANCY AND LACTATION

TPM Literature

None.

Current Evidence

Mastic is not recommended in woman who are pregnant or breastfeeding. In theory, mastic causes fetal injury or death (Ulbricht, 2010).

DRUG INTERACTIONS

ACE inhibitors: Additive effects may be observed in concomitant use with ACE inhibitors; caution is advised (Ulbricht, 2010).

METHOD OF ADMINISTRATION

TPM Literature

Mastic powder or decoction is administered orally. The smoke may be collected and used topically. Rubbing mastic powder or mastic oil on the teeth or chewing mastic gum is used in periodontal problems. In topical application, it may be used as a compress, oil, or powder (Aghili Khorasani 1771).

Current Evidence

Mastic gum can be used as powder/decoction/extract/lyophilized aqueous extract for oral intake or topical use. It may also be used as chewing gum.

DOSAGE

For oral use (adults 18 years or older): 1–2 g per day mastic gum powder (Committee on Herbal Medicinal Products, 2016). However, in an RCT on healthy subjects, a daily dose of 5 g of mastic powder for 18 months was reported to be safe and well tolerated (Triantafyllou et al., 2007). 150 mL of 10% aqueous resin decoction per day is also suggested (Duke, 2008).

For topical use (adolescents above 12 years, adults, and elderly): Semi-solid preparations containing 9–11% of the powdered herbal substance to be applied as a thin layer on the affected area up to three times daily (Committee on Herbal Medicinal Products, 2016).

REFERENCES

Abidi A, Kourda N, Ennigrou S, et al. Effect of *Pistacia lentiscus* oil on experimental pulmonary fibrosis. Tunis Med. 2016;94(7):401–406.

Aghili Khorasani MH 1771. *Makhzan-al-Adviah* (*The treasury of drugs*) (rewritten by Shams Ardakani MR, Rahimi R, Farjadmand F, 1st ed.). Tehran: Tehran University of Medical Sciences; 2009.

Aksoy A, Duran N, Koksal F. In vitro and in vivo antimicrobial effects of mastic chewing gum against *Streptococcus mutans* and mutans streptococci. Arch Oral Biol. 2006;51(6):476–481.

Aksoy A, Duran N, Toroglu S, Koksal F. Short-term effect of mastic gum on salivary concentrations of cariogenic bacteria in orthodontic patients. Angle Orthod. 2007;77(1):124–128.

Ammari M, Othman H, Hajri A, et al. *Pistacia lentiscus* oil attenuates memory dysfunction and decreases levels of biomarkers of oxidative stress induced by lipopolysaccharide in rats. Brain Res Bull. 2018;140:140–147.

Avicenna 1025. *Al-Qanoon fi al-Tibb* (*The canon of medicine*) (rewritten by Masoudi A, ed.). Tehran: Almaei; 2015.

Biria M, Eslami G, Taghipour E, Baghban AA. Effects of three mastic gums on the number of mutans streptococci, lactobacilli and pH of the saliva. J Dent (Tehran, Iran). 2014;11(6):672–679.

Boelens MH, Jimenez R. Chemical composition of the essential oils from the gum and from various parts of *Pistacia lentiscus* L. (mastic gum tree). Flavour Fragr J. 1991;6(4):271–275.

Committee on Herbal Medicinal Products (HMPC). *European Union herbal monograph on Pistacia lentiscus L., resina (mastic)*. Amsterdam: European Medical Agency; 2016.

Dabos KJ, Sfika E, Vlatta LJ, et al. Is chios mastic gum effective in the treatment of functional dyspepsia? A prospective randomised double-blind placebo-controlled trial. J Ethnopharmacol. 2010;127(2):205–209.

Dabos KJ, Sfika E, Vlatta LJ, Giannikopoulos G. The effect of mastic gum on *Helicobacter pylori*: A randomized pilot study. Phytomedicine. 2010;17(3–4):296–299.

De Pooter HL, Schamp NM, Aboutabl EA, et al. Essential oils from the leaves of three pistacia species grown in Egypt. Flavour Fragr J. 1991;6(3):229–232.

Duke AJ. *Handbook of medicinal herbs*. 2nd ed. Ann Arbor: University of Michigan; 2008.

Gioxari A, Kaliora AC, Papalois A, et al. *Pistacia lentiscus* resin regulates intestinal damage and inflammation in trinitrobenzene sulfonic acid-induced colitis. J Med Food. 2011;14(11):1403–1411.

Kaliora AC, Stathopoulou MG, Triantafillidis JK, et al. Chios mastic treatment of patients with active Crohn's disease. World J Gastroenterol. 2007;13(5):748–753.

Kannt A, Papada E, Kammermeier C, et al. Mastiha (*Pistacia lentiscus*) improves gut microbiota diversity, hepatic steatosis, and disease activity in a biopsy-confirmed mouse model of advanced non-alcoholic steatohepatitis and fibrosis. Mol Nutr Food Res. 2019;63(24):1900927.

Kishimoto R, Kato N, Koike M, et al. Topical treatment with mastic (resin from *Pistacia lentiscus*) elicits anti-inflammatory and anti-pruritic responses by modulating keratinocyte activation in a mouse model of allergic dermatitis. Phytomedicine. 2021;91:153679.

Kontogiannis C, Georgiopoulos G, Loukas K, et al. Chios mastic improves blood pressure haemodynamics in patients with arterial hypertension: Implications for regulation of proteostatic pathways. Eur J Prev Cardiol. 2019;26(3):328–331.

Kottakis F, Kouzi-Koliakou K, Pendas S, et al. Effects of mastic gum *Pistacia lentiscus* var. Chia on innate cellular immune effectors. Eur J Gastroenterol Hepatol. 2009;21(2):143–149.

Koutsoudaki C, Krsek M, Rodger A. Chemical composition and antibacterial activity of the essential oil and the gum of *Pistacia lentiscus* var. chia. J Agric Food Chem. 2005;53(20):7681–7685.

Magiatis P, Melliou E, Skaltsounis AL, et al. Chemical composition and antimicrobial activity of the essential oils of *Pistacia lentiscus* var. chia. Planta Med. 1999;65(08):749–752.

Moudi Z, Edozahi M, Emami SA, et al. Effects of mastic oleoresin on wound healing and episiotomy pain: A mixed methods study. J Ethnopharmacol. 2018;214:225–231.

Naouar MS, Mekki LZ, Charfi L, et al. Preventive and curative effect of *Pistacia lentiscus* oil in experimental colitis. Biomed Pharmacother. 2016;83:577–583.

Ostovan M, Fazljou SM, Khazraei H, et al. The anti-inflammatory effect of *Pistacia lentiscus* in a rat model of colitis. J Inflamm Res. 2020:369–376.

Papada E, Amerikanou C, Torović L, et al. Plasma free amino acid profile in quiescent inflammatory bowel disease patients orally administered with mastiha (*Pistacia lentiscus*): A randomised clinical trial. Phytomedicine. 2019;56:40–47.

Papada E, Forbes A, Amerikanou C, et al. Antioxidative efficacy of a *Pistacia Lentiscus* supplement and its effect on the plasma amino acid profile in inflammatory bowel disease: A randomised, double-blind, placebo-controlled trial. Nutrients. 2018;10(11):1779.

Papada E, Gioxari A, Amerikanou C, et al. Regulation of faecal biomarkers in inflammatory bowel disease patients treated with oral mastiha (*Pistacia lentiscus*) supplement: A double-blind and placebo-controlled randomised trial. Phytother Res. 2019;33(2):360–369.

Papanicolaou D, Melanitou M, Katsaboxakis K. Changes in chemical composition of the essential oil of Chios "mastic resin" from *Pistacia lentiscus* var. Chia tree during solidification and storage. Dev Food Sci. 1995; 37:303–310.

Spyridopoulou K, Tiptiri-Kourpeti A, Lampri E, et al. Dietary mastic oil extracted from *Pistacia lentiscus* var. chia suppresses tumor growth in experimental colon cancer models. Sci Rep. 2017;7(1):3782.

Takahashi K, Fukazawa M, Motohira H, et al. A pilot study on antiplaque effects of mastic chewing gum in the oral cavity. J Periodontol. 2003;74(4):501–505.

Triantafyllou A, Chaviaras N, Sergentanis TN, et al. Chios mastic gum modulates serum biochemical parameters in a human population. J Ethnopharmacol. 2007;111(1):43–49.

Ulbricht CE. *Mosby's natural standard herb & supplement guide*. St. Louis: Elsevier; 2010.

29 *Plantago major* L.

Maryam Kabiri and Mohammad M. Zarshenas

Scientific name: *Plantago major* L.
Family: Plantaginaceae
Common names:

- **English:** Greater plantain, broadleaf plantain, waybread
- **Persian:** *bārtang*, *bārhang*
- **Arabic:** *lisān al-ḥaml*

Medicinal part(s): Seeds, leaves (Figure 29.1)
Temperament (nature): Cold and dry in the second degree. The seed's dryness is more than that of the leaves
Major chemical constituents:

- **Flavonoids:** Luteolin, apigenin, baicalein, hispidulin, plantaginin, scutellarin, nepetin
- **Alkaloids:** Indicain, plantagonin
- **Terpenoids:** Loliolid, ursolic acid, oleanolic acid, sitosterol acid, 18β-glycyrrhetinic
- **Caffeic acid derivatives:** Plantamajoside, acteoside
- **Iridoid glycosides:** Aucubin, majoroside
- **Fatty acids:** Lignoceric acid, palmitic acid, stearic acid, oleic acid, linoleic acid, linolenic acid, myristic acid, arachidic acid, behenic acid
- **Polysaccharides:** Xylose, arabinose, galacturonic acid (Adom et al., 2017)

THERAPEUTIC USE

TPM Literature

The plant (leaves) is useful for preventing and treating hemoptysis, bleeding, epistaxis, and epilepsy when taken orally. Ear discomfort has been found to respond favorably to topical administration of fresh leaves juice as ear or nasal drops. Toothache, aphthous lesions, and oral problems may benefit from using leaf juice as a mouthwash. Seeds have been used to treat bleeding and leaves have been used to treat ascites due to hot dystemperament, asthma, dyspnea, respiratory lesions, and lung ulcers. Oral use of the leaves juice has been known as a tonic for liver, spleen, and kidney and may be effective for liver obstruction (also for seeds), bleeding hemorrhoids, urinary tract discomfort, and menorrhagia. The decoction of leaves and seeds is recommended for diarrhea and dysentery as well as gastrointestinal bleeding. Leaves and seeds in macerated form are recommended for dysuria. It has been topically applied for skin infections (Aghili Khorasani 1771; Avicenna 1025).

DOI: 10.1201/b22971-29

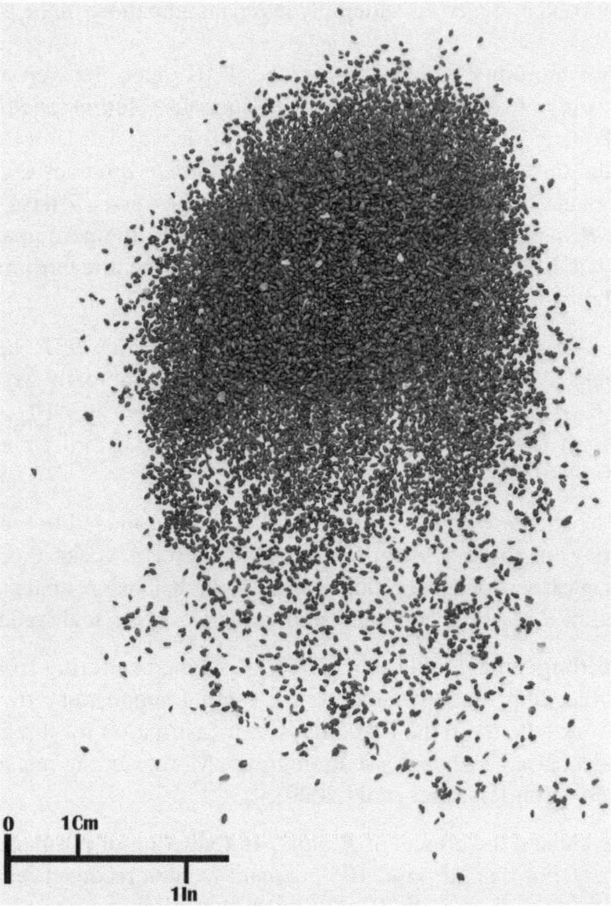

FIGURE 29.1 Greater plantain seeds.

Current Evidence

Clinical Evidence

Wound: A topical formulation from aerial parts of *P. major* was investigated in 130 patients with stage 1 pressure ulcer during a triple-blind RCT for 14 days. The findings indicated a significant difference in recovery of the damage between the test and control groups (Ghiasian et al., 2021).

In an open-label RCT, the impact of hydroalcoholic extract from *P. major* leaves was studied in 100 patients with diabetic foot ulcers or pressure ulcers. Patients randomly received *P. major* 10% topical gel extract once daily along with dressing and regular wound care or just dressing with routine wound care for 2 weeks. The results showed that the application of the extract gel led to a significantly greater reduction in wound size as compared to the control group at both the first week and also at the end of the protocol. Additionally, a higher number of patients in the drug group (32 out of 50, 64%) achieved complete wound healing compared to the control group (20 out of 44, 20.45%) (Ghanadian et al., 2022).

Mucositis: In an RCT, the efficacy of syrup made from *P. major* seeds was investigated in 46 cancer patients with radiation-induced mucositis for 7 weeks. Mucositis severity was substantially lower in the intervention group than in the placebo group. Moreover, during the radiotherapy period, patients in the intervention group experienced considerably less pain than those in the placebo group (Soltani et al., 2020).

In another trial, 45 solid tumor patients with grade II–III mucositis were randomized to one of three treatments, consisting of sodium bicarbonate 5% aqueous solution together with: an additional dose of sodium bicarbonate 5% aqueous solution, *P. major* leaves extract, or chlorhexidine 0.12%. The results showed that 68% (n=34) of patients achieved grade 0 mucositis, with those using the double sodium bicarbonate rinse healing in 5 days on average versus 7 days for the chlorhexidine group and 7 days for *P. major* group. The pain experienced by the participants lessened over the 14 days of treatment, but differences in pain intensity between the three groups did not show statistical significance (Cabrera-Jaime et al., 2018).

NAFLD: In an RCT, 74 patients with NAFLD were given either 2 g of *P. major* seeds or placebo twice daily for 12 weeks. All patients were instructed to follow the daily exercise and food modification suggestions. *P. major* group showed significant reduction in ALT, AST, TAG, waist circumference, and grade of fatty liver in ultrasonography compared to the placebo group (Jazayeri et al., 2021).

Colitis: In an RCT, 51 patients with ulcerative colitis were randomized to receive roasted *P. major* seeds (3,600 mg per day) or roasted wheat flour as placebo for 8 weeks. According to the results, abdominal tenderness, gastroesophageal reflux, gastric pain, distension, anal pain, and blood in stool significantly decreased in *P. major* group compared to the placebo (Baghizadeh et al., 2021).

Heavy menstrual bleeding: In a double-blind RCT, 60 women suffering from uterine leiomyoma and heavy menstrual bleeding randomly received a vaginal suppository from the leaf extract of *P. major* or placebo every 8 hours in the first 3 days of menstruation for three menstruation cycles. The mean blood loss decreased in the intervention group. Moreover, the mean of bleeding duration improved in the *P. major* group (Navaei et al., 2020).

Labor: A study has evaluated the effects of *P. major* in reduction of postpartum hemorrhage as an emergency in midwifery. For this purpose, 105 pregnant women received rectal suppositories (one at the starting point and five doses with 30 min intervals) following removal of the placenta and embryonic membranes. In both groups, infusion of 30 units' oxytocin in 1,000 mL crystalloids was given after delivery as per the hospital routine practice. Average bleeding rate at the end of the first 4 hours after delivery was significantly decreased in *P. major* group compared to placebo (Zahra et al., 2022).

Chronic bronchitis: An old study without precise information about the dose and route of administration, reported the positive effect of *P. major* on the subjective complaints as well as some indices of external respiration. As a result, it was indicated that in 80% of cases, a quick effect on subjective complaints and objective findings was found. The preparation was well tolerated and did not show any toxic effects on gastrointestinal tract, liver, kidneys, hemopoiesis (Matev Angelova et al., 1982).

Preclinical Evidence

Wound: The wound-healing activities of three different doses (0.01, 0.1, and 1.0 mg/mL) of aqueous extract and ethanolic extract from dried leaves of *P. major* were investigated in *ex vivo* porcine wound-healing model. The results showed that both extracts enhanced wound-healing activity. Furthermore, it was reported that ethanolic extract in concentration of 1.0 mg/mL had the maximum wound-healing activity when compared to the other samples. The same concentration of *P. major* aqueous extract resulted in improved wound-healing activity, but not to the same extent as ethanolic ones (Zubair et al., 2016).

Peptic ulcer: The results of evaluating antiulcer activity of *P. major* leaves on alcohol and aspirin-induced stomach ulcers showed that a combination of methanolic and aqueous extracts considerably reduced ulcer formation by 40% compared to the control group. Methanolic extract decreased ulcer formation by 29%, while the aqueous extract prevented ulcer formation by 37% (Atta and Mouneir, 2005).

Diarrhea: The effects of methanolic extract of *P. major* leaves were evaluated on castor oil-induced diarrhea and gastrointestinal movement in rats as well as the motility of duodenum isolated from newly slaughtered rabbits. *P. major* methanolic extract at dose of 1.6 mg/mL produced a transient stimulation followed by inhibition of duodenal motility (Atta and Mouneir, 2005).

Inflammation: The anti-inflammatory activity of various *P. major* leaf extracts including aqueous, methanolic and ethanolic extracts all of them at dose of 1,000 mg/kg was evaluated in acetaminophen-induced liver damage in rats. The extracts significantly reduced the proinflammatory cytokine levels and significantly increased the 11β-hydroxysteroid dehydrogenase type 1 enzyme activity (Hussan et al., 2015).

Pain: The antinociceptive activity of *P. major* leaves and seeds methanolic extracts was studied in an acetic acid-induced writhing and tail-flick tests. The results demonstrated that a 400 mg/kg oral dose of seed extract demonstrated a stronger antinociceptive activity against acetic acid-induced writhes compared to leaf extract at the same dose (Atta and El-Sooud, 2004).

ADVERSE REACTIONS

TPM Literature

The plant may be harmful to the lung, respiratory system, and spleen. Administration with honey or mastic gum could decline these unwanted effects (Aghili Khorasani 1771).

Current Evidence

Although *P. major* is a safe plant, it might cause side effects such as nausea, vomiting, diarrhea, anorexia, bloating, hypersensitivity, and dermatitis. In more acute situations of overdosing, life-threatening anaphylaxis can ensue (Nazarizadeh et al., 2013).

CONTRAINDICATIONS

TPM Literature

None.

Current Evidence

The plant is contraindicated in subjects with gastrointestinal obstruction or fecal impaction as well as in patients with difficulty swallowing due to the risk of esophageal obstruction (Gruenwald et al., 2007).

PREGNANCY AND LACTATION

TPM Literature

None.

Current Evidence

Although no detrimental constituents have been detected, the herb has not been examined in human pregnancy. As a result, it can be administered, but only with caution (Gardner and McGuffin, 2013; Kennedy et al., 2016).

DRUG INTERACTIONS

Warfarin: Great plantain leaves contain large amounts of vitamin K. So, it can be assumed to interact with warfarin and reduce its effects theoretically. However, no clinical evidence has been available yet (WebMD, January 2024).

METHOD OF ADMINISTRATION

TPM Literature

Distillate water of the aerial parts is recommended orally. The leaf juice can be used as an eye- or eardrop or as a mouthwash. Also, the leaf juice can be used topically as a lotion. The seeds can be taken orally or in the form of enema (Aghili Khorasani 1771).

Current Evidence

The leaf juice can be used orally or topically. The leaves can also be taken as an infusion (Spiteri, 2011; Therapeutic Research Faculty, 2013).

DOSAGE

Generally, 2–4 g of the herb can be used daily (Spiteri, 2011; Therapeutic Research Faculty, 2013). According to RCTs, 2–3.6 g per day of the major plantain seeds can be used orally.

REFERENCES

Adom MB, Taher M, Mutalabisin MF, et al. Chemical constituents and medical benefits of Plantago major. Biomedi Pharmacother. 2017;96:348–360.

Aghili Khorasani MH 1771. *Makhzan-al-Adviah* (*The treasury of drugs*) (rewritten by Shams Ardakani MR, Rahimi R, Farjadmand F, 1st ed.). Tehran: Tehran University of Medical Sciences; 2009.

Atta AH, El-Sooud KA. The antinociceptive effect of some Egyptian medicinal plant extracts. J Ethnopharmacol. 2004;95(2–3):235–238.

Atta AH, Mouneir SM. Evaluation of some medicinal plant extracts for antidiarrhoeal activity. Phytother Res. 2005;19(6):481–485.

Avicenna 1025. *Al-Qanoon fi al-Tibb* (*The canon of medicine*) (rewritten by Masoudi A, ed.). Tehran: Almaei; 2015.

Baghizadeh A, Davati A, Heidarloo AJ, et al. Efficacy of *Plantago major* seed in management of ulcerative colitis symptoms: A randomized, placebo controlled, clinical trial. Complement Ther Clin Pract. 2021;44:101444.

Cabrera-Jaime S, Martínez C, Ferro-García T, et al. Efficacy of *Plantago major*, chlorhexidine 0.12% and sodium bicarbonate 5% solution in the treatment of oral mucositis in cancer patients with solid tumour: A feasibility andomized triple-blind phase III clinical trial. Eur J Oncol Nurs. 2018;32:40–47.

Gardner Z, McGuffin M. *Botanical safety handbook*. Boca Raton: Taylor & Francis; 2013.

Ghanadian M, Soltani R, Homayouni A, et al. The effect of *Plantago major* hydroalcoholic extract on the healing of diabetic foot and pressure ulcers: A randomized open-label controlled clinical trial. Int J Low Extrem Wounds. 2022:15347346211070723.

Ghiasian M, Niroomandi Z, Dastan D, et al. Clinical and phytochemical studies of *Plantago major* in pressure ulcer treatment: A randomized controlled trial. Complement Ther Clin Pract. 2021;43:101325.

Gruenwald J, Brendler T, Jaenicke C. *PDR for herbal medicines*. Montvale: Thomson Reuters; 2007.

Hussan F, Mansor AS, Hassan SN, et al. Anti-inflammatory property of *Plantago major* leaf extract reduces the inflammatory reaction in experimental acetaminophen-induced liver injury. Evid-Based Complement Altern Med. 2015;2015:347861.

Jazayeri SF, Ghods R, Hashem Dabaghian F, Shojaii A, Moravej SA, Khadem E, Seyedian SS. The efficacy of plantago major seed on liver enzymes in nonalcoholic fatty liver disease: A randomized double-blind clinical trial. Evid-Based Complement Altern Med. 2021;2021:6693887.

Kennedy DA, Lupattelli A, Koren G, Nordeng H. Safety classification of herbal medicines used in pregnancy in a multinational study. BMC Complement Altern Med. 2016;16(1):102.

Matev M, Angelova I, Koĭchev A, et al. Clinical trial of a *Plantago major* preparation in the treatment of chronic bronchitis. Vutreshni Bolesti. 1982;21(2):133–137.

Navaei F, Ebrahimzadeh MA, Formi EN, et al. The effect of *Plantago major* vaginal supp on heavy menstrual bleeding patients with uterine leiomyoma: A double-blind randomized clinical trial. Pak J Med Health Sci. 2020;14(3):1678–1685.

Nazarizadeh A, Mikaili P, Moloudizargari M, et al. Therapeutic uses and pharmacological properties of *Plantago major* L. and its active constituents. J Basic Appl Sci Res. 2013;3(9):212–221.

Samuelsen AB. The traditional uses, chemical constituents and biological activities of Plantago major L. A review. J Ethnopharmacol. 2000;71(1-2):1–21.

Soltani GM, Hemati S, Sarvizadeh M, et al. Efficacy of the *Plantago major* L. syrup on radiation induced oral mucositis in head and neck cancer patients: A randomized, double blind, placebo-controlled clinical trial. Complement Ther Med. 2020;51:102397.

Spiteri M. *Herbal monographs including herbal medicinal products and food supplements*. Malta: University of Malta; 2011.

Therapeutic Research Faculty. *Natural medicines: Comprehensive database*. 13th ed. Stockton: Pharmacist's Letter; 2013.

Zahra K, Kimiya D, Nahid G, et al. The effects of rectal suppositories of *Plantago major* and *Anetheum graveolens* on postpartum hemorrhage: A randomized triple blinded clinical trial. J Herb Med. 2022;31:100526.

Zubair M, Nybom H, Lindholm C, et al. Promotion of wound healing by *Plantago major* L. leaf extracts: Ex-vivo experiments confirm experiences from traditional medicine. Nat Prod Res. 2016;30(5):622–624.

30 *Plantago ovata* Forssk., *Plantago psyllium* L.

Maryam Kabiri and Mohammad M. Zarshenas

Scientific name: *Plantago ovata* Forssk., *Plantago psyllium* L.
Family: Plantaginaceae
Common names:

- **English:** Blond plantain, blond psyllium, ispagol, ispaghula
- **Persian:** *'espağūl, 'esfarzeh, 'esparzeh*
- **Arabic:** *bizr al-qaṭūnah*

Medicinal part(s): Seeds, seed husk (Figure 30.1)
Temperament (nature): Seed husk is cold in the third degree and wet in the first to second degree
Major chemical constituents:

- **Psyllium seed:**
  - **Mucilage (20–30%):** Chiefly arabinoxylans and glacturonosidorhamnoses
  - Fatty oil
  - **Iridoids:** Aucubin
- **Psyllium seed epidermis:**
  - Mucilage (parent substance arabinoxylans) (Gruenwald et al., 2007)

THERAPEUTIC USE

TPM Literature

Seeds of the herb are recommended for thirst relief. It is an anti-inflammatory agent either generally or in the GI tract, laxative, and a remedy for pleuritis, yellow bile-related disorders, and modification of humoral balance in the body. Topical application of the mucilage or the crushed seeds with rose water is helpful for the relief of hot-tempered headaches. Topical use of the mucilage is also recommended as an emollient for hair and in hair split ends and breakage (trichoptilosis and trichorrhexis nodosa), especially when mixed with sweet violet oil. Oral intake of the seed decoction is a demulcent for the respiratory tract and chest pain. The seeds macerated in hot water and mixed with sugar or oxymel can be orally taken as a laxative. On the other hand, roasted seeds that are rubbed with rose oil have antidiarrheal effects due to astringent properties. Furthermore, oral intake of the seeds has soothing effects on GI ulcers and is thus useful in colitis and cramps. It is recommended for pediatric intestinal ulcers, especially in combination with sweet almond oil. It is also an antipyretic agent. In the form of a poultice, mixed with vinegar and rose oil, it is used for hot-tempered joint pains, gout, and decrease in local inflammations such as mastoiditis, lymphadenopathy, nerve and skin complications (Aghili Khorasani 1771; Avicenna 1025).

DOI: 10.1201/b22971-30

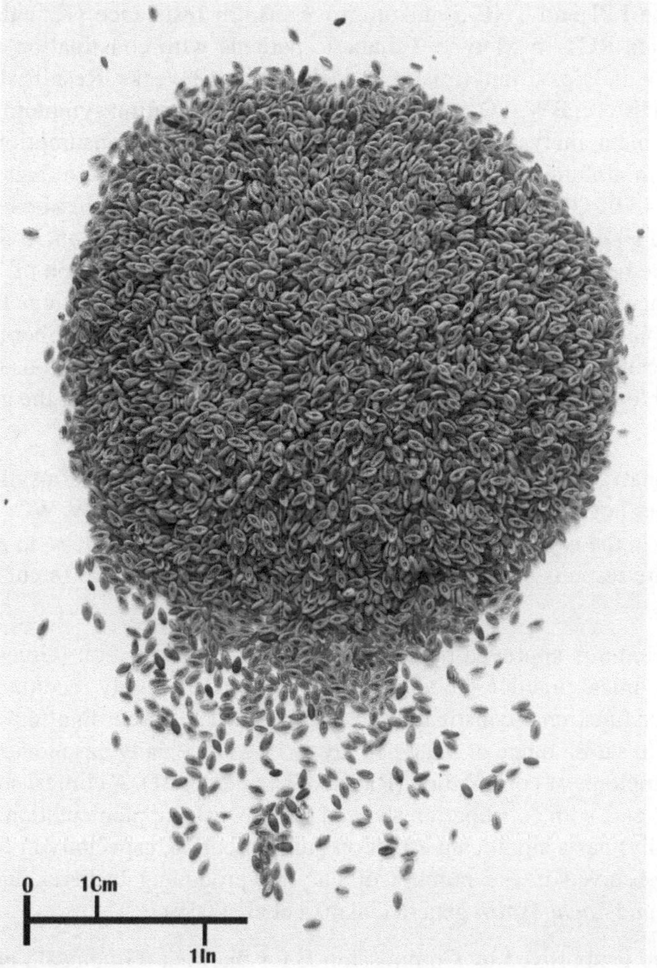

FIGURE 30.1 Psyllium seeds.

Current Evidence

Clinical Evidence

Hypercholesterolemia and hypertriglyceridemia: Psyllium seed is approved by Commission E for hypercholesterolemia. According to a systematic review and meta-analysis on 28 RCTs, *P. ovata* with a median daily dose of 10.2 g and treatment period of 8 weeks can significantly reduce LDL-C, non-HDL-C, and ApoB (Jovanovski et al., 2018). Also, another meta-analysis including three RCTs demonstrated that addition of psyllium husk with a daily dosage of 7–15 g to therapeutic regimen of hyperlipidemic patients under treatment with statins for 4–12 weeks has a significant effect on lowering LDL-C, similar to doubling the dose of statins (Brum et al., 2018). In a placebo-controlled RCT in 51 hypercholestrolemic children and adolescents, 8-week oral intake of psyllium (7 g daily) caused a significant reduction of TC and LDL-C (Ribas et al., 2015). In another placebo-controlled RCT on 113 obese adolescents, 7-week supplementation with *P. psyllium* (10 g daily) resulted in a significant decrease in small dense LDL-C and IL-6 (González et al., 2021).

Type 2 diabetes: An open-labeled RCT in 37 type 2 diabetic patients showed that daily intake of 7 g psyllium powder for 2 weeks along with a moderate-carbohydrate low-calorie diet can significantly reduce FPI and TNF-α and improve insulin resistance (Kamalpour et al., 2018). A placebo-controlled RCT in 51 type 2 diabetic patients with constipation assessed the therapeutic effect of 10 g daily psyllium (mixed in cookies) for 12 weeks. Results showed a significant reduction of FBS, HbA1c, BW, TC, and TAG, as well as constipation symptoms (Noureddin et al., 2018). Based on a meta-analysis including eight RCTs, psyllium consumption with a daily dose of 10–15 g and a minimum treatment duration of 8 weeks causes significant decrease in FBS, HbA1c, TAG, and LDL-C in diabetic patients; though, the effects were not significant regarding TC, BW, BMI, and HDL-C (Xiao et al., 2020). Another meta-analysis on 35 RCTs demonstrated that psyllium intake before meals has a significant effect on the reduction of FBS and HbA1c in type 2 diabetic patients, while it showed a less potent effect on prediabetic patients, and no effect on euglycemic subjects (Gibb et al., 2015). Overall, psyllium dietary fibers have been widely utilized as pharmaceutical supplements and food additives in processed foods to help with weight control and lower blood cholesterol levels in hyperlipidemia and regulate the glucose level in diabetic patients.

Obesity: A meta-analysis of 22 RCTs assessing the antiobesity effects of psyllium concluded that this supplement does not have a significant effect on the reduction of BW, WC, and BMI; however, high heterogeneity in the type of psyllium preparation, dosage, and follow-up period, sample size, and study design are responsible for controversial results reported in different RCTs (Darooghegi et al., 2020).

Constipation: Psyllium is approved by Commission E for constipation (Gruenwald et al., 2007). Also, a review of clinical practice guidelines showed that it is highly recommended as a suitable treatment option for functional constipation (Dai et al., 2019). According to a meta-analysis on 9 RCTs, psyllium with a dose range of 3.5 g per day to 11 g twice daily has moderate evidence (grade B) to reduce the symptoms of constipation (Rao and Brenner, 2021). A clinical study in eight healthy subjects and 16 patients with constipation showed that 1-week supplementation with psyllium husk (7 g three times daily) has a significant effect on gut microbiota, especially in constipated patients. An increase was observed in the number of butyrate-producing bacteria, including *Roseburia*, *Faecalibacterium*, and *Lachnospira* genera (Jalanka et al., 2019).

Diarrhea: Psyllium is approved by Commission E for diarrhea (Gruenwald et al., 2007). A pilot clinical study in 60 cancerous patients with radiotherapy-induced diarrhea showed that psyllium can significantly reduce the incidence and duration of diarrhea, as well as the need for conventional antidiarrheal medication (Murphy et al., 2000). Psyllium has also been studied in diarrhea in hospitalized patients receiving enteral nutrition; however, a meta-analysis on three RCTs mentioned the antidiarrheal effect of psyllium in these patients is not yet completely confirmed (Kaewdech et al., 2022).

Prebiotic potential effects: In a clinical study, 11 healthy women consumed 7.0 g per day of psyllium seed husk for 1 month, and the viability of *Bifidobacteria* in their feces was monitored at different intervals. The results showed that although fecal counts increased significantly in 6 out of the 11 women, the average fecal content of viable *Bifidobacteria* was not significantly affected. *In vitro*, tests were carried out on *Bifidobacteria* strains isolated from treated women, but they failed to confirm the prebiotic potential of undigested psyllium seed husk. However, after exposure to simulate the gastric and pancreatic juices that mimicked physical and chemical changes during human gut transit, *Bifidobacteria* isolates were able to metabolize psyllium seed husk as a source of carbon in a sugar-deprived growth medium. The study concludes that psyllium seed husk can only be metabolized by *Bifidobacteria* after partial hydrolysis and that the bifidogenic potential of psyllium seed husk is more noticeable in healthy women with low levels of fecal *Bifidobacteria* before treatment (Elli et al., 2008).

Hypertension: A 6-month intervention with 3.5 g of psyllium powder, three times daily in 141 overweight hypertensive patients showed a significant reduction in SBP (about 2 mmHg) and DBP, as well as LDL-C, TAG, ApoB, FBS, FPI, HOM-IR, HbA1c, and BMI compared with baseline values (Cicero et al., 2007). On the other hand, a 12-week RCT supplementation with *P. ovata* fiber (7 g three times daily) in overweight/obese subjects caused no significant effect on blood pressure compared with placebo (Pal et al., 2012). A meta-analysis including 11 RCTs suggests that psyllium consumption has a significant effect on the reduction of systolic blood pressure, with higher potency in subsets of hypertensive patients and a treatment period longer than 8 weeks (Clark et al., 2020).

Dry eye: In a placebo-controlled RCT on 68 patients with dry eye, 6-week treatment with a *P. ovata* mucilage 1% solution as an ophthalmic drop (four times daily) caused a significant improvement in patient's symptoms based on Ocular Surface Disease Index score (Haji-Ali-Nili et al., 2019).

Chemotherapy-induced oral mucositis: In a placebo-controlled crossover RCT on 28 breast cancer patients under chemotherapy, *P. ovata* husk was administered in the form of a mouthwash containing 0.5 of the husks in 30 mL of water, mixed with three drops of vinegar. Treatments were used three times daily from the first day of chemotherapy up to 2 weeks. Herbal mouthwash showed a significant improvement in mucositis and pain severity, xerostomia grade, and quality of life, in comparison to placebo (Hasheminasab et al., 2020).

Colitis: An open-label multicenter RCT on 102 patients with colitis compared the effect of psyllium seeds (10 g, twice daily) with mesalamine (500 mg, three times daily) or mesalamine and psyllium for 12 months. In addition to a significant increase in fecal butyrate in psyllium-treated patients, psyllium showed a similar effect to mesalamine in maintenance of remission in these patients. The combination of psyllium and mesalamine was numerically but not statistically better than each individual treatment (Fernández-Bañares et al., 1999).

Changes in levodopa pharmacokinetics: The use of *P. ovata* husk therapy could potentially improve gastrointestinal symptoms in patients with Parkinson's disease. However, it is important to investigate whether this therapy affects the pharmacokinetics of levodopa, which is critical for maintaining constant plasma concentrations and reducing clinical fluctuations. The purpose of this RCT was to evaluate the impact of *P. ovata* husk on levodopa pharmacokinetics in well-controlled Parkinson's patients. The study involved 18 volunteers who received either *P. ovata* husk or a placebo in addition to their usual levodopa/carbidopa oral dose. Levodopa pharmacokinetics and various biochemical parameters were assessed on days 0, 14, and 35. The results showed that while C_{max} levels were similar across all treatments, the administration of *P. ovata* husk resulted in a reduction in levodopa concentration peaks and more stable concentrations. No significant differences were found in TC or TAG levels. Overall, the administration of *P. ovata* husk led to smoothing and homogenization of levodopa absorption, resulting in more stable and higher concentrations, which could benefit Parkinson's patients (Fernandez-Martinez et al., 2014).

Preclinical Evidence

Wound: In a rat model of second-degree burn wound, topical application of *P. ovata* seed powder for 3 weeks showed a significantly better wound healing compared with negative control and similar to silver sulfadiazine as the positive control (Jalilimanesh et al., 2021). Also, there are several attempts to formulate psyllium fiber together with other natural/synthetic polymers and antibiotics or wound-healing agents as wound-dressing plasters; however, most of these novel formulations are still under development (Shaikh et al., 2021).

Colitis: An animal study evaluated the effect of a diet enriched with 0.5% or 5% psyllium fiber in DSS-induced colitis in germ free and specific pathogen free mice. Results showed a significant improvement in the severity of intestinal inflammation via microbiota-dependent and microbiota-independent mechanisms (Llewellyn et al., 2018). Another study in DSS-induced colitis in mice also showed that a diet containing 5% *P. ovata* husk can alleviate colitis symptoms and inflammation (Lin et al., 2020). *P. ovata* fiber supplementation with 5–10% dietary concentration could also cause an improvement in colitis symptoms and colonic microbiota (Ogata et al., 2017). Additionally, in high fructose-induced acute colitis, psyllium could highly prevent colitis symptoms and tumorigenesis via modification of gut microbiota (Nishiguchi et al., 2021).

Inflammation in GI: In an animal study, transgenic rats were fed a fiber-rich diet supplemented with psyllium seeds for 13 weeks, and their colonic inflammatory status was evaluated. According to the results, psyllium improved the intestinal cytoarchitecture and decreased the levels of proinflammatory mediators such as NO, leukotriene B4, and TNF-α. The colonic contents of fiber-treated rats showed a significant increase in the production of SCFA, particularly butyrate, and propionate, compared to untreated rats. *In vitro*, studies demonstrated that butyrate and propionate acted synergistically to inhibit TNF-α production. Therefore, dietary fiber supplementation improved colonic damage in rats with transgenic colitis by increasing SCFA production, which inhibited the production of proinflammatory mediators (Rodrıguez-Cabezas et al., 2003).

Metabolic syndrome: Four groups of adult obese Zucker rats were given different diets for 10 weeks. These diets included a standard diet, a diet supplemented with cellulose, a diet supplemented with methylcellulose, and a diet supplemented with *P. ovata* husks. The rats that were given the *P. ovata* husks-supplemented diet showed improvements in hyperlipidemia, hyperinsulinemia, hyperleptinemia, increased TNF-α, and reduced adiponectin secretion by adipose tissue. Additionally, these rats had a lower hepatic lipid content and activation of the signaling pathway of AMP-protein kinase in the liver. Rats that were given the methylcellulose-supplemented diet showed improvements in body weight, hyperlipidemia, circulating free fatty acids concentration, and adipose tissue secretion of adiponectin and TNF-α. However, only the cellulose-supplemented diet reduced circulating levels of free fatty acids. The study found that soluble dietary fibers, such as those in *P. ovata* husks, were more effective in treating metabolic syndrome than insoluble fiber (Galisteo et al., 2010).

ADVERSE REACTIONS

TPM Literature

Oral use of crushed seeds may cause severe complications and even death due to the release and adhesion of toxic compounds to the lumen's internal side; thus, for oral use, only the intact (uncrushed) seeds or the seed husk should be administered (Aghili Khorasani 1771).

Current Evidence

In oral ingestion, psyllium should be taken with enough amount of liquid; otherwise, it may cause choking or GI obstruction.

Allergic reactions including wheezing, sneezing, chest congestion, skin rash, rhinitis, and asthma have been reported, mostly due to respiratory exposure to psyllium powder. Also, anaphylaxis is reported for oral use of psyllium (Khalili et al., 2003; Gruenwald et al., 2007). There may be a cross-sensitivity in people with a history of allergy to *Plantago lanceolata* L. pollen, grass pollen, or melon (Ulbricht, 2010).

CONTRAINDICATIONS

TPM Literature

None.

Current Evidence

Psyllium is a bulk laxative. Accordingly, patients suffering from obstruction of the GI tract, fecal impaction, and abnormal narrowing of the intestine should avoid it. Moreover, in case of difficulty swallowing or esophageal stenosis, especially in the elderly, psyllium should be avoided due to the risk of esophageal obstruction.

Due to its blood sugar-lowering effect, psyllium should be avoided in uncontrolled diabetes (Gruenwald et al., 2007). Due to the inhibition of pancreatic lipase, psyllium is contraindicated in patients with exocrine pancreatic insufficiency.

PREGNANCY AND LACTATION

TPM Literature

According to TPM, any substance which is mucilaginous, including psyllium, is contraindicated during pregnancy.

Current Evidence

FDA has categorized over-the-counter psyllium preparations as generally safe (category B) during pregnancy. Psyllium is generally safe on lactating mothers (Anderson, 2021).

DRUG INTERACTIONS

Due to the high content of mucilage, psyllium can delay absorbance of other drugs, and thus, conventional drugs should be taken 1 hour before or several hours after psyllium.

Due to the blood sugar-lowering effect, dose adjustment is necessary when used along with insulin and oral antihyperglycemic drugs (Gardner and McGuffin, 2013).

METHOD OF ADMINISTRATION

TPM Literature

Only intact (uncrushed) psyllium seeds should be used for oral intake. The seeds may be macerated in water, rose water, or oxymel for oral use. It can also be prepared as a decoction. For the antidiarrheal effect, the seeds should be roasted (heated without oil or water) and then rubbed with rose oil. The mucilage or hydrated seeds are topically used for hair and skin care. Crushed seeds may also be used topically (Aghili Khorasani 1771).

Current Evidence

Psyllium seeds should be mixed with enough water or juice, i.e., at least 250 mL of liquid for each 3–5 g of husk or 7 g of seeds (Gruenwald et al., 2007).

DOSAGE

Adults: 2.5–7.5 g, up to three times daily.
Children (6–12 years): 2 g, up to three times daily (Gruenwald et al., 2007).

REFERENCES

Aghili Khorasani MH 1771. *Makhzan-al-Advиah* (*The treasury of drugs*) (rewritten by Shams Ardakani MR, Rahimi R, Farjadmand F, 1st ed.). Tehran: Tehran University of Medical Sciences; 2009.

Anderson PO. Laxative and cathartic use during breastfeeding. Breastfeed Med. 2021;16(9):675–677.

Avicenna 1025. *Al-Qanoon fi al-Tibb* (*The canon of medicine*) (rewritten by Masoudi A, ed.). Tehran: Almaei; 2015.

Brum J, Ramsey D, McRorie J, et al. Meta-analysis of usefulness of psyllium fiber as adjuvant antilipid therapy to enhance cholesterol lowering efficacy of statins. Am J Cardiol. 2018;122(7):1169–1174.

Cicero AF, Derosa G, Manca M, et al. Different effect of psyllium and guar dietary supplementation on blood pressure control in hypertensive overweight patients: A six-month, randomized clinical trial. Clin Exp Hypertens. 2007;29(6):383–394.

Clark CC, Salek M, Aghabagheri E, Jafarnejad S. The effect of psyllium supplementation on blood pressure: A systematic review and meta-analysis of randomized controlled trials. Korean J Intern Med. 2020;35(6):1385–1399.

Dai L, Zhong LL, Ji G. Irritable bowel syndrome and functional constipation management with integrative medicine: A systematic review. World J Clin Cases. 2019;7(21):3486.

Darooghegi Mofrad M, Mozaffari H, Mousavi SM, et al. The effects of psyllium supplementation on body weight, body mass index and waist circumference in adults: A systematic review and dose-response meta-analysis of randomized controlled trials. Crit Rev Food Sci Nutr. 2020;60(5):859–872.

Elli M, Cattivelli D, Soldi S, et al. Evaluation of prebiotic potential of refined psyllium (*Plantago ovata*) fiber in healthy women. J Clin Gastroenterol. 2008;42:S174–176.

Fernandez-Banares F, Hinojosa J, Sanchez-Lombrana JL, et al. Randomized Clinical Trial of Plantago Ovata Seeds (Dietary Fiber) As Compared With Mesalamine in Maintaining Remission in Ulcerative Colitis. Am J Gastroenterol. 1999;94(2):427–433.

Fernandez-Martinez MN, Hernandez-Echevarria L, Sierra-Vega M, et al. A randomised clinical trial to evaluate the effects of *Plantago ovata* husk in Parkinson patients: Changes in levodopa pharmacokinetics and biochemical parameters. BMC Complement Altern Med. 2014;14(1):1–10.

Galisteo M, Morón R, Rivera L, et al. *Plantago ovata* husks-supplemented diet ameliorates metabolic alterations in obese Zucker rats through activation of AMP-activated protein kinase: Comparative study with other dietary fibers. Clin Nutr. 2010;29(2):261–267.

Gardner Z, McGuffin M. *Botanical safety handbook*. Boca Raton: Taylor & Francis; 2013.

Gibb RD, McRorie Jr JW, Russell DA, et al. Psyllium fiber improves glycemic control proportional to loss of glycemic control: A meta-analysis of data in euglycemic subjects, patients at risk of type 2 diabetes mellitus, and patients being treated for type 2 diabetes mellitus. Am J Clin Nutr. 2015;102(6):1604–1614.

González AP, Flores-Ramírez A, Gutiérrez-Castro KP, et al. Reduction of small dense LDL and Il-6 after intervention with Plantago psyllium in adolescents with obesity: a parallel, double blind, randomized clinical trial. Eur J Pediatr. 2021;180(8):2493–2503.

Gruenwald J, Brendler T, Jaenicke C. *PDR for herbal medicines*. Montvale: Thomson Reuters; 2007.

Haji-Ali-Nili N, Khoshzaban F, Karimi M, et al. Effect of a natural eye drop, made of *Plantago ovata* mucilage on improvement of dry eye symptoms: A randomized, double-blind clinical trial. Iran J Pharm Res. 2019;18(3):1602–1611.

Hasheminasab FS, Hashemi SM, Dehghan A, et al. Effects of a *Plantago ovata*-based herbal compound in prevention and treatment of oral mucositis in patients with breast cancer receiving chemotherapy: A double-blind, randomized, controlled crossover trial. J Integr Med. 2020;18(3):214–221.

Jalanka J, Major G, Murray K, et al. The effect of psyllium husk on intestinal microbiota in constipated patients and healthy controls. Int J Mol Sci. 2019;20(2):433.

Jalilimanesh M, Azhdari M, Mirjalili A, et al. The comparison of clinical and histopathological effects of topical psyllium (*Plantago ovata*) powder and silver sulfadiazine on second-degree burn wound healing in rats. World J Plast Surg. 2021;10(1):96–103.

Jovanovski E, Yashpal S, Komishon A, et al. Effect of psyllium (*Plantago ovata*) fiber on LDL cholesterol and alternative lipid targets, non-HDL cholesterol and apolipoprotein B: A systematic review and meta-analysis of randomized controlled trials. Am J Clin Nutr. 2018;108(5):922–932.

Kaewdech A, Sripongpun P, Wetwittayakhlang P, Churuangsuk C. The effect of fiber supplementation on the prevention of diarrhea in hospitalized patients receiving enteral nutrition: A meta-analysis of randomized controlled trials with the GRADE assessment. Front Nut. 2022;9:1008464.

Kamalpour M, Ghalandari H, Nasrollahzadeh J. Short-term supplementation of a moderate carbohydrate diet with psyllium reduces fasting plasma insulin and tumor necrosis factor-α in patients with type 2 diabetes mellitus. J Diet Suppl. 2018;15(4):507–515.

Khalili B, Bardana JE, Yunginger JW. Psyllium-associated anaphylaxis and death: A case report and review of the literature. Ann Allergy Asthma Immunol. 2003;91(6):579–584.

Lin CY, Lee AH, Chiu KK, et al. *Saccharomyces cerevisiae* fermentation product did not attenuate clinical signs, but psyllium husk has protective effects in a murine dextran sulfate sodium-induced colitis model. Curr Dev Nutr. 2020;4(11):nzaa159.

Llewellyn SR, Britton GJ, Contijoch EJ, et al. Interactions between diet and the intestinal microbiota alter intestinal permeability and colitis severity in mice. Gastroenterology. 2018;154(4):1037–1046.

Murphy J, Stacey D, Crook J, et al. Testing control of radiation induced diarrhea with a psyllium bulking agent: A pilot study. Can Oncol Nurs J. 2000;10(3):96–100.

Nishiguchi R, Basu S, Staab HA, et al. Dietary interventions to prevent high-fructose diet-associated worsening of colitis and colitis-associated tumorigenesis in mice. Carcinogenesis. 2021;42(6):842–852.

Noureddin S, Mohsen J, Payman A. Effects of psyllium vs. placebo on constipation, weight, glycemia, and lipids: A randomized trial in patients with type 2 diabetes and chronic constipation. Complement Ther Med. 2018;40:1–7.

Ogata M, Ogita T, Tari H, et al. Supplemental psyllium fibre regulates the intestinal barrier and inflammation in normal and colitic mice. Br J Nutr. 2017;118(9):661–672.

Pal S, Khossousi A, Binns C, et al. The effects of 12-week psyllium fibre supplementation or healthy diet on blood pressure and arterial stiffness in overweight and obese individuals. Br J Nutr. 2012;107(5):725–734.

Rao SS, Brenner DM. Efficacy and safety of over-the-counter therapies for chronic constipation: An updated systematic review. Am J Gastroenterol. 2021;116(6):1156–1181.

Ribas SA, Cunha DB, Sichieri R, da Silva LC. Effects of psyllium on LDL-cholesterol concentrations in Brazilian children and adolescents: A randomised, placebo-controlled, parallel clinical trial. Br J Nutr. 2015;113(1):134–141.

Rodrıguez-Cabezas ME, Galvez J, Camuesco D, et al. Intestinal anti-inflammatory activity of dietary fiber (*Plantago ovata* seeds) in HLA-B27 transgenic rats. Clin Nutr. 2003;22(5):463–471.

Shaikh MA, Gilhotra R, Pathak S, et al. Current update on psyllium and alginate incorporate for interpenetrating polymer network (IPN) and their biomedical applications. Int J Biol Macromol. 2021;191:432–444.

Ulbricht CE. *Mosby's natural standard herb & supplement guide*. St. Luis. Elsevier, 2010.

Xiao Z, Chen H, Zhang Y, et al. The effect of psyllium consumption on weight, body mass index, lipid profile, and glucose metabolism in diabetic patients: A systematic review and dose–response meta-analysis of randomized controlled trials. Phytother Res. 2020;34(6):1237–1247.

31 *Quercus infectoria* Oliv., *Quercus brantii* Lindl.

Mozhgan MehriArdestani

Scientific name: *Quercus infectoria* Oliv., *Quercus brantii* Lindl.
Family: Fagaceae
Common names:

- **English:** Oak gall
- **Persian:** *māzū*
- **Arabic:** *'afiṣ*

Medicinal part: Gall (Figure 31.1)
Temperament (nature): Cold in the first degree and dry in the second degree
Major chemical constituents:

- ***Q. infectoria* gall:**
  - **Tannins (50–70%):** Gallotannins, ellagitannins
  - **Phenolic acids:** Gallic acid, catechin hydrate, caffeic acid, ellagic acid, *p*-hydroxybenzoic acid, vanillic acid
  - **Flavonoids:** Amentoflavone and isocryptomerin
  - **Triterpenoids:** Roburic acid, nyctanthic acid, methyl-oleanolate, methyl-betulate
  - **Steroids:** β-sitosterol (Elham et al., 2020)
  - **Fatty acid:** Oleic acid, palmitic acid, linoleic acid, stearic acid (Başyiğit et al., 2020)

In limited studies on *Q. brantii* gall, the presence of flavonoids and gallic acid has been confirmed (Noori et al., 2015; Khanavi et al., 2014).

THERAPEUTIC USE

TPM Literature

Oak gall is generally a very potent astringent agent. The powdered oak gall controls nosebleed. Ocular administration of its decoction is effective in blepharitis and epiphora. The use of its decoction in the form of mouthwash, especially with vinegar, as well as rubbing its powder on the teeth strengthens the teeth and gums and is useful for gingivitis and periodontitis by preventing dental infections. Moreover, in the same medicinal forms, it is useful in the treatment of aphthous stomatitis, dental cavities, toothache, oral wounds, sialorrhea, and prevents tooth decay. Oral consumption of its ground powder with water has been suggested for chronic diarrhea, intestinal ulcers, hypermenorrhea, and vaginal discharge. Topical decoction (especially with vinegar) is used in early stages of the erysipelas, early stages of psoriasis, melasma, alopecia, and vitiligo. Sprinkling the oak gall powder on the healed wound can reduce the size of the keloid scars. Poultice of oak gall is

DOI: 10.1201/b22971-31

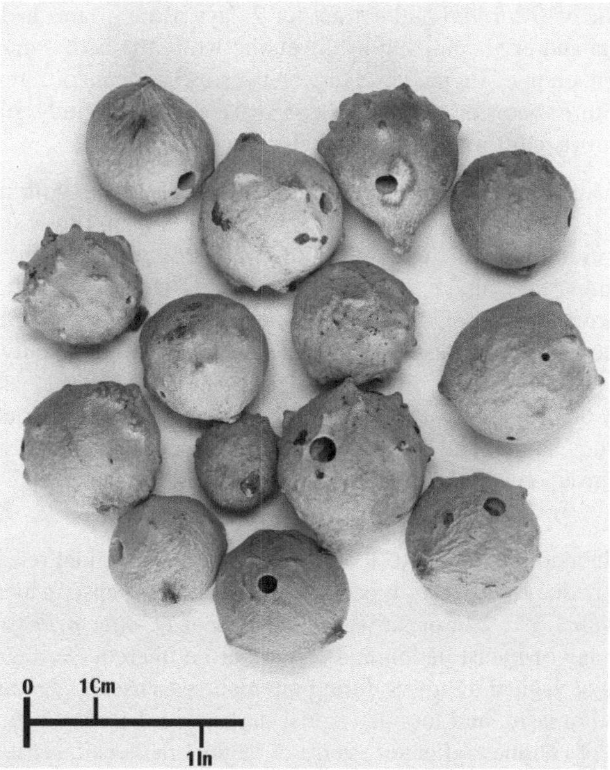

FIGURE 31.1 Oak gall.

effective on inflammation and prevents the progression of wounds, acne, and anal swellings. Oak gall is used for bone fracture healing in the form of poultice. Oak gall decoction is a dying agent for gray hairs. Also, its topical preparation eliminates malodorous sweat and heavy perspiration (Aghili Khorasani 1771; Avicenna 1025).

CURRENT EVIDENCE

Clinical Evidence

Gingivitis: In a clinical study in 35 patients with gingivitis, *Q. infectria* gall powder was topically applied twice a day, in the morning and before bedtime which could reduce the size of plaques and gingival progress after 2 weeks of treatment (Alhamadani et al., 2020). In a double-blind RCT in 20 cases of chronic gingivitis, 7-day administration of *Q. infectoria* gall mouthwash (200 g of gall powder macerated in 600 mL of water) could significantly reduce plaque index and gingival index in comparison with baseline (Choudhary et al., 2015).

Vaginitis: In an RCT on 84 women with bacterial vaginosis, patients were treated with either *Q. infectoria* gall cream (methanolic extract 2.5%) or metronidazole. For each group, 5 g of the product was applied intravaginally for 5 consecutive days, and all the signs and symptoms were assessed after 4–7 days from treatment completion. Bacterial vaginosis was treated in 82.1% patients in the herbal intervention group and in 87.5% patients in metronidazole group (Afzali et al., 2020). In another study, 89 women with vaginal candidiasis randomly received clotrimazole vaginal cream

(1%) or vaginal douche of *Q. brantii* gall extract for 7 days. Both groups had significant improvement of vaginal edema and erythema, and dyspareunia; while the herbal intervention had a more significant effect on reduction of vaginal discharge. Also, no significant difference was seen in terms of colony count of cultures between the two groups at the end of the study, suggesting similar efficacy for oak gall cream vs. clotrimazole (Moshfeghy et al., 2018).

Diabetic foot ulcer: An RCT was performed in 51 diabetic patients with ulcers (Wagner Ulcer Classification grades 1–3), who received standard wound treatment (normal saline solution) plus *Q. infectoria* gall solution (ethanolic extract diluted as a 30% w/v solution) or the standard solution alone for 3 months. Percentage reduction in wound size was significantly greater in the herbal intervention group than the control since week 4. During week 4, rapid wound healing with 60% wound size reduction was observed in oak gall group vs. only 30% in the control group. Approximately 90% reduction in wound size was revealed in the oak gall group by week 8 compared with only 60% in the control group. By the end of the third month, the reduction was 91.51% and 76% in the oak gall and the control group, respectively. Furthermore, 80.77% of the patients in the study group achieved complete wound healing vs. only 20% in the control group (Chokpaisarn et al., 2020).

Vaginal relaxation: In a double-blind RCT on 120 women with vaginal relaxation who were candidate for colporrhaphy due to different types of pelvic organ prolapse, patients were divided into four groups treated with 1.5%, 2%, or 2.5% vaginal gels of *Q. infectoria* gall extract or placebo, 3 days after the final day of menstruation and 5 min before intercourse. Significant improvement was observed in sense of vaginal tightness during intercourse, sense of vaginal lubrication, sense of sexual satisfaction and orgasm, and loss of vaginal dryness in the intervention groups. Moreover, lack of orgasm, sense of calmness after sex, sense of vaginal mass exit, sense of air outflow during intercourse, loss of libido, and urinary incontinence were significantly decreased in patients treated with 2.5% oak gall gel vs. other groups (Lorzadeh et al., 2016).

Preclinical Evidence

Wound: In an excision wound model in diabetic mice, 5% and 10% *Q. infectoria* gall ointment were topically assessed as a wound healing treatment. Compared with control treatment, oak gall showed a significant improvement of wound healing, collagen deposition, and reepithelialization, as well as a reduction in inflammatory markers, i.e., IL-6 and TNF-α. Moreover, a significant decrease in MDA, along with an improvement of total antioxidant capacity, VEGF, and Bcl-2 were reported (Dardmah et al., 2021).

Colitis: In TNBS-induced colitis in rats, *Q. brantii* gall powder and hydroethanolic extract were orally administered with a 500 mg/kg dose for 10 days. Macroscopic and microscopic scores, LPO, TAP, IL-1β, TNF-α, and MPO were significantly improved by both gall extract and powder and reached close to normal levels (Khanavi et al., 2014).

Peptic ulcer: The hydroalcoholic extract of *Q. brantii* gall was evaluated orally at doses of 250, 500, and 1,000 mg/kg in ethanol-induced peptic ulcer in rats. After 14 days of treatment, oak gall extract showed a significant improvement in ulcer healing, especially with the 1,000 mg/kg dose with respect to the thickness of ulcerated mucosa which was similar to the normal mucosa (Azizi et al., 2014).

ADVERSE REACTIONS

TPM Literature

It is harmful for throat and gum acacia, and tragacanth can ameliorate its damage. Ingestion with soft-boiled eggs can prevent this adverse event (Aghili Khorasani 1771).

Current Evidence

No health hazards are known in conjunction with the proper external administration of designated therapeutic dosages (Gruenwald et al., 2007).

In an acute toxicity study using *Q. infectoria* aqueous extract, three doses of 5, 7.5, and 10 g/kg were administered via enema to ICR mice. An experiment using the maximum tolerance dose, i.e., 10 g/kg, was also performed. Data were gathered for 14 days. Chronic toxicity was also evaluated on Wistar rats for over 180 consecutive days with 0.2, 0.8, and 2 g/kg of the extract. No death, adverse effect, or behavioral abnormalities were observed during the studies. After the administration of enema at study beginning, all the animals reacted with anal spasms. Their behaviors returned to normal several days later (Iminjan et al., 2014).

In two studies using vaginal cream and gel of oak gall extract, no side effect was reported (Afzali et al., 2020; Lorzadeh et al., 2016).

CONTRAINDICATIONS

TPM Literature

None.

Current Evidence

None.

PREGNANCY AND LACTATION

TPM Literature

None.

Current Evidence

None.

DRUG INTERACTIONS

Vancomycin: The combination of extracts from *Q. infectoria* gall and vancomycin displayed an additive bactericidal effect (Basir et al., 2012).

METHOD OF ADMINISTRATION

TPM Literature

Oak gall is recommended to be used orally as powder or decoction for internal purposes. It can also be used as a mouthwash or dental powder. It may be dropped in ear and nose.

For topical administration, oak gall decoction, sprinkle, or poultice of its powder can be used (Aghili Khorasani 1771; Avicenna 1025).

Current Evidence

Preparations of the whole, cut, and powdered drug are recommended for internal and external applications (Gruenwald et al., 2007).

DOSAGE

Most modern references suggest local use of oak gall. Up to 3 g of the gall can be orally used (Ministry of Health & Family Welfare, Government of India, 2007).

REFERENCES

Afzali E, Siahposh A, Haghighi-Zadeh MH, Farajzadeh A, Abbaspoor Z. The effect of Quercus (oak gal) vaginal cream versus metronidazole vaginal gel on bacterial vaginosis: A double-blind randomized controlled trial. Complement Ther Med. 2020;52:102497.

Aghili Khorasani MH 1771. *Makhzan-al-Adviah* (*The treasury of drugs*) (rewritten by Shams Ardakani MR, Rahimi R, Farjadmand F, 1st ed.). Tehran: Tehran University of Medical Sciences; 2009.

Alhamadani AH, Saeed HA, Khayoon HA. Clinical study on the therapeutic effects of *Quercus infectoria* galls as oral powder in gingivitis and plaque patients. Indian J Forensic Med Toxicol. 2020;14:744–748.

Avicenna 1025. *Al-Qanoon fi al-Tibb* (*The canon of medicine*) (rewritten by Masoudi A, ed.). Tehran: Almaei; 2015.

Azizi S, Ghasemi Pirbalouti A, Amirmohammadi M. Effect of hydro-alcoholic extract of Persian oak (*Quercus brantii*) in experimentally gastric ulcer. Iran J Pharm Res. 2014;13(3):967–974.

Basri DF, Khairon R. Pharmacodynamic interaction of *Quercus infectoria* galls extract in combination with vancomycin against MRSA using microdilution checkerboard and time-kill assay. Evid-Based Complement Alternat Med. 2012;2012:493156.

Başyiğit B, Sağlam H, Köroğlu K, Karaaslan M. Compositional analysis, biological activity, and food protecting ability of ethanolic extract of *Quercus infectoria* gall. J Food Process Preserv. 2020;44(9):e14692.

Cheng YY, Zhao J, Tse HF, et al. Plant natural products calycosin and GA synergistically attenuate neutrophil infiltration and subsequent injury in isoproterenol-induced myocardial infarction: A possible role for leukotriene B4 12-hydroxydehydrogenase? Oxid Med Cell Longev. 2015;2015:434052.

Chokpaisarn J, Chusri S, Voravuthikunchai SP. Clinical randomized trial of topical *Quercus infectoria* ethanolic extract for the treatment of chronic diabetic ulcers. J Herb Med. 2020;21:100301.

Choudhary A, Smitha C, Suresh D, Basu S. Clinical evaluation of efficacy of *Quercus infectoria* and *Mimusops elengi* Linn. Herbal preparation in inhibition of gingivitis. Adv Hum Biol. 2015;5(3):68–76.

Dardmah F, Farahpour MR. *Quercus infectoria* gall extract aids wound healing in a streptozocin-induced diabetic mouse model. J Wound Care. 2021;30(8):618–625.

Elham A, Arken M, Kalimanjan G, Arkin A, Iminjan M. A review of the phytochemical, pharmacological, pharmacokinetic, and toxicological evaluation of *Quercus infectoria* galls. J Ethnopharmacol. 2021;12(273):113592.

Gruenwald J, Brendler T, Jaenicke C. *PDR for herbal medicines*. Montvale: Thomson Reuters; 2007.

Haghdoost F, Baradaran Mahdavi MM, Zolfaghari B, et al. The effect of *Quercus brantii* gall extract on burn wound healing in rat. Iran J Basic Med Sci. 2016;19(10):1144–1150.

Iminjan M, Amat N, Li XH, et al. Investigation into the toxicity of traditional Uyghur medicine *Quercus infectoria* galls waterextract. PLoS ONE. 2014;9:1–8.

Kaur G, Athar M, Alam MS. *Quercus infectoria* galls possess antioxidant activity and abrogates oxidative stress-induced functional alterations in murine macrophages. Chem-Biol Interact. 2008;171(3):272–282.

Khanavi M, Sabbagh-Bani-Azad M, Abdolghaffari AH, et al. On the benefit of galls of *Quercus brantii* Lindl. in murine colitis: The role of free gallic acid. Arch Med Sci. 2014;10(6):1225–1234.

Lodhi G, Singh HK, Pant KK, Rao CV, Hussain Z. Hepatoprotective effects of *Quercus infectoria* gall extract against carbon tetrachloride treated liver injury in rats. Int J Appl Res Nat Prod. 2012;5(3):17–22.

Lorzadeh N, Sepavand F, Soleimaninezhad M, Kazemirad N. The effect of extract of oak gall for vaginal tightening and rejuvenation in women with vaginal relaxation. Open J Obstet Gynecol. 2016;6(13):879–887.

Ministry of Health & Family Welfare, Government of India. *Unani pharmacopoeia of India*. Part 1, Vol. 3. New Delhi: Rakmo Press; 2007.

Moshfeghy Z, Asadi K, Akbarzadeh M, et al. *Quercus brantii* Lindl. vaginal douche versus clotrimazole on vaginal candidiasis: A randomized clinical trial. J Pharmacopuncture. 2018;21(3):185–194.

Noori M, Talebi M, Ahmadi T. Comparative studies of leaf, gall and bark flavonoids in collected *Quercus brantii* Lindl.(Fagaceae) from Lorestan Province, Iran. Int J Plant Res. 2015;5:42–49.

32 *Rheum palmatum* L.

Babak Daneshfard

Scientific name: *Rheum palmatum* L.
Family: Polygonaceae
Common names:

- **English:** Chinese rhubarb, ornamental rhubarb
- **Persian:** *rīvand-e čīnī*
- **Arabic:** *rāvand*

Medicinal part(s): Root and rhizome (Figure 32.1)
Temperament (nature): Hot and dry in the second degree
Major chemical constituents:

- **Anthracene derivatives (3–12%):** Glucosides of rheum emodin, aloe-emodin, rhein, chrysophanol, physcion (totally 60–80%), 8,8'-diglucosides of dianthrones (10–25%), sennosides A and B
- **Tannins:** Gallotannins, galloyl glucose, galloyl saccharose, lindleyin, isolindleyin
- Flavonoids (2–3%)
- Naphthohydroquinone glycosides (Gruenwald et al., 2007)

THERAPEUTIC USE

TPM Literature

Rhubarb has been recommended for chronic productive cough, asthma, hemoptysis, and dyspnea. It is also beneficial for the treatment of hemorrhoid, scorpion bite and other cold-nature toxins, and oral lesions. It is used for treating cold dystemperament of stomach, spleen, and liver, as well as obstructive jaundice. Rhubarb can alleviate painful uterine, bladder, and kidney. Due to laxative properties, it is used for cleansing the stomach and intestines from waste material and is recommended in dysentery. It is also a potent diuretic and, therefore, can be used in urinary hesitancy and urolithiasis. Its topical application in combination with astringent agents is helpful to relieve pain and swelling of the traumatized parts of the body (Aghili Khorasani 1771). In topical application, it is useful for skin spots and melasma (Avicenna 1025).

Current Evidence

Clinical Evidence

Respiratory diseases: Rhubarb can improve microcirculation, reduce tissue edema, and decrease inflammatory exudation and necrosis. Results of a meta-analysis including eight RCTs revealed that its combination with routine treatment of ARDS could ameliorate the arterial blood gas and cytokine levels in addition to decreasing the mortality and mechanical ventilation time (Yang et al., 2017).

DOI: 10.1201/b22971-32

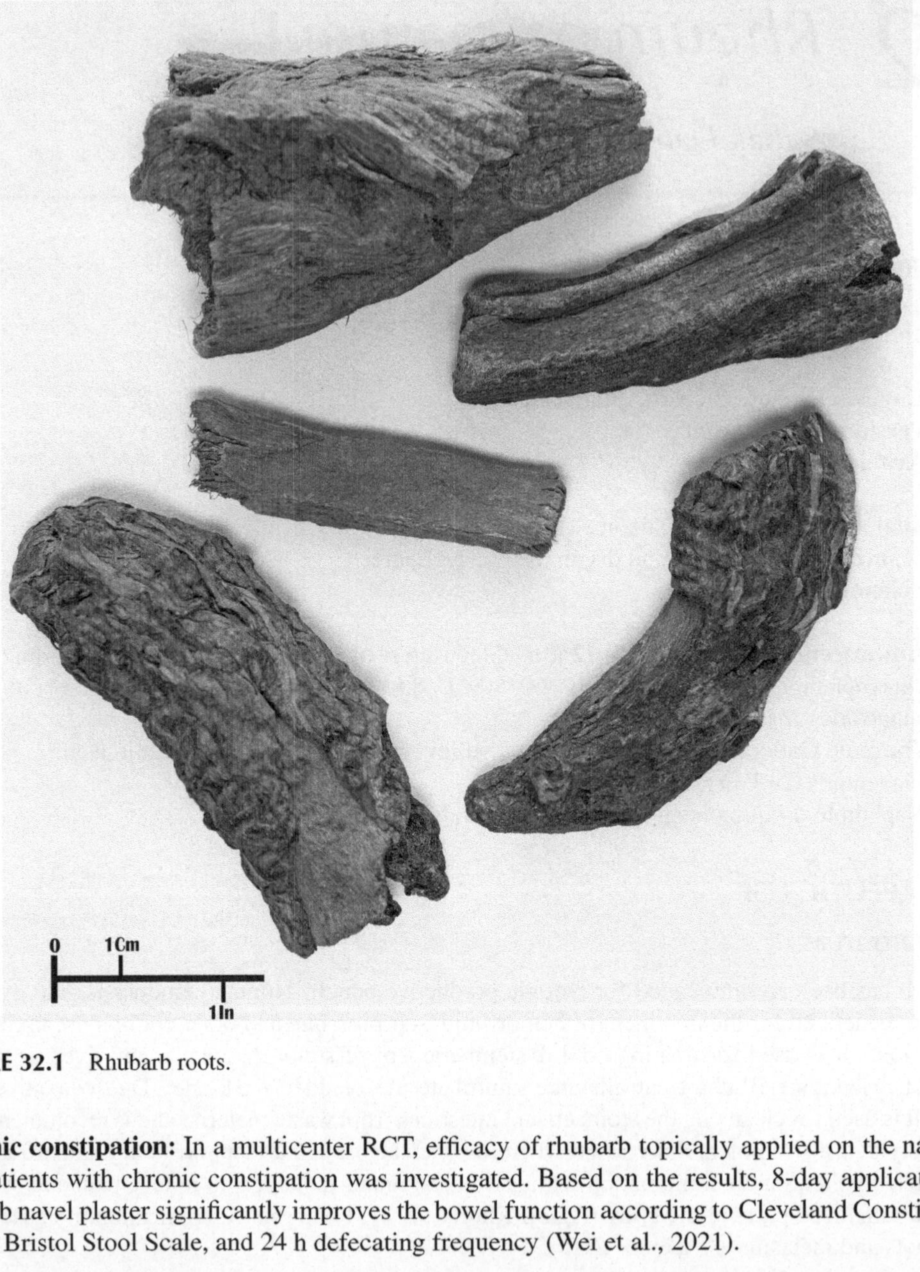

FIGURE 32.1 Rhubarb roots.

Chronic constipation: In a multicenter RCT, efficacy of rhubarb topically applied on the navel of 374 patients with chronic constipation was investigated. Based on the results, 8-day application of rhubarb navel plaster significantly improves the bowel function according to Cleveland Constipation Score, Bristol Stool Scale, and 24 h defecating frequency (Wei et al., 2021).

Intestinal obstruction: Effect of topical *Rheum officinale* powder at Shenque (CV 8) acupoint was investigated in 58 patients with incomplete intestinal obstruction. In this clinical trial, control group received enema and laxative drugs, while intervention groups received enema and topical rhubarb at CV8 point. At the end of study, the time of gas passing, intensity of abdominal bloating, and defecation was significantly decreased in the intervention group (Yu, 2016).

Sepsis: A four-arm RCT assessed the effect of rhubarb, ulinastatin, or their combination in 75 septic patients for a period of 5 days in comparison to a control group who only received a basic treatment. Rhubarb was administered to patients as 12 g of a commercial granule preparation via oral/nasal feeding. While all three interventions could significantly improve APACHE II score, WBC, lactic acid, and CRP, only rhubarb plus ulinastatin could significantly decrease procalcitonin level (Meng et al., 2020).

Pancreatitis: In an RCT on 126 patients with severe acute pancreatitis, addition of rhubarb to early enteral nutrition as a solution of 15 g plant powder in 100 mL warm water was evaluated. The patients received rhubarb preparation via a nasojejunal tube once or twice daily for 5–7 days. Addition of rhubarb caused a significant decrease in APACHE II score, high fever, abdominal pain period, ICU and hospital stay period, as well as normalizing bowel movements. Furthermore, markers of systemic inflammation, including CRP, IL-6, WBC, and IL-11 were significantly modulated in those received rhubarb vs. control group (Wan et al., 2014). A meta-analysis including 11 RCTs also confirmed that addition of rhubarb to early enteral nutrition for a period of 7–14 days in severe acute pancreatitis significantly reduce abdominal symptoms (pain, distension, bowel sounds), ICU and hospital stay, APACHE II score, WBC, CRP, and IL-6, in comparison to the patients only received early enteral nutrition (Chen et al., 2020).

Acute nonvaricose upper gastrointestinal bleeding: A meta-analysis including 14 RCTs compared the effect of rhubarb powder solution spray, as a traditional hemostatic herbal intervention, under gastroscope compared with norepinephrine as the standard care for the management of acute nonvaricose upper gastrointestinal bleeding. According to the results, a concentration of 0.1–0.15 g/mL of rhubarb solution has a significantly higher hemostatic effect vs. norepinephrine at 24–48 h, respectively; whereas the effect of lower concentrations (e.g., 0.031 g/mL) is similar to norepinephrine (Liu et al., 2020).

Chronic kidney disease: An RCT including patients with stage 3 and 4 chronic kidney disease assessed the effects of 12-week supplementation with rhubarb capsule (350 mg, three times daily) on the renal parameters. In comparison to the control group which only received conservative treatment, addition of rhubarb to the conservative treatment in the intervention groups caused a larger improvement of clinical symptoms, FBS, blood urea and creatinine, and 24-h total urine protein. Moreover, hemoglobin, GFR, and 24-h total urine volume were significantly increased by rhubarb vs. control (Khan et al., 2014).

Preclinical Evidence

Acute liver failure: In a d-galactosamine/LPS-induced mouse model of liver failure, intraperitoneal injection of rhubarb (1.5 g/kg) reduced liver enzymes and inflammatory factors through NF-κB signaling pathway (Zhang et al., 2015). In another study, the effect of rhubarb extract on thioacetamide-induced hepatic encephalopathy was investigated in rats. Rhubarb decreased endotoxin concentrations and the staging of hepatic encephalopathy in addition to improvement of neuroreflexes and liver function (Zhang et al., 2002).

Chronic kidney disease: The effect of ether, *n*-butanol, and ethyl acetate rhubarb extracts with a dose range of 200–800 mg/kg was investigated in a rat model of chronic kidney disease. Adenine was used in this study to induce chronic tubulointerstitial nephropathy. All extracts, especially ethyl acetate extract, improved renal injury by attenuating upregulation of profibrotic proteins, including connective tissue growth factor, α-SMA, collagen-1, TGF-β1, PAI-1, and fibronectin (Zhang et al., 2016).

ADVERSE REACTIONS

TPM Literature

It is harmful on the anus. To prevent the side effects, it should be used together with gum Arabic. It may also be harmful for children and people who are generally weak (Aghili Khorasani 1771).

Current Evidence

As an anthranoid laxative, it can cause gastrointestinal spasm. Long-term use of rhubarb may also lead to loss of electrolytes (especially potassium), nephropathy, cardiac arrhythmia, inhibition of intestinal motility, hyperaldosteronism, enhancement of the effect of cardioactive steroids, accelerated bone deterioration, and edema (Gruenwald et al., 2007). Red-brown or bright yellow discoloration of the urine can also occur after consumption of this medicinal herb. Other reported side effects include loss of appetite, nausea, and vomiting. Cirrhosis and intestinal damage are reported in case of overdose or long-term use. Allergic reactions such as tachypnea and asthma, flushing, pruritus, and papular rashes are reported in large doses. The fresh herb causes a more severe toxicity (Gardner and McGuffin, 2013).

Due to the controversial results of current literature on the hepatotoxic or hepatoprotective properties of rhubarb, it is suggested to be used in lower doses and short periods as long-term use results in the accumulation of rhubarb phytochemicals and exacerbates the toxicity (Zhuang et al., 2020).

CONTRAINDICATIONS

TPM Literature

None.

Current Evidence

Rhubarb is contraindicated in patients with intestinal obstruction, abdominal pain of unknown origin, acute inflammatory intestinal disease such as appendicitis, and during menstruation. It also should not be used for more than 8 consecutive days and by children under 12 years old (Gardner and McGuffin, 2013).

PREGNANCY AND LACTATION

TPM Literature

As it can harm children, it seems not to be applicable during pregnancy and especially lactation.

Current Evidence

Rhubarb is not recommended for use during pregnancy or lactation unless under supervision of a physician (Gardner and McGuffin, 2013).

DRUG INTERACTIONS

As rhubarb can decrease gastrointestinal transit time, the reduction of absorption of orally administered drugs should be considered as a possible consequence. It can also interact with potassium-losing drugs (such as thiazide diuretics and corticosteroids) or herbs like licorice and lead to electrolyte imbalance due to low level of potassium. Another interaction of this medicinal herb is with antiarrhythmic drugs and botanicals containing cardiac glycosides. Their effect could be increased due to hypokalemia (Gardner and McGuffin, 2013).

METHOD OF ADMINISTRATION

TPM Literature

Rhubarb dried root is used in the form of decoction. It can be also prepared as a lozenge or sublingual pill for respiratory disorders. In addition, its dried powder is used topically as a poultice or in combination with other drugs in the form of tablet or syrup (Aghili Khorasani 1771).

Current Evidence

Dried roots and rhizome can be taken directly (Gardner and McGuffin, 2013), or as an infusion (Gruenwald et al., 2007).

DOSAGE

Daily dosage as a laxative (maximum 1–2 weeks) is 1–2 g of dried powder with sufficient liquid. As an appetizer, daily dose of 0.1–0.2 g is recommended (Gruenwald et al., 2007). Some references suggest the maximum dose to be 10 g daily (Gardner and McGuffin, 2013).

REFERENCES

Aghili Khorasani MH 1771. *Makhzan-al-Adviah* (*The treasury of drugs*) (rewritten by Shams Ardakani MR, Rahimi R, Farjadmand F, 1st ed.). Tehran: Tehran University of Medical Sciences; 2009.

Avicenna 1025. *Al-Qanoon fi al-Tibb* (*The canon of medicine*) (rewritten by Masoudi A, ed.). Tehran: Almaei; 2015.

Bahtiar A, Setyowati HT, Mahanani RR, et al. Rhaponticin contained *Rheum officinale* root extract improved postmenopause symptom of ovariectomized rat. J Adv Pharm Technol Res. 2021;12(2):175.

Chen X, Yang K, Jing G, et al. Meta-analysis of efficacy of rhubarb combined with early enteral nutrition for the treatment of severe acute pancreatitis. J Parenter Enter Nutr. 2020;44(6):1066–1078.

Gardner Z, McGuffin M. *Botanical safety handbook*. Boca Raton: Taylor & Francis; 2013.

Gruenwald J, Brendler T, Jaenicke C. *PDR for herbal medicines*. Montvale: Thomson Reuters; 2007.

Ji SM, Li LS, Ji DX. Effects of baoshen pill in treating chronic renal failure with long-term hemodialysis. Zhongguo Zhongxiyi jiehe zazhi = Chin J Integr Med. 1993;13(2):71–73.

Khan IA, Nasiruddin M, Haque SF, Khan RA. Evaluation of rhubarb supplementation in stages 3 and 4 of chronic kidney disease: a randomized clinical trial. Int J Chronic Dis. 2014;789340.

Liu JT, Wu J, Wang HR, et al. Spraying rhubarb powder solution under gastroscope in the treatment of acute non-varicose upper gastrointestinal bleeding: A systematic review and meta-analysis of randomized controlled trials. Complement Ther Med. 2020;52:102476.

Meng F, Du C, Zhang Y, et al. Protective effect of rhubarb combined with ulinastatin for patients with sepsis. Medicine. 2020;99(7):e18895.

Song H, Wang Z, Zhang F. Investigation of urinary interleukin-6 level in chronic renal failure patients and the influence of *Rheum palmatum* in treating it. Zhongguo Zhongxiyi Jiehe Zazhi = Chin J Integr Med. 2000;20(2):107–109.

Wan B, Fu H, Yin J, Xu F. Efficacy of rhubarb combined with early enteral nutrition for the treatment of severe acute pancreatitis: A randomized controlled trial. Scand J Gastroenterol. 2014;49(11):1375–1384.

Wei L, Luo Y, Zhang X, et al. Topical therapy with rhubarb navel plasters in patients with chronic constipation: Results from a prospective randomized multicenter study. J Ethnopharmacol. 2021;264:113096.

Yang TZ, Liu Y, Liu YY, et al. The use of *Rheum Palmatum* L. in the treatment of acute respiratory distress syndrome: A meta-analysis of randomized, controlled trials. Afr J Tradit Complement Altern Med. 2017;14(2):334–347.

Yu M. Clinical study on Da Huang (*Rheum officinale*) powder application at Shenque (CV 8) for incomplete intestinal obstruction. Shanghai J Acup Mox. 2016:541–542.

Zhang Q, Cheng H, Wang C, et al. Preventive and therapeutic effects of extract from *Rheum palmatum* on hepatic encephalopathy in rats with acute liver failure. J Chinese Med Mater. 2002;25(8):573–575.

Zhang RZ, Qiu H, Wang N, et al. Effect of *Rheum palmatum* L. on NF-κB signaling pathway of mice with acute liver failure. Asian Pac J Trop Med. 2015;8(10):841–847.

Zhang ZH, Vaziri ND, Wei F, et al. An integrated lipidomics and metabolomics reveal nephroprotective effect and biochemical mechanism of *Rheum officinale* in chronic renal failure. Sci Rep. 2016;6(1):22151.

Zhuang T, Gu X, Zhou N, et al. Hepatoprotection and hepatotoxicity of Chinese herb Rhubarb (Dahuang): How to properly control the "General (Jiang Jun)" in Chinese medical herb. Biomed Pharmacother. 2020;127:110224.

33 *Rosa damascena* Herrm.

Zohreh Abolhassanzadeh

Scientific name: *Rosa damascena* Herrm.
Family: Rosaceae
Common names:

- **English:** Damask rose, Persian rose
- **Persian:** *gol-e sorḫ*
- **Arabic:** *ward al-aḥmar*

Medicinal part(s): Flowers, especially petals (Figure 33.1)
Temperament (nature): Dry in the second degree, cold in the first to second degree
Major chemical constituents:

- **Essential oil:** β-citronellol, nonadecane, geraniol, nerol
- **Flavonoids:** Kaempferol
- Anthocyanins
- **Terpenes** (Boskabady et al., 2011; Davoodi et al., 2017; Bikmoradi et al., 2016)

THERAPEUTIC USE

TPM Literature

Damask rose is considered as a general tonic for body, as well as a cardiotonic and antidepressant, both in oral consumption and as aromatherapy. The fresh petals are purgative while the dried ones are astringent. The extract of damask rose is useful for headache, eyesore and earache as drop. Dropping the dry petals decoction is used for thickening of upper eyelid. The mouthwash of the decoction is also useful for strengthening the teeth and gums. Smelling and eating the petals is tonic especially for the heart and brain and is useful for hot-tempered palpitations, as well as fainting due to heart weakness. The fine powder of the petals applied for ameliorating oral aphthous, wound, and small pox scars. Damask rose is a tonic for lungs, stomach, liver, GI tract, kidneys, and uterine. Dry powder of rose petals is recommended for vaginal discharge and odor, and for tightening the vagina. The poultice of the petals is applied for dyspepsia caused by moist dystemperament of GI tract, swollen anus, warts, abrasion, limbs fractures, and wounds. Administration of rose decoction as enema is beneficial for intestinal ulcers. The embrocation in bath is used to eliminate sweat odor and to scent the body. Rose oil, prepared by macerating or boiling rose petals in sesame oil base, can be used topically or orally and has similar therapeutic applications in addition to its use for earache, insomnia, intestinal ulcers, spasmodic pain in bowels, potent wound healing effects, and as a demulcent. Rose water which is produced from hydrodistillation of petals is another widely used preparation of damask rose. It is used for palpitation, pain in liver and spleen, cramps, faint and as a general tonic. In addition to rose petals, the buds are also used for therapeutic purposes, especially in case a higher astringent effect is needed (Aghili Khorasani 1771; Avicenna 1025).

DOI: 10.1201/b22971-33

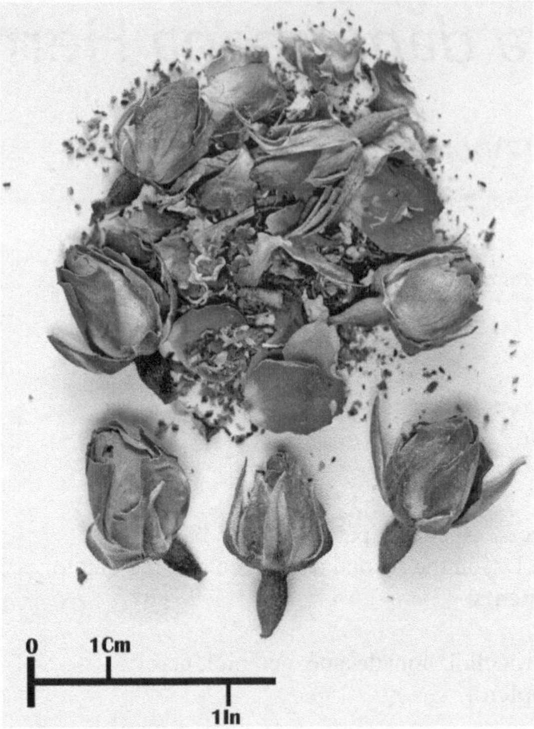

FIGURE 33.1 Damask rose buds and petals.

Current Evidence

Clinical Evidence

Pain: Considerable pain relief was reported in a study using preemptive inhalation of damask rose essential oil in patients who suffering from deep burn wounds (Bikmoradi et al., 2016). In another work on 92 pregnant women before cesarean section, the pain score was significantly decreased in patients who received rose oil capsules compared to placebo group (Gharabaghi et al., 2011). This remarkable diminution in pain was also observed in another investigation on children from 3 to 6 years old using rose essential oil aromatherapy after operation (Marofi et al., 2015). In an RCT on 120 pregnant women, topical application of rose oil two times a day for 1 month, improved low back pain in comparison with those who received almond oil or no intervention (Shirazi et al., 2016). Also, a systematic review and meta-analysis evaluated 11 RCTs showed that damask rose in oral use may have a nonsignificant effect on the improvement of acute pain, while no such effect is observed for topical use. It should be noted that due to the high heterogeneity of the included studies regarding the dosage form and route of administration of damask rose preparations, the study suggested further clinical trial to obtain a more reliable conclusion in this regard (Koohpayeh et al., 2022).

PMS: A placebo-controlled RCT in three groups of 40 women compared the effects of omega-3 capsules 500 mg per day, oral rose oil 30 drops per day, or distilled water 30 drops per day as placebo, during luteal phase for three consecutive cycles. Results showed that tension, depression fatiguability, decreased libido, lack of concentration, crying, suicidal thoughts and increased appetite in rose oil group were significantly lower than the other groups. But physical symptoms including edematous extremities, breast tenderness, bloating and palpitation in omega-3 group were significantly lower than the other groups. Headache and forgetfulness did not show any meaningful difference between groups (Jamalian et al., 2013). In another study, 395 students were randomized to receive three different oils including 4% concentration of damask rose essential oil, 0.5% concentration of *Citrus aurantium* blossom essential oil, or sweet almond oil as aromatherapy 1 week before menstruation (for 5 days) twice a day in two consecutive cycles. Mental symptoms were decreased in all three groups which was significant in both *C. aurantium* and damask rose groups. The score of physical symptoms was decreased in all three groups but it was only significant in the damask rose group. The reduction of effect of symptoms on social function was also only significant in damask rose group (Heydari et al., 2019).

Dysmenorrhea: In a crossover RCT in 92 single women with primary dysmenorrhea, rose capsules, administered every 6 h for 3 days in two menstrual cycles, showed a similar efficacy to mefenamic acid in relieving dysmenorrhea (Bani et al., 2014). In another RCT on three groups of 25 female students, applying self-massage with rose oil, self-massage with almond oil, and self-massage alone in the first day of menstruation in two subsequent cycles, the baseline pain reduced in the first cycle but this reduction was not significant between groups. In the second cycle, the menstrual pain was significantly lower in the rose oil group than in the other two groups (Sadeghi Aval Shahri et al., 2015). Topical administration of rose essential oil 10 drops twice daily to 110 students in the first 3 days of menstruation of two subsequent cycles, demonstrated significant decrease of menstrual related pain compared to placebo (Ataollahi et al., 2016). In another double-blind RCT, 105 university students randomly assigned into one of the four groups: fish oil 1,000 mg per day (n = 26), damask rose extract 1,000 mg per day (n = 27), fish oil and damask rose extract concurrently, with the same dose (n = 27), and control group (n = 25) for 60 days. Supplementation with rose extract significantly reduced severity of bloating and sweat but fish oil supplementation had no significant effect on primary dysmenorrhea symptoms. The concurrent use of these two interventions significantly decreased severity of diarrhea, weakness, dizziness, and feeling cold (Davaneghi et al., 2017).

Oral aphthous stomatitis: In a double-blind RCT, using the mouthwash containing the aqueous extract of damask rose for 2 weeks on 50 patients with recurrent oral aphthous, a better effect of extract on pain and inflammation like size and number of the ulcers, were observed in days 4 and 7 (Hoseinpour et al., 2011). Another double-blind RCT on 100 people randomized in two groups of rose extract and diphenhydramine applied topically 10 drops on a swap four times a day for 1 week, revealed that the severity of pain and burning in the rose extract treated group in the second, fourth, and seventh days after treatment were similar to diphenhydramine group (Khatibi et al., 2017).

Respiratory effect: In an RCT on 60 preterm neonates, application of two drops of 10% rose distillate five times as aromatherapy from 6:00 a.m. to 6:00 p.m. in the second day of birth could reduce the occurrence of apnea attacks, bradycardia and improve O_2 saturation compared to control group (Aghagoli et al., 2016).

Drug-induced sexual dysfunctions: In a placebo-controlled RCT, 60 male patients with major depressive disorder using selective serotonin-reuptake inhibitors, randomly received 2 mL per day of rose essential oil or placebo, orally, for 2 months. Depression symptoms were reduced in both groups but more in rose oil group. In addition, sexual dysfunction was ameliorated in rose oil group (Farnia et al., 2015a). A similar study conducted by the same research group but on 50 female patients, showed that this decrease is less significant in females with similar problems (Farnia et al., 2015b). In another double-blind RCT on 50 male patients with opium use disorder under methadone maintenance therapy, decrease in sexual dysfunction and increase in testosterone levels were reported after using 2 mL of rose oil daily for 8 weeks (Farnia et al., 2017).

Sleep quality: A systematic review and meta-analysis of 10 RCTs on the effect of damask rose on improvement of adults' sleep quality showed that the inhalation and oral intake of this plant could improve some sleep-related outcomes. The pooled analysis of seven effect sizes revealed that inhalation aromatherapy with damask rose significantly improved sleep quality. Most RCTs had fair methodological quality (Ghorbani Rami et al., 2021). Also, in an unblinded placebo-controlled RCT on 80 operating room staff with anxiety and poor sleep quality during COVID-19 pandemic, aromatherapy with damask rose essential oil (10 minutes inhalation on morning shift, followed by 30 nights using five drops of the products next to the pillow) could significantly improve Pittsburgh sleep quality index and Spielberger state anxiety inventory compared with placebo (paraffin oil) (Mahdood et al., 2022).

Anxiety, stress, and depression: A systematic review and dose–response meta-analysis of 32 RCTs of damask rose on state anxiety, stress and depression revealed significant reduction in anxiety, depression, and stress but no effect on trait anxiety (Rasooli et al., 2021).

Relaxing effect: The study on 20 female university students using 0.2 μL of rose essential oil aromatherapy by an artificial air chamber for 90 seconds, presented a significant decrease in oxyhemoglobin concentration in the right prefrontal cortex and an increase in "comfortable," "relaxed," and "natural" feelings compare to control group who inhaled unimpregnated air with same device (Igarashi et al., 2014). Another investigation reported the relaxing effect of self-massage of 1 mL of rose essential oil (20%) on human autonomic parameters including breathing rate, blood O_2 saturation, SBP, and emotional responses on 40 healthy volunteers (both male and female) after transdermal absorption (Hongratanaworakit, 2009).

Constipation: In a single-arm clinical trial study on 35 pregnant women (14–34 weeks) with constipation diagnosed on the basis of Rome IV criteria, daily oral administration of damask rose products containing 750 mg of dried petals and 1,250 mg of white rock candy as a fine powder 30 minutes after breakfast with 25 mL of rose water for 4 weeks, could significantly improve constipation signs including straining, lumpy, and hard stools, a sensation of incomplete evacuation, a sensation of anorectal obstruction, manual facilitation maneuvers, and less than three spontaneous bowel movements per week (Nili et al., 2021). Also, in a double-blind RCT, 100 pediatric patients (above 1 year old) with functional constipation were randomized to receive PEG or a sweetened damask rose decoction (0.1 g rose petals and 0.85 g brown sugar per each 1 mL of the decoction) for 4 weeks. A cure rate of 100% was observed in damask rose-treated patients vs. 91.7% in PEG-treated group. Damask rose decoction showed a statistically similar efficacy to PEG for the management of pediatric functional constipation (Imanieh et al., 2022).

GERD: In a double-blind controlled RCT in 70 subjects with GERD, rose oil softgel capsules (rose oil in sesame oil base, prepared as per TPM instructions) with a dose of 2 capsules 3 times per day showed a similar efficacy to omeprazole during 1 month of intervention (Mehraban et al., 2021).

Colitis: According to a pilot placebo-controlled RCT in 40 patients with ulcerative colitis, rose oil was administered as 1,000 mg softgel capsules (2 capsules 3 times per day) for 2 months; however, no significant difference was observed between the outcomes of rose oil and placebo groups (Tavakoli et al., 2019).

Preclinical Evidence

Alzheimer's disease: In an aluminum chloride-induced rat model of Alzheimer's disease, oral administration of aqueous extract of damask rose (500 and 1,000 mg/kg) for 8 weeks could significantly improve spatial memory, CAT, and GSH levels. It also significantly reduced LPO and AchE activity (Hejaziyan et al., 2023).

Ulcerative colitis: In a study on acetic acid-induced colitis, using damask rose hydroalcoholic extract (250, 500 and 1,000 mg/kg orally, or 125, 250 and 500 mg/kg i.p.) in rats 2 h before colitis induction and 4 successive days, resulted in considerable improvement of colitis symptoms as well as antioxidant effect against MPO (Latifi et al., 2015).

Cardiac effects: In a study on hyperlipidemic rabbits that used 1.5 g/kg methanolic extract of damask rose orally for 45 days, the serum level of TC, LDL-C, TAG and the plaque formation was numerically, but not statistically, decreased (Gholamhoseinian et al., 2012). In a similar investigation, the left ventricular systolic pressure was increased in extract group (Joukar et al., 2013). Another study on 32 normotensive rats received 250, 500, or 1,000 mg/kg hydroalcoholic extract, i.p., demonstrated the hypotensive effect but no remarkable effect on heart rate was revealed (Baniasad et al., 2015).

Hepatotoxicity: Oral intake of 250–1,000 mg/kg of damask rose aqueous extract in acetaminophen-induced oxidative stress in rats inverted biochemical parameters including AST, ALT, ALP, LDH, albumin, bilirubin, urea and creatinine, hepatic LPO, and GSH levels as well as histopathological parameters (Sharma et al., 2013).

ADVERSE REACTIONS

TPM Literature

It reduces libido and causes thirst. Consumption with anise can decrease the side effects (Aghili Khorasani 1771).

Current Evidence

Using 1,440 mg/kg/day of damask rose infusion for 10 days in dogs resulted in inconsequential nephrotoxic and hepatotoxic effects (Akbari et al., 2013). In one study, rats with intraabdominal adhesion after laparotomy that were treated with 3 mL of 5% of ethanolic extract of damask rose (locally applied on the peritoneal wounds) were found all dead, while rats treated with 1% extract showed an improvement in wound healing (Karimi et al., 2016). In a clinical study, one case of allergic rhinitis in a pregnant woman after topical use of rose oil was reported (Shirazi et al., 2016). Small hairs on rose hip can cause irritation in the mouth, throat, and other areas (Gardner and McGuffin, 2013). Headache, frequent sneezing, and nausea were reported after aromatherapy with damask rose oil (Heydarirad et al., 2019).

CONTRAINDICATIONS

TPM Literature

None.

Current Evidence

None.

PREGNANCY AND LACTATION

TPM Literature

Damask rose is considered as a fetus-protective plant in TPM and its products can be used during pregnancy and lactation (Aghili Khorasani 1780).

Current Evidence

None.

DRUG INTERACTIONS

None.

METHOD OF ADMINISTRATION

TPM Literature

For oral administration, petals can be used as powder or decoction. The decoction is also recommended for oral cavity diseases. Rose water can be used orally or via inhalation for aromatherapy. Fresh petals can also be used for aromatherapy and oral intake. Liquid dosage forms of the plant can be used as drops in eyes or nose. Also, a mixture of rose petals with sugar or honey in the form of jam or electuary is popular for oral use (Aghili Khorasani 1771).

For topical administration, dried or fresh plant material can be used as a poultice, fine powder, or oil. Rose oil is processed in two ways according to TPM literatures. In the first, fresh petals are soaked in sesame or olive oil in sunlight; whenever the color of petals changes to white, the petals are replaced with fresh ones. This procedure is repeated seven times. This oil is called pure raw rose oil. In the second way, juice of fresh petals is mixed with sesame or olive oil on mild heat till the aqueous part evaporates. This oil is called heated rose oil. Rose oil may be used topically for massage or orally.

For rectal administration the decoction is used as enema. Damask rose dry powder as a pessary can be used for vaginal drug delivery (Aghili Khorasani 1771).

Current Evidence

Rose hip, bud, and petals are used as herbal teas or food additives. The essential oil is used for aromatherapy.

DOSAGE

5–10 g daily (Gruenwald et al., 2007).

REFERENCES

Aghagoli S, Salimi A, Salimi M, et al. Aromatherapy with *Rosa damascenes* in apnea, bradycardia and Spo2 of preterm infants: A randomized clinical trial. Int J Pediatr. 2016;4(6):1911–1918.

Aghili Khorasani MH 1771. *Makhzan-al-Adviah* (*The treasury of drugs*) (rewritten by Shams Ardakani MR, Rahimi R, Farjadmand F, 1st ed.). Tehran: Tehran University of Medical Sciences; 2009.

Aghili Khorasani MH 1780. *Khulasat al Hikmah* (rewritten by Nazem E). Tehran: Esmailian; 2006.

Akbari M, Kazerani HR, Kamrani A, Mohri M. A preliminary study on some potential toxic effects of Rosa damascena Mill. *Iran J Vet Res*. 2013;14(3):232236.

Ataollahi M, Amir Ali Akbari S, Mojab F, Roshanaie G. Effects of aromatherapy by rosaceous on the severity and systemic symptoms of primary dysmenorrhea. Adv Nurs Midwifery. 2016;89:59–67.

Bani S, Hasanpour S, Mousavi Z, et al. The effect of *Rosa damascena* extract on primary dysmenorrhea: A double-blind cross-over clinical trial. Iran Red Crescent Med J. 2014;16(1):e14643.

Baniasad A, Khajavirad A, Hosseini M, et al. Effect of hydro-alcoholic extract of *Rosa damascena* on cardiovascular responses in normotensive rat. Avicenna J Phytomed. 2015;5(4):319–324.

Bikmoradi A, Harorani M, Roshanaei G, et al. The effect of inhalation aromatherapy with damask rose (*Rosa damascena*) essence on the pain intensity after dressing in patients with burns: A clinical randomized trial. Iran J Nurs Midwifery Res. 2016;21(3):247–254.

Boskabady MH, Shafei MN, Saberi Z, Amini S. Pharmacological effects of *Rosa damascena*. Iran J Basic Med Sci. 2011;14(4):295–307.

Davaneghi S, Tarighat Esfanjani A, Safaiyan A, Fardiazar Z. Effective reduction of primary dysmenorrheal symptoms through concurrent use of n-3 fatty acids and *Rosa damascena* extract (RDE). Prevent Care Nurs Midwif J. 2017;2:33–40.

Davoodi I, Rahimi R, Abdollahi M, et al. Promising effect of *Rosa damascena* extract on high-fat diet-induced nonalcoholic fatty liver. J Tradit Complement Med. 2017;7(4):508–514.

Farnia V, Hojatitabar S, Shakeri J, et al. Adjuvant *Rosa Damascena* has a small effect on SSRI-induced sexual dysfunction in female patients suffering from MDD. Pharmacopsychiatry. 2015a;48(4–5):156–163.

Farnia V, Shirzadifar M, Shakeri J, et al. *Rosa damascena* oil improves SSRI-induced sexual dysfunction in male patients suffering from major depressive disorders: Results from a double-blind, randomized, and placebo-controlled clinical trial. Neuropsychiatr Dis Treat. 2015b;11:625–635.

Farnia V, Tatari F, Alikhani M, et al. *Rosa Damascena* oil improved sexual function and testosterone in male patients with opium use disorder under methadone maintenance therapy: Results from a double-blind, randomized, placebo-controlled clinical trial. Drug Alcohol Depend. 2017;176:117–125.

Gardner Z and McGuffin *M. American Herbal Products Association's Botanical Safety Handbook*. London and New York: Taylor & Francis. 2013; 747–748.

Gharabaghi PM, Tabatabei F, Fard SA, et al. Evaluation of the effect of preemptive administration of *Rosa damascena* extract on post-operative pain in elective cesarean sections. Afr J Pharm Pharmacol. 2011;5(16):1950–1955.

Gholamhoseinian A, Shahouzehi B, Joukar S, Iranpoor M. Effect of *Quercus infectoria* and *Rosa damascena* on lipid profile and atherosclerotic plaque formation in rabbit model of hyperlipidemia. Pak J Biol Sci. 2012;15(1):27–33.

Ghorbani Rami MS, Nasiri M, Aghili Nasab MS, et al. Effect of *Rosa damascena* on improvement of adults' sleep quality: A systematic review and meta-analysis of randomized controlled trials. Sleep Med. 2021;87:8 19.

Gruenwald J, Brendler T, Jaenicke C. *PDR for herbal medicines*. Thomson Reuters; 2007.

Hejaziyan LB, Hosseini SM, Taravati A, et al. Effect of *Rosa damascena* extract on rat model Alzheimer's disease: A histopathological, behavioral, enzyme activities, and oxidative stress study. Evid-Based Complement Altern. 2023;2023.

Heydari N, Abootalebi M, Tayebi N, et al. The effect of aromatherapy on mental, physical symptoms, and social functions of females with premenstrual syndrome: A randomized clinical trial. J Fam Med Prim Care. 2019;8(9):2990–2996.

Heydarirad G, Keyhanmehr AS, Mofid B, et al. Efficacy of aromatherapy with *Rosa damascena* in the improvement of sleep quality of cancer patients: A randomized controlled clinical trial. Compl Ther Clin Pract. 2019; 35:57–61.

Hongratanaworakit T. Relaxing effect of rose oil on humans. Nat Prod Commun. 2009;4(2):291–296.

Hoseinpour H, Peel SA, Rakhshandeh H, et al. Evaluation of *Rosa damascene* mouthwash in the treatment of recurrent aphthous stomatitis: A randomized, doubleblinded, placebo-controlled clinical trial. Quintessence Int. 2011;42(6):483–491.

Igarashi M, Ikei H, Song C, Miyazaki Y. Effects of olfactory stimulation with rose and orange oil on prefrontal cortex activity. Complement Ther Med. 2014;22(6):1027–1031.

Imanieh MH, Honar N, Mohagheghzadeh A, et al. *Rosa damascena* together with brown sugar mitigate functional constipation in children over 12 months old: A double-blind randomized controlled trial. J Ethnopharmacol. 2022;298:115582.

Joukar S, Askarzadeh M, Shahouzehi B, et al. Assessment of safety and therapeutic efficacy of *Rosa damascena* L. and *Quercus infectoria* on cardiovascular performance of normal and hyperlipidemic rabbits: Physiologically based approach. J Toxicol. 2013;2013:769143.

Karimi M, Yazdan AS, Parsaei P, et al. The effect of ethanol extract of rose (*Rosa damascena*) on intra-abdominal adhesions after laparotomy in rats. Wounds: Compend Clin Res Pract. 2016;28(5):167–174.

Khatibi M, Mohammadian S, Arezoobakhsh M. The comparison of the effectiveness of rose extract and diphenhydramine on aphthus ulcers in oral mucosa. J Res Dent Sci. 2017;14(2):70–76.

Koohpayeh SA, Hosseini M, Nasiri M, Rezaei M. Effects of topical application and oral intake of *Rosa Damascena* on acute pain in adults: A systematic review and meta-analysis. Oman Med J. 2022;37(5):1–4.

Latifi G, Ghannadi A, Minaiyan M. Anti-inflammatory effect of volatile oil and hydroalcoholic extract of *Rosa damascena* Mill. on acetic acid-induced colitis in rats. Res Pharm Sci. 2015;10(6):514–522.

Mahdood B, Imani B, Khazaei S. Effects of inhalation aromatherapy with *Rosa damascena* (Damask rose) on the state anxiety and sleep quality of operating room personnel during the COVID-19 pandemic: A randomized controlled trial. J Perianesth Nurs. 2022;37(4):493–500.

Marofi M, Sirousfard M, Moeini M, Ghanadi A. Evaluation of the effect of aromatherapy with *Rosa damascena* Mill. on postoperative pain intensity in hospitalized children in selected hospitals affiliated to Isfahan University of Medical Sciences in 2013: A randomized clinical trial. Iran J Nurs Midwifery Res. 2015;20(2):247–254.

Mehraban MS, Shirzad M, Ahmadian-Attari MM, et al. Effect of rose oil on Gastroesophageal Reflux Disease in comparison with omeprazole: A double-blind controlled trial. Complement Ther Clin Pract. 2021;43:101361.

Nili N, Hadavand S, Emadi F, et al. Evaluation of the effect of *Rosa damascena* Mill. product on constipation during pregnancy: A single-arm clinical trial. Int J Women's Health Reprod Sci. 2021;9(1):11–16.

Rasooli T, Nasiri M, Kargarzadeh Aliabadi Z. et al. *Rosa Damascena* Mill. for treating adults' anxiety, depression, and stress: A systematic review and dose-response meta-analysis of randomized controlled trials. Phytother Res. 2021;35(12):6585–6606.

Sadeghi Aval Shahr H, Saadat M, Kheirkhah M, Saadat E. The effect of self-aromatherapy massage of the abdomen on the primary dysmenorrhoea. J Obstet Gynaecol. 2015;35(4):382–385.

Sharma M, Shakya A, Sharma N, et al. Therapeutic efficacy of *Rosa damascena* Mill. on acetaminophen-induced oxidative stress in albino rats. J Environ Pathol Toxicol Oncol. 2012;31(3):193–201.

Shirazi M, Mohebitabar S, Bioos S, et al. The effect of topical *Rosa damascena* (rose) oil on pregnancy-related low back pain: A randomized controlled clinical trial. J Evid-Based Complement Alternat Med. 2016:2156587216654601.

Tavakoli A, Shirzad M, Taghavi A, et al. Efficacy of Rose Oil Soft Capsules on Clinical Outcomes in Ulcerative Colitis: A Pilot Randomized, Double-Blinded, Placebo-Controlled Clinical Trial. Galen Med J. 2019;8:e1307.

34 *Senna alexandrina* Mill.

Roja Rahimi and Nafiseh Hosseini Yekta

Scientific name: *Senna alexandrina* Mill. (syn. *Senna angustifolia* (Vahl) Batka)
Family: Fabaceae
Common names:

- **English:** Tinnevelly senna, Indian senna
- **Persian:** *senā-ye makkī*

Medicinal part(s): Leaf (Figure 34.1)
Temperament (nature): Hot in the second degree and dry in the first degree
Major chemical constituents:

- **Anthraquinone glycosides (2.5–3.5%):** Sennosides A, B, C, and D, palmidin A, rhein anthrone, aloe-emodin glycosides
- Naphthalene glycosides
- **Mucilage:** Arabinose, galactose, galacturonic acid
- **Others:** Flavonoids, volatile oil, and resins (Williamson et al., 2013)

THERAPEUTIC USE

TPM Literature

Senna is a purgative of phlegm, black bile, and yellow bile from the body. It is a cleanser of brain and so is useful for epilepsy, migraine and chronic headache, as well as psychosis. Senna is also used for respiratory tract disorders including pleurisy and asthma. It also purges waste materials from skin and is used for the treatment of skin disease including alopecia areata, ichthyosis, pruritis, dermatitis, and chronic rash. Senna is also applied for musculoskeletal disorders including osteoarthritis, sciatica, gout, and backache (Aghili Khorasani 1771).

Current Evidence

Clinical Evidence

Laxative effects: In a multicenter double-blind RCT on a group of 90 patients with idiopathic chronic constipation, senna (1 g daily) was compared with Magnesium oxide (1.5 g daily) and placebo. The results showed significant improvement of the frequency of bowel movements as well as constipation quality of life (Morishita et al., 2021). Another crossover RCT in children aged 2–14 years old reported that 3-week administration of senna (0.45–0.9 mg/kg, once daily) significantly repaired anorectal malformations and constipation compared with PEG (Santos-Jasso et al., 2017). A systematic review and meta-analysis considering three RCTs compared the effect of senna and PEG in constipation of children. The study suggested PEG to be a better laxative in children since it causes less pain vs. senna; however, due to the limited number of RCTs and high heterogenicity of the current studies, future high-quality clinical studies are still needed (Watanabe et al., 2021).

DOI: 10.1201/b22971-34

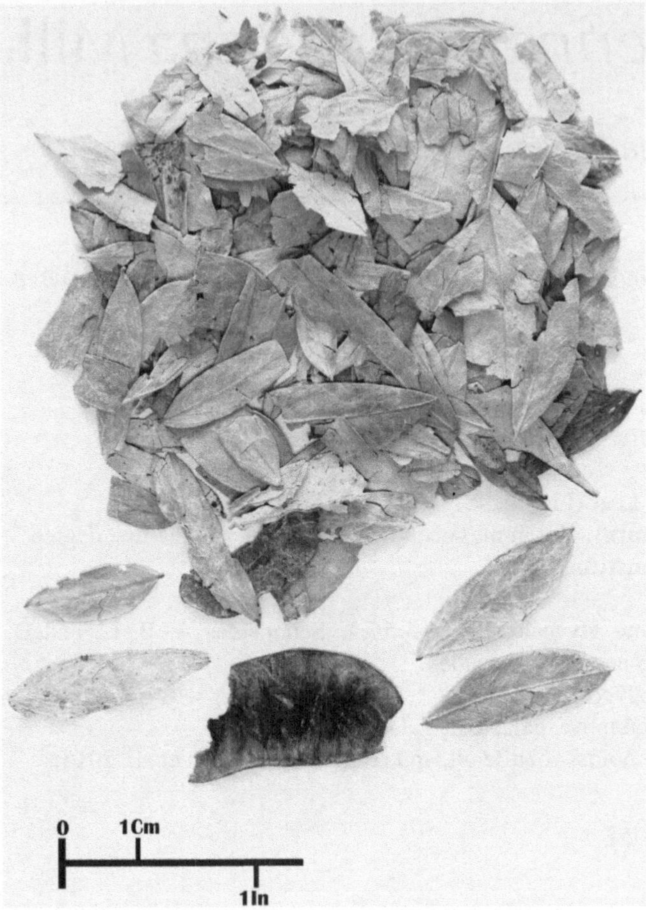

FIGURE 34.1 Senna leaves (top) and pod (bottom).

Senna improved constipation-related symptoms and constipation quality of life in 43 patients with opioid-induced constipation with a similar efficacy to lubiprostone (Marciniak et al., 2014). Furthermore, senna extract (40 mg/kg) showed acceptable effectiveness and safety in 82 patients with chemotherapy-induced constipation (Tao et al., 2012).

Bowel preparation for colonoscopy: In a double-blind RCT, 320 patients were randomized to receive PEG or C-Lax® syrup. PEG solution was prepared from 5×70 g sachets in 20×250 mL water (250 mL every 15 minutes), prescribed 24 h before the colonoscopy. In the other group 3×60 mL C-Lax syrup glasses (each containing 90 mg sennoside B) was given in two divided doses (1.5 glasses of 250 mL every 12 hours), 24 h before the colonoscopy. There was no significant difference between C-Lax syrup and PEG solution in cleansing colon (Khorasanynejad et al., 2017).

Type 2 diabetes: Twenty male Yemeni patients with type 2 diabetes mellitus (FBS 130–150 mg/100 mL) received three types of interventions for 10 days with 2 weeks washout period between each two successive interventions. The three interventions were two placebo tablets daily for 10 days, fenugreek seeds 6 g daily for 10 days, and a macerate of 200 mg of senna leaves daily for 10 days, respectively. The results showed that senna leaves lowered the FBS by 14.3%, fenugreek seeds by 12%, while placebo tablets did not change this parameter in the patients (Al-adhal, 2009).

In a clinical study, 50 patients with type 2 diabetes and constipation received senna leaves infusion thrice a week in the first month, twice in a week in corresponding second and third months and once in a week from fourth to sixth month. These patients were compared with 50 healthy subjects. The results demonstrated the higher levels of serum hepatic enzymes in diabetic patients which were normalized after 6 months of treatment with senna. The diabetic patients were found to have high FBS and altered lipid profile with vulnerability to skin infection, particularly in the pelvic regions, backside, legs, etc. which were reversed to normal after 6 months of senna leaves treatments. The neurological symptoms like sustaining pain in legs was also recovered with the treatment. The stools quality also changed to normal. The Gpx decreased in red blood cells of diabetics by 20–30%, was normalized after 6 months of treatment with senna leaves extract. The GSH level found to be decreased in diabetics by 15–20% (Kumar et al., 2019). In spite of the reported data, further high-quality studies are needed to support this therapeutic effect for senna.

Hypertension: Thirty male Yemeni patients with mild hypertension received three types of interventions for 10 days with 2 weeks washout period between each two successive interventions. The three interventions were two placebo tablets for 1 week, two tablets of bisacodyl 10 mg for 1 week, and boiled infusion of 200 mg of senna leaves daily for 1 week, respectively. The results showed that senna leaves caused 12.3% decrease in SBP and 8.4% decrease in DBP, whereas the pulse rate was not changed significantly. Placebo and bisacodyl tablets did not change these measurements in the investigated patients (El Adhal, 2006). Though, future studies are needed to confirm the antihypertensive properties of senna.

Preclinical Evidence

None.

ADVERSE REACTIONS

TPM Literature

The common adverse events following the use of senna are gastrointestinal problems including abdominal cramps and nausea. Using with almond oil and *Rosa damascena* can ameliorate its adverse events. Also, senna infusion has fewer side effects than the leaf powder (Aghili Khorasani 1771).

Current Evidence

Spasmodic gastrointestinal complaints, discoloration of the urine, hemorrhoidal congestion. Prolonged use and overdose can result in diarrhea, extreme loss of electrolytes, especially potassium (hypokalemia has several signs and symptoms including hypertension, weakness and fatigue, muscle cramps and spasms, heart palpitations, tingling and numbness, breathing difficulties), damage to the GI surface epithelium, and impairment of bowel function by damage to autonomic nerves. Anatomic alteration of the colon is seen secondary to chronic use of senna (more than three times weekly for 1 year or longer). Abuse of senna has also been associated with melanosis coli, but recovery occurs 8–11 months after withdrawal. Prolonged use may lead to cardiac arrhythmias, nephropathies, edema, and accelerated bone deterioration. Senna abuse has also resulted in tetany and hypogammaglobulinemia. Finger clubbing has been also reported from senna use which was reversible upon discontinuation of the drug (Gruenwald et al., 2007). Hypersensitivity reactions (pruritus, urticaria, anaphylaxis) are reported, as well (Irazábal et al., 2021). Some reports suggest the association between anthraquinone laxatives use and colorectal cancer. However, the result form a meta-analysis showed that the use of anthraquinone laxatives is not associated with the development of colorectal cancer (Lombardi et al., 2022). Acute hepatitis, pancytopenia and portal vein thrombosis have been reported from chronic use of senna (Haoudar et al., 2021; Soyuncu et al., 2008).

CONTRAINDICATIONS

TPM Literature

Since senna is a potent purgative, it should not be used without almond oil and *Rosa damascena* (Aghili Khorasani 1771).

Current Evidence

The herb should not be administered in the presence of intestinal obstruction, acute inflammatory intestinal diseases, or appendicitis. Moreover, it should not be used individually as a laxative agent for more than 2 weeks (Gruenwald et al., 2007). It is contraindicated in children under 12 years of age (HMPC, 2018).

PREGNANCY AND LACTATION

TPM Literature

None.

Current Evidence

The use during pregnancy is contraindicated because of experimental data concerning a genotoxic risk of several anthranoids, e.g., emodin and aloe-emodin.

Use during lactation is contraindicated because after administration of anthranoids, active metabolites such as rhein were excreted in breastmilk in small amounts (HMPC, 2018).

DRUG INTERACTIONS

Senna has been predicted to interact with a number of drugs that lower potassium (such as the corticosteroids, potassium-depleting diuretics, licorice root), or drugs where the effects become potentially harmful when potassium is lowered (such as digoxin and other antiarrhythmic drugs). The long-term use of senna with these medications is contraindicated. Senna may slightly reduce quinidine levels (Williamson et al., 2013; HMPC, 2018).

METHOD OF ADMINISTRATION

TPM Literature

As a purgative, it is used as decoction with almond oil and *Rosa damascena* flowers. For skin disorders, it is also used topically. For musculoskeletal disorders, its powder with honey is used for 3–7 consecutive days (Aghili Khorasani 1771).

Current Evidence

Its infusion as well as various pharmaceutical preparations, including tablet and syrup, are used orally (Gruenwald et al., 2007).

DOSAGE

Single dose: Herbal preparation equivalent to 10–30 mg hydroxyanthracene derivatives, calculated as sennoside B, to be taken once daily at night. The correct individual dose is the smallest required to produce a comfortable soft-formed motion (HMPC, 2018).

To prepare an infusion, hot water (not boiling) should be added to 0.5–2 g of comminuted drug for 10 minutes. Also, the leaves can be macerated in cold water for 10–12 hours, then strained (Gruenwald et al., 2007).

REFERENCES

Aghili Khorasani MH 1771. *Makhzan-al-Adviah* (*The treasury of drugs*) (rewritten by Shams Ardakani MR, Rahimi R, Farjadmand F, 1st ed.). Tehran: Tehran University of Medical Sciences; 2009.

Al-adhal A. The effect of *Cassia angustifolia* (senna) leaves on the fasting blood sugar in a sample of mild diabetic Yemeni patients. Yemeni J Med Sci. 2009;3:1–6.

Committee on Herbal Medicinal Products (HMPC). *European Union herbal monograph on Senna alexandrina Mill. (Cassia senna L.; Cassia angustifolia Vahl) 1, folium.* EMA/HMPC/625849/2015. London: European Medical Agency; 2018.

El Adhal A, Olwan AA. Effect of *Cassia angustifolia* [Senna] leaves on the blood pressure and the pulse rate in a sample of mild hypertensive Yemeni patients. Arab J Pharm Sci 2006;3(2):47–56.

Gruenwald J, Brendler T, Jaenicke C. *PDR for herbal medicines*. Montvale: Thomson Reuters; 2007.

Haoudar A, Chekhlabi N, El Kettani C, Dini N. Acute hepatitis and pancytopenia in a child with chronic abuse of senna. Cureus. 2021;13(1):e12436.

Irazábal B, Sánchez de Vicente J, Galán C, et al. Anaphylaxis due to senna (*Cassia angustifolia*). J Investig Allergol Clin Immunol. 2021;31(1):71–73.

Khorasanynejad R, Norouzi A, Roshandel G, Besharat S. Bowel preparation for a better colonoscopy using polyethylene glycol or C-lax: A double blind randomized clinical trial. Middle East J Dig Dis. 2017;9(4):212–217.

Kumar R, Gupta B. Beneficial effects of cassia angustifolia (senna leaves) treatment improves constipation, liver functions and defense of red blood cells in type 2 diabetic patients. Clin Gastroenterol 2019;68(S1):A111–A112.

Lombardi N, Crescioli G, Maggini V, et al. Anthraquinone laxatives use and colorectal cancer: A systematic review and meta-analysis of observational studies. Phytother Res. 2022;36(3):1093–1102.

Marciniak CM, Toledo S, Lee J, et al. Lubiprostone vs senna in postoperative orthopedic surgery patients with opioid-induced constipation: A double-blind, active-comparator trial. World J Gastroenterol. 2014;20(43):16323–16333.

Morishita D, Tomita T, Mori S, et al. Senna versus magnesium oxide for the treatment of chronic constipation: A randomized, placebo-controlled trial. Am J Gastroenterol. 2021;116(1):152–161.

Santos-Jasso KA, Arredondo-García JL, Maza-Vallejos J, Lezama-Del Valle P. Effectiveness of senna vs polyethylene glycol as laxative therapy in children with constipation related to anorectal malformation. J Pediatr Surg. 2017;52(1):84–88.

Soyuncu S, Cete Y, Nokay AE. Portal vein thrombosis related to *Cassia angustifolia*. Clin Toxicol (Phila). 2008;46(8):774–777.

Tao LM, Xiong JP, Liu TX. A crossover control study of prophylactic treatment of chemotherapy-induced constipation by senna extract. Zhongguo Zhong Xi Yi Jie He Za Zhi. 2012;32(1):47–49.

Watanabe J, Kotani, K., Polyethylene glycol versus senna for bowel preparation for colonoscopy in children: Updated evidence by a systematic review and meta-analysis. Cureus. 2021;13(9):e17813.

Williamson E, Driver S, Baxter K (eds.). *Stockley's herbal medicines interactions*. London: Pharmaceutical Press; 2013.

35 *Syzygium aromaticum* (L.) Merr. & L.M.Perry

Zahra Taghipour

Scientific name: *Syzygium aromaticum* (L.) Merr. & L.M.Perry (Syn. *Eugenia caryophyllata* Thunb.)
Family: Myrtaceae
Common names:

- **English:** Clove
- **Persian:** *mīḫak*
- **Arabic:** *qaranful*

Medicinal part(s): Flower buds (Figure 35.1)
Temperament (nature): Hot and dry in the third degree
Major chemical constituents:

- **Volatile oil (15–21%):** Eugenol (70–90%), eugenyl acetate (aceteugenol, up to 17%), β-caryophyllene (5–12%)
- **Flavonoids:** Astragalin, hyperoside, quercetin derivatives
- **Tannins (10%):** Ellagitannins including eugenin
- **Triterpenes:** Oleanolic acid (1%), crataegolic acid (maslic acid, 0.15%)
- **Steroids:** Sterols, including β-sitosterol (Brendler et al., 2007)

THERAPEUTIC USE

TPM Literature

Clove is a potent detoxifying agent and antidepressant. It can be used as a brain tonic and can strengthen the mind. It is useful for headaches due to cold and wet dystemperament and other neurological disorders due to phlegmatic or melancholic disorders including stroke, hemiplegia, facial palsy, and numbness by oral or topical administration. Moreover, it has been applied for recurrent catarrh. Chewing clove buds strengthens gums, relieves toothache, eliminates bad breath, and freshens the mouth. Clove improves eyesight, recovers eye pannus and blurred vision, both orally and topically. Oral administration of clove buds improves productive cough, dyspnea due to thick phlegm, as well as dysrhythmia due to cold dystemperament. Moreover, it can ameliorate psychological disorders including panic, anxiety, and obsession.

Oral consumption of clove strengthens gastrointestinal tract and liver and improves digestion. It is recommended for flatulence, nausea, vomiting, hiccup, belching, and diarrhea. Moreover, clove has libido-enhancing properties. It is useful for uterine and renal disorders due to cold dystemperament and eliminates urinary incontinence and strangury. Continuity of eating about 3 g of clove per day except during menstruation warms uterine and reduces infertility in women. Applying clove as a

 DOI: 10.1201/b22971-35

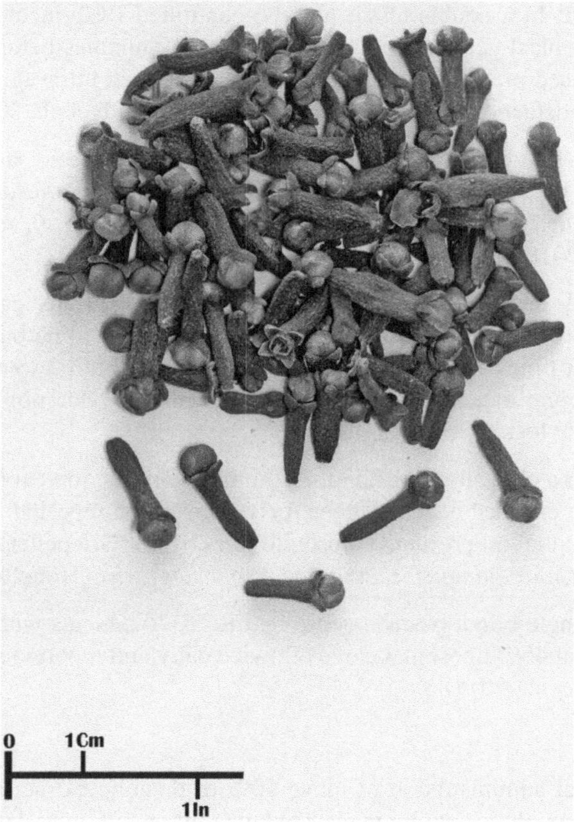

FIGURE 35.1 Clove buds.

poultice relieves pain caused by cold dystemperament and helps detoxification (Aghili Khorasani 1771; Avicenna 1025).

Current Evidence

Clinical Evidence

Anal fissure: In a single-blind RCT including 55 patients (30 patients in intervention and 25 patients in control group), a topical clove cream containing 1% clove oil was administered three times daily for 6 weeks. There was a significant healing effect on chronic anal fissure by improving resting anal pressure and other anorectal manometric pressures in comparison with 5% lignocaine cream (Elwakeel et al., 2007). In another double-blind RCT including 35 patients in each group with chronic anal fissure, applying one gram, twice a day of a topical gel containing clove extract for 6 weeks, versus topical diltiazem (2%), significantly reduced pain and improved wound healing, but did not significantly affect recurrence rate (Tavakoli-Dastjerdi et al., 2019).

Anesthesia: In a single-blind RCT in 73 adult volunteers under experimentally induced pain by needle sticks, applying topical clove gel (fine powder of clove in glycerin with ratio 2:3) demonstrated local anesthetic effect similar to 20% benzocaine gel (Alqareer et al., 2006).

Premature ejaculation: In a double-blind, placebo-controlled RCT including two groups of 11 participants, applying topical gel containing 1% clove oil, 10 minutes before the intercourse for a period of 8 weeks reduced premature ejaculation score, increased intravaginal ejaculation latency time, and intercourse satisfaction compared to placebo (Olounabadi et al., 2021).

Detoxification: In a double-blind, crossover RCT including 16 male social drinkers, daily intake of one 250 mg capsule of clove bud hydroethanolic extract has shown faster elimination of blood acetaldehyde with significant decrease in oxidative stress, LPO, CRP, IL-6, and increase in GSH and SOD (Mammen et al., 2018).

Radiotherapy-induced oral mucositis: In a single-blind RCT in patients suffering from radiotherapy-induced oral mucositis, gargling 10 mL of clove-based herbal mouthwash vs. clear water for 1 minute, four times a day at the onset of radiotherapy until 2 weeks after completion or until radiation-induced oral mucositis subsided, has shortened the duration of grade ≥2 mucositis and reduced body weight loss (Kong et al., 2016).

Mosquito repellent: In a clinical trial using three human subjects, topical pure clove essential oil was applied to the skin exposed to mosquitoes for 1 minute and repeated every 30 minutes until the first bite. Clove essential oil prevented mosquito bites by 100% repellent activity for 2–4 hours against *Aedes aegypti*, *Culex quinquefasciatus* and *Anopheles dirus* (Trongtokit et al., 2005).

Hyperhidrosis: In a single-blind, placebo-controlled RCT, 40 patients with palmar hyperhidrosis were treated with topical 45% liposomal clove oil twice daily and reported significant reduction in sweating rate (Ibrahim et al., 2018).

Preclinical Evidence

Anxiety: Intraperitoneal administration of clove 50% methanolic extract by doses 100 and 200 mg/kg to rats showed anxiolytic activity in elevated plus-maze and light–dark model (Tiwari et al., 2014). Moreover, oral administration of clove 70% hydroethanolic extract at two doses of 100 and 200 mg/kg for 14 days reduced stress in rats (Singh et al., 2009).

Depression: Acute administration of clove essential oil by gavage exerted antidepressant-like effects in the forced swimming test (200 mg/kg) and tail suspension test (100 and 200 mg/kg). Long-term oral treatment with clove essential oil significantly increased sucrose preference (50, 100, and 200 mg/kg), as well as the protein levels of hippocampal p-ERK, p-CREB, and brain-derived neurotrophic factor in mice exposed to chronic unpredictable mild stress (Liu et al., 2015). In another study, intraperitoneal administration of clove essential oil in doses of 0.025, 0.05, and 0.1 mL/kg/day for 3 weeks significantly decreased the immobility time in animal models of depression (Mehta et al., 2013).

Memory impairment: Administration of clove oil (0.025, 0.05, 0.1 mL/kg, intraperitoneal injection) for 3 weeks in scopolamine-induced memory impairment in mice reversed learning and memory by increasing acquisition latency and retention latency in elevated plus-maze (Halder et al., 2011). Another animal study using the same animal model confirmed the memory enhancing properties of clove essential oil (0.1, 0.025, and 0.05 mL/kg) (Halder et al., 2012). Clove essential oil (0.05 and 0.1 mL/kg) could also improve cognitive performance in a rat model of intracerebroventricular colchicine-induced cognitive dysfunction, evidenced by reducing transfer latency and increased time spent in target quadrant in Morris water maze task, decreased AchE activity and oxidative damage (Kumar et al., 2016). Also, neuroprotective effect of acute oral administration of 200 mg/kg of clove aqueous extract is demonstrated against oxidative damages induced by $AlCl_3$ in rat brains for 14 consecutive days (Kassab et al., 2014).

Seizures: In mouse model of PTZ-induced seizures, the anticonvulsant effect of different clove extracts was observed. The minimal clonic seizure and generalized tonic-clonic seizure latency was significantly extended by single injection of clove aqueous and ethanolic extract at a dose range of 50, 100, 250, and 500 mg/kg (Hosseini et al., 2012). In an animal study, intraperitoneal clove essential oil at the doses of 0.05, 0.075, and 0.1 mL/kg exhibited anticonvulsant activity against tonic seizures induced by maximal electroshock in male mice (Pourgholami et al., 1999).

Arthritis: In an animal study using Freund's complete adjuvant-induced arthritis in rats, topical 1.2% clove essential oil in a lipid nanocarrier inhibited serum lysosomal enzymes and proinflammatory cytokines TNF-α and IL-6, and improved hind leg function (Shakeel et al., 2021).

Pain: In a mouse model of pain using tail-flick test and formalin-induced pain, intraperitoneal administration of clove essential oil with a dose range of 0.1, 0.025, and 0.05 mL/kg could reduce pain response by a predominantly peripheral action via the involvement of opioid receptors (Halder et al., 2012). In an animal study, subcutaneous administration of clove essential oil at doses 100 and 200 mg/kg produced analgesia compared to vehicle in the acute corneal pain through involvement of opioidergic and cholinergic systems. In addition, topical administration at the dose of 50 and 200 μg per eye in rats with acute corneal pain, significantly decreased corneal sensitivity (Khalilzadeh et al., 2016). In another study, administration of clove oil intraperitoneally at a dose of 33 mg/kg, significantly decreased acetic acid-induced writhing movements compared with aspirin injection (100 mg/kg), increased the reaction latency to pain compared with morphine (5 mg/kg), and showed anti-inflammatory activity by suppressing the increase in paw edema compared with control group (Taher et al., 2015). In another animal study, intraperitoneal injection of 0.1 mL/kg of clove essential oil significantly reduced pain response in the tail-flick and formalin tests (Halder et al., 2012). Moreover, aqueous extract of clove in doses of 50, 100, and 200 mg/kg demonstrated analgesic effect in mice in hot plate test in comparison to normal saline (Kamkar Asl et al., 2013). Intraperitoneal injection of ethanolic extracts of clove in doses of 50, 100, and 200 mg/kg exerted a significant protective effect on acetic acid-induced abdominal constriction in mouse (Tanko et al., 2008).

Neurotoxicity: Administration of ethanolic extract of clove with the dose of 100 mg/kg in chloride-induced neurotoxicity in mice for 60 days, restored memory impairment, decreased acetylcholinesterase activity, decreased oxidative stress, and prevented histopathological alteration (Kadri et al., 2019). Also, in $AlCl_3$-induced neurotoxicity in mice, 500 mg/kg of clove ethanolic extract for 21 days improved the neuronal structural damage (Amber et al., 2018).

Peptic ulcer: In ethanol-induced gastric injury in rats, oral administration of 250 mg/kg of clove aqueous extract for 3 days showed gastroprotective effect by increasing PGE2 compared with negative control (Jin et al., 2016). In another study using the same animal model, single oral dose of 100 mg/kg of clove polyphenol-rich extract exhibited antiulcerogenic activity against stomach ulcers in rats (Issac et al., 2015). Single oral administration of 100 and 250 mg/kg of clove essential oil exhibited gastroprotective activity by enhancing mucus production in both ethanol and indomethacin-induced peptic ulcer models in rats (Santin et al., 2011).

Hyperlipidemia: Daily oral administration of 40 mg/kg of clove essential oil during 1 month showed lipid-lowering activity in both plasma and liver in high-fructose-fed induced metabolic syndrome in rats (Al-Okbi et al., 2014).

Adding 0.5 g/100 g of ethanolic extract of clove to mice diet for 3 weeks exhibited hypoglycemic effects on genetically diabetic KK-A^y mice (Kuroda et al., 2012). It is in agreement with another study which showed hypoglycemic effect of clove by adding its powder to the diet of STZ-induced diabetes in rats through 15 weeks (Shukri et al., 2010).

Hepatotoxicity: In CCl_4-induced liver injury in rats, oral gavage of 70% ethanolic extract of clove in a dose of 100 mg/kg three times a week for 5 weeks, decreased AST and ALT, as well as inflammatory markers such as TGF-β level (Abdelrahman et al., 2018). In another study in the same animal model, oral 100 and 200 mg/kg of clove essential oil for 8 weeks could reduce AST, ALT, and ALP, and ameliorate central lobular necrosis, hepatic lipidosis, and hepatic fibrosis (El-Hadary et al., 2016). In paracetamol-induced hepatotoxicity in rabbit, oral administration of 100 mg of grinded clove bud for 20 days could decrease ALT, AST and GGT (Kazi et al., 2017). Also, in the hepatotoxicity induced by *Catha edulis* in rat, oral administration of 0.74 g/kg of clove aqueous extract for 6 weeks, reversed liver damage by decreasing ALT, AST, ALP activities, as well as bilirubin and albumin levels (Saad et al., 2015).

Nephrotoxicity: In levofloxacin-induced nephrotoxicity in rats, oral administration of clove oil at the dose of 10 mg/kg for 28 days could ameliorate renal histopathological damage (Fiqardina et al., 2022).

Aphrodisiac: Intracavernosal injection of a single dose of 1 μM clove essential oil restored erectile responses in STZ-induced diabetic rats by inducing remarkable relaxation in the cavernosal smooth muscle (Yilmaz-Oral et al., 2020). In another animal study oral administration of clove ethanolic extract at the dose of 250 and 500 mg/kg, once a day for 7 days, significantly improved sexual behavior in male rats in comparison with sildenafil (Tajuddin et al., 2004).

ADVERSE REACTIONS

TPM Literature

It may be harmful to the kidneys and intestines and thus is recommended to be taken with gum Arabic (Aghili Khorasani 1771).

Current Evidence

No health hazards or side effects are known with the proper administration of therapeutic dosages. Clove essential oil in concentrated form may be irritating to the mucosa (Brendler et al., 2007). Clove oil should be used with caution orally. Repeated application of clove oil as a toothache remedy may damage the gingival tissue (Barnes et al., 2007) as reported in a clinical trial (Alqareer et al., 2006). In a clinical trial, applying clove cream 5% for anal fissure led to severe itching in 2 of 30 patients (Elwakeel et al., 2007).

CONTRAINDICATIONS

TPM Literature

None.

Current Evidence

Undiluted clove oil should not be used on the skin (Barnes et al., 2007).

PREGNANCY AND LACTATION

TPM Literature

None.

Current Evidence

There are no known problems with the use of clove in food amounts during pregnancy or lactation (Barnes et al., 2007).

DRUG INTERACTIONS

None.

METHOD OF ADMINISTRATION

TPM Literature

It could be chewed for oral cavity disorders, orally or topically for eye disorders, and topically for pain. For uterine disorders, it can be used orally or intravaginally. For other diseases, it can be used orally as decoction, syrup, or raw plant powder (Aghili Khorasani 1771).

Current Evidence

Clove oil can be used orally for gastrointestinal disorders and topically as an analgesic or as undiluted essential oil for dental antiseptic (Brendler et al., 2007). Clove powder or decoction may be taken orally (Gardner and McGuffin, 2013).

DOSAGE

Clove buds: 120–300 mg as powder or 1–5 g as a decoction.
Clove oil: 0.05–0.2 mL (Barnes et al., 2007).

Aqueous solution corresponding to 1–5% essential oil can be used externally in mouthwashes (Brendler et al., 2007).

REFERENCES

Abdelrahman MT, Maina EN, Elshemy HA. Clove (*Syzygium aromaticum*) and honey extracts significantly reduce inflammatory cytokines and liver function enzymes in experimental rats fed on carbon tetrachloride (CCl4). J Radiat Res Appl Sci. 2018;11(4):416–422.

Aghili Khorasani MH 1771. *Makhzan-al-Adviah* (*The treasury of drugs*) (rewritten by Shams Ardakani MR, Rahimi R, Farjadmand F, 1st ed.). Tehran: Tehran University of Medical Sciences; 2009.

Al-Okbi SY, Mohamed DA, Hamed TE, Edris AE. Protective effect of clove oil and eugenol microemulsions on fatty liver and dyslipidemia as components of metabolic syndrome. J Med Food. 2014;17(7):764–771.

Alqareer A, Alyahya A, Andersson L. The effect of clove and benzocaine versus placebo as topical anesthetics. J Dent. 2006;34(10):747–750.

Amber S, Shah SA, Ahmed T, Zahid S. *Syzygium aromaticum* ethanol extract reduces AlCl3-induced neurotoxicity in mice brain through regulation of amyloid precursor protein and oxidative stress gene expression. Asian Pac J Trop Med. 2018;11(2):123–130.

Avicenna 1025. *Al-Qanoon fi al-Tibb* (*The canon of medicine*) (rewritten by Masoudi A, ed.). Tehran: Almaei; 2015.

Barnes J, Anderson LA, Phillipson JD. *Herbal medicines*, vol. 4. London: Pharmaceutical Press; 2007.

El-Hadary AE, Ramadan MF. Potential protective effect of cold-pressed *Coriandrum sativum* oil against carbon tetrachloride-induced hepatotoxicity in rats. J Food Biochem. 2016;40(2):190–200.

Elwakeel HA, Moneim HA, Farid M, Gohar AA. Clove oil cream: A new effective treatment for chronic anal fissure. Color Dis. 2007;9(6):549–552.

Fiqardina A, Djabir YY, Santoso A, et al. The nephroprotective effect of clove oil (*Oleum Caryophylli*) against levofloxacin toxicity in rats. Iran J Toxicol. 2022;16(1):27–34.

Gardner Z, McGuffin M. *Botanical safety handbook*. Boca Raton: Taylor & Francis; 2013.

Halder S, Mehta AK, Kar R, et al. Clove oil reverses learning and memory deficits in scopolamine-treated mice. Planta Med. 2011;77(8):830–834.

Halder S, Mehta AK, Mediratta PK, et al. Acute effect of essential oil of *Eugenia caryophyllata* on cognition and pain in mice. Naunyn Schmiedebergs Arch Pharmacol. 2012;385(6):587–593.

Hosseini M, Jafarianheris T, Seddighi N, et al. Effects of different extracts of *Eugenia caryophyllata* on pentylenetetrazole-induced seizures in mice. J Chinese Integr Med. 2012;10(12):1476–1481.

Ibrahim IM, Abdel Kareem IM, Alghobashy MA. Evaluation of topical liposome incorporated clove oil in the treatment of idiopathic palmar hyperhidrosis: Single-blinded placebo-controlled study. J Cosmet Dermatol. 2018;17(6):1084–1089.

Issac A, Gopakumar G, Kuttan R, et al. Safety and anti-ulcerogenic activity of a novel polyphenol-rich extract of clove buds (*Syzygium aromaticum* L). Food Funct. 2015;6(3):842–852.

Jin SE, Lee M-Y, Shin I-S, et al. *Syzygium aromaticum* water extract attenuates ethanol-induced gastric injury through antioxidant effects in rats. Mol Med Rep. 2016;14(1):361–366.

Kadri Y, Nciri R, Bardaa S, et al. *Syzygium aromaticum* alleviates cerium chloride-induced neurotoxic effect in the adult mice. Toxicol Mech Methods. 2019;29(1):26–34.

Kamkar Asl M, Nazariborun A, Hosseini M. Analgesic effect of the aqueous and ethanolic extracts of clove. Avicenna J Phytomed. 2013;3(2):186–192.

Kassab RB, Bauomy AA. The neuroprotective efficency of the aqueous extract of clove (*Syzygium aromaticum*) in aluninium-induced neurotoxicity. Int J Pharm Sci. 2014;6(5):503–508.

Kazi S, Ansari MA, Memon AR, et al. Reversal of paracetamol induced hepatotoxicity in animals model: Clove, an alternative medicine beyond the spices. J Liaquat Univ Med Heal Sci. 2017;16(3):154–157.

Khalilzadeh E, Hazrati R, Saiah GV. Effects of topical and systemic administration of *Eugenia caryophyllata* buds essential oil on corneal anesthesia and analgesia. Res Pharm Sci. 2016;11(4):293–302.

Kong M, Hwang D-SS, Yoon SW, et al. The effect of clove-based herbal mouthwash on radiation-induced oral mucositis in patients with head and neck cancer: A single-blind randomized preliminary study. Onco Targets Ther. 2016;9:4533–4538.

Kumar A, Aggrawal A, Pottabathini R, et al. Possible neuroprotective mechanisms of clove oil against icv-colchicine induced cognitive dysfunction. Pharmacol Reports. 2016;68(4):764–772.

Kuroda M, Mimaki Y, Ohtomo T, et al. Hypoglycemic effects of clove (*Syzygium aromaticum* flower buds) on genetically diabetic KK-A^y mice and identification of the active ingredients. J Nat Med. 2012;66(2):394–399.

Liu B, Luo L, Liu XL, et al. Essential oil of *Syzygium aromaticum* reverses the deficits of stress-induced behaviors and hippocampal p-ERK/p-CREB/brain-derived neurotrophic factor expression. Planta Med. 2015;81(3):185–192.

Mammen RR, Natinga Mulakal J, Mohanan R, et al. Clove bud polyphenols alleviate alterations in inflammation and oxidative stress markers associated with binge drinking: A randomized double-blinded placebo-controlled crossover study. J Med Food. 2018;21(11):1188–1196.

Mehta AK, Halder S, Khanna N, et al. The effect of the essential oil of *Eugenia caryophyllata* in animal models of depression and locomotor activity. Nutr Neurosci. 2013;16(5):233–238.

Olounabadi ARS, Khayyamfar F, Kamalinejad M, et al. Effect of topical clove (*Syzygium aromaticum* (L.) Merr. & L.M.Perry) gel on premature ejaculation: A pilot randomized double-blind placebo-controlled clinical trial. Tradit Integr Med. 2021;6(3):236–248.

Pourgholami MH, Kamalinejad M, Javadi M, et al. Evaluation of the anticonvulsant activity of the essential oil of *Eugenia caryophyllata* in male mice. J Ethnopharmacol. 1999;64(2):167–171.

Saad EA, Toson EA, Ahmed GM. Clove or green tea administration antagonizes khat hepatotoxicity in rats. Int J Pharm Pharm Sci. 2015;7(6):72–76.

Santin JR, Lemos M, Klein-Júnior LC, et al. Gastroprotective activity of essential oil of the *Syzygium aromaticum* and its major component eugenol in different animal models. Naunyn Schmiedebergs = Arch Pharmacol. 2011;383(2):149–158.

Shakeel F, Alam P, Ali AA, et al. Investigating antiarthritic potential of nanostructured clove oil (*Syzygium aromaticum*) in fca-induced arthritic rats: Pharmaceutical action and delivery strategies. Molecules 2021;26(23):7327.

Shukri R, Mohamed S, Mustapha NM. Cloves protect the heart, liver and lens of diabetic rats. Food Chem. 2010;122(4):1116–1121.

Singh AK, Dhamanigi SS, Asad M. Anti-stress activity of hydro-alcoholic extract of *Eugenia caryophyllus* buds (clove). Indian J Pharmacol. 2009;41(1):28–31.

Taher YA, Samud AM, El-Taher FE, et al. Experimental evaluation of anti-inflammatory, antinociceptive and antipyretic activities of clove oil in mice. Libyan J Med. 2015;10(1):28685.

Tajuddin A, Ahmad S, Latif A, et al. Effect of 50% ethanolic extract of *Syzygium aromaticum* (L.) Merr. & Perry. (clove) on sexual behaviour of normal male rats. BMC Complement Altern Med. 2004;4(1):1–7.

Tanko Y, Mohammed A, Okasha MA, et al. Anti-nociceptive and anti-inflammatory activities of ethanol extract of *Syzygium aromaticum* flower bud in Wistar rats and mice. African J Tradit Complement Altern Med. 2008;5(2):209–212.

Tavakoli-Dastjerdi S, Motavasselian M, Emami SA, et al. Efficacy of a combination of herbal gel versus topical diltiazem (2%) in chronic anal fissure healing: A randomized double-blind clinical trial. J HerbMed Pharmacol. 2019;8(2):139–145.

Tiwari P, Verma R, Ahirwar D, et al. Evaluation of anxiolytic effect of *Syzygium aromaticum*: A traditional herb of India. Asian Pacific J Trop Dis. 2014;4(S1):S77–80.

Trongtokit Y, Rongsriyam Y, Komalamisra N, et al. Comparative repellency of 38 essential oils against mosquito bites. Phyther Res. 2005;19(4):303–309.

Yilmaz-Oral D, Onder A, Gur S, et al. The beneficial effect of clove essential oil and its major component, eugenol, on erectile function in diabetic rats. Andrologia. 2020;52(6):1–8.

36 *Terminalia chebula* Retz.

Ayeh Naghizadeh

Scientific name: *Terminalia chebula* Retz.
Family: Combretaceae
Common names:

- **English:** Chebulic myrobalan, tropical almond, black myrobalan, true myrobalan, haritaki
- **Persian:** *halīleh*
- **Arabic:** *'ihlīlağ*

Medicinal part(s): Fruit (Figure 36.1)
Temperament (nature): Cold in the first degree and dry in the second degree
Major chemical constituents:

- **Tannins (20–45%):** Gallotannins, including terchebulin, terflavin A, punicalagin, corilagin, chebulic acid, and chebulagic acid
- **Monosaccharides/oligosaccharides (9%):** D-glucose, D-fructose, saccharose
- **Phenolic acid derivatives:** Gallic acid, ellagic acid, methyl/ethyl gallate, ferulic acid
- **Flavonoids:** Rutin, quercetin, luteolin
- **Alpha-hydroxy acids:** Quinic acid, shikimic acid (Nigam et al., 2020; Gruenwald et al., 2007)

THERAPEUTIC USE

TPM Literature

According to the degree of ripeness, chebulic myrobalan fruit is named black (unripe), yellow (partially ripe), or Kabolian (completely ripe) which act as purgative of black bile, bile, and phlegm humors, respectively. This fruit can reinforce the senses and memory. It is recommended for several diseases of the nervous system including headaches, melancholy, epilepsy, tremors, depression, obsessive disorder, and amnesia, either by itself or in combination with sugar, honey, or other herbs as jam or electuary. It sharpens brain and is useful in true vertigo and dizziness. Persistent use of chebulic myrobalan prevents graying of hair. Used topically, burnt powder of this fruit helps stop bleeding, and also strengthens the teeth and gingiva. A strong beneficial effect on the gingiva is also regarded for keeping the fruit in the mouth. In *The canon of medicine*, it is also recommended for palpitations, and splenic pain. Chebulic myrobalan is a tonic for the stomach and the liver, as well. Chebulic myrobalan is an astringent and used to treat diarrhea. It is also beneficial for hemorrhoids (Aghili Khorasani 1771; Avicenna 1025).

Current Evidence

Clinical Evidence

Schizophrenia: In a double-blind, placebo-controlled RCT in 54 patients with chronic schizophrenia, chebulic myrobalan fruit powder was administered as six 500 mg capsules (also containing

DOI: 10.1201/b22971-36

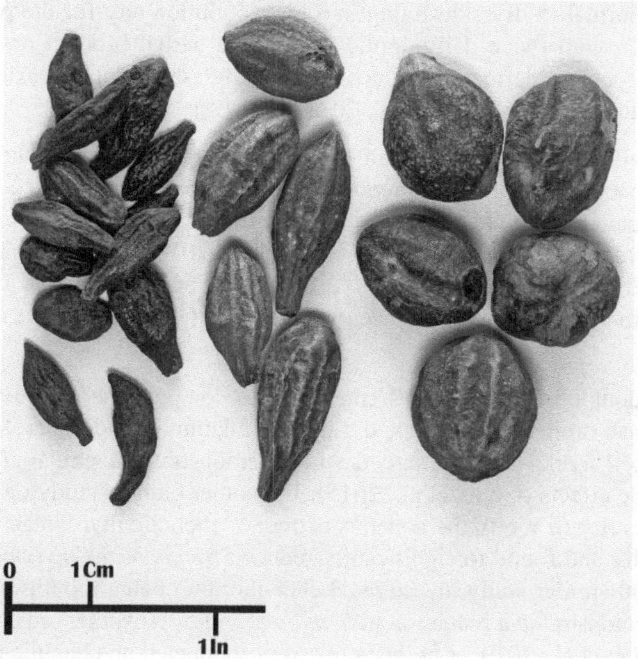

FIGURE 35.1 Clove buds.

10% sweet almond oil as coregent) for 4 weeks. Considering Screen for Cognitive Impairments in Psychiatry (SCIP) and the relevant subscales of the Positive and Negative Syndrome Scale (PANSS), significant improvements were observed in cognitive impairment, negative and positive symptoms of the patients under treatment with the herbal capsule without a notable side effect (Banazadeh et al., 2022).

Type 2 diabetes: In a placebo-controlled RCT, the effect of chebulic myrobalan with the doses of 250 and 500 mg per day on endothelial dysfunction and biomarkers of oxidative stress has been studied in 60 type 2 diabetic patients. Upon 12 weeks of intervention, significant improvement of HbA1c, lipid parameters, refractive index and NO, GSH, MDA, and hs-CRP were observed, especially with the higher dose (Pingali et al., 2020).

Joint pain: In an RCT on 105 overweight, apparently healthy subjects, a standardized aqueous extract of chebulic myrobalan fruit was administered in 250 or 500 mg twice daily doses for 12 weeks. Both doses improved modified Knee Injury & Osteoarthritis Outcomes Score (mKOOS) global scores, knee discomfort with activity/exercise, knee soreness following leg extension resistance exercise, and overall whole-body joint function, as well as a significant reduction of TNF-α compared with placebo. No significant difference was found between the two doses (Lopez et al., 2017).

Hyperuricemia: The efficacy and tolerability of chebulic myrobalan on reduction of serum uric acid levels has been clinically investigated in 110 hyperuricemic patients. This RCT showed that aqueous extract of chebulic myrobalan with a dosage of 500 mg twice a day for 24 weeks can significantly reduce uric acid in patients with hyperuricemia compared with placebo; however, it was not as potent as the control drug febuxostat (Usharani et al., 2016).

Skin damage: A topical standardized oil-in-water emulsion containing 1% chebulic myrobalan extract was investigated for the ability to reverse visible signs of pollution-induced skin damage in 52 females with normal to dry skin living in a high-pollution city for the past 5 years. After 8 weeks of intervention with twice daily application of the herbal product or placebo, significant improvements were found in dermatologist scores and self-assessments for skin texture, hydration, tone, firmness and radiance (Randhawa et al., 2021).

Pain: In a double-blind, placebo-controlled RCT, the analgesic activity and safety of a single 1,000 mg dose of chebulic myrobalan aqueous extract was investigated in 12 healthy participants using a mechanical pain model which resulted in a significant increase in both pain threshold force and time, and pain tolerance force and time (Pokuri et al., 2016). The same dosage has also been assessed in a hot air pain model in healthy 12 human participants, which indicated significant increase in mean pain threshold and tolerance time compared to both baseline and placebo (Kumar et al., 2015).

Dental plaque: A double-blind RCT was conducted to compare the effectiveness of a chebulic myrobalan mouthwash on dental plaque and gingival inflammation compared with chlorhexidine 0.2% and placebo for 4 weeks in 90 volunteers which demonstrated a similar effectiveness to chlorhexidine with no side effects (Gupta et al., 2015). In another clinical study on 8–12-year-old children with high caries risk ($n = 60$), the aqueous extract of chebulic myrobalan was investigated for anticariogenic activity and found to significantly reduce *Streptococcus mutans* counts (Palit et al., 2016). A more recent similar study investigated chebulic myrobalan mouthwash in 8–15-year-old children and also demonstrated a reduction in *S. mutans* and improvement in oral hygiene after 15–30 days of use (Mishra et al., 2019). Another study was conducted on chebulic myrobalan ethanolic extract formulated as a mouthwash in 60 children which also showed a reduction in *S. mutans* count as early as 5 minutes after rinsing, which continued up to 6 hours post rinsing among 80% of the children (Nayak et al., 2012).

Preclinical Evidence

GI disorders: In a study on hydroalcoholic extract of chebulic myrobalan fruit, pretreatment with doses of 200 and 500 mg/kg resulted in significant reduction in lesion index, total affected area, and percentage of lesion in aspirin, ethanol, and cold restraint stress-induced ulcer models (Sharma et al., 2011). In another study, an orally administered chebulic myrobalan extract (100 mg/kg/day) for 15 days showed prokinetic activity and could significantly increase gastric emptying in rats (Tamhane et al., 1997). This is while an aqueous extract of dried chebulic myrobalan (200–800 mg/kg) has been demonstrated to reduce diarrhea, inhibits intestinal transit, and decrease the volume of enteropooling in a dose-dependent manner (Sheng et al., 2016).

Neuroprotection: An animal study on a middle cerebral artery occlusion model of stroke in rats showed that administration of chebulic myrobalan ameliorates neurological defects. Using metabolomics technology, this study attributed this effect to pathways of energy metabolism (glycolysis and the tricarboxylic acid cycle), amino acid metabolism, and glycerophospholipid metabolism (Liu et al., 2018). Moreover, oral chebulic myrobalan extract in 100 and 200 mg/kg doses for 2 weeks has been demonstrated to exert antidepressant and anxiolytic activities, with the higher dose also causing significant reduction in MAO-A activity in the mouse brain (Mani et al., 2021).

Learning and memory impairment: Administration of chebulic myrobalan extract in 100 or 200 mg/kg doses for 14 days, has been demonstrated to reverse scopolamine-induced learning and memory deficits. These effects are exerted via reduced hippocampal AchE activities and increased choline acetyltransferase and Ach levels (Kim et al., 2018). Chebulic myrobalan can also reverse methamphetamine-induced memory and learning deficits, and reduce oxidative stress in the hippocampus and serum of mice (Zeng et al., 2022).

Seizure: Oral administration of chebulic myrobalan extract (1,000 mg/kg) has significant anticonvulsant activity in animal models, and can attenuate seizure-induced oxidative stress and cognitive impairment. It also potentiates the anticonvulsant effect of subtherapeutic doses of phenytoin and valproate (Kumar et al., 2018).

Organ toxicity: Chebulic myrobalan has been investigated in a number of studies regarding cardioprotective activity. Pretreatment of rats with chebulic myrobalan extract stabilizes the lysosomal membrane and ameliorates LPO, thereby protecting the heart against isoproterenol-induced damages (Suchalatha and Devi, 2005; Suchalatha and Shyamala Devi, 2004). Also, doses of 300 mg/kg have been associated with significant reduction in troponin and ameliorate toxicity induced by doxorubicin (Manikandan et al., 2022).

This fruit can also protect the liver against injuries and oxidative damage (Lee et al., 2005). An investigation on the effect of chebulic myrobalan methanolic extract on iron overload showed that it can reduce iron-induced hepatic toxicity and possibly be beneficial as an iron-chelating drug (Sarkar et al., 2012). Moreover, pretreatment with chebulic myrobalan aqueous extract could efficiently ameliorate acute and severe liver injury via inhibition of oxidative stress and inflammation (Choi et al., 2015). Another study found that chebulic myrobalan administration for 15 days can attenuate diazinon-induced oxidative stress in the liver (Ahmadi-Naji et al., 2017).

Chebulic myrobalan extract has been demonstrated to suppress kidney damage induced by nickel and ferric nitrilotriacetic acid and prevent carcinogenesis due to these chemical substances in animal models (Prasad et al., 2006; Prasad et al., 2007). Furthermore, oxidative and histological damage in a cisplatin-induced nephrotoxicity model were ameliorated with chebulic myrobalan pretreatment (Kalra et al., 2019).

Protective effects of chebulic myrobalan on the skin have also been investigated. Topical application of chebulic myrobalan extract is beneficial in protecting the skin against photodamage (Yakaew et al., 2016). Chemically induced skin tumorigenesis is also inhibited by chebulic myrobalan via upregulation of endogenous cytoprotective mechanisms and downregulation of inflammatory mediators (Majed et al., 2015).

Chebulic myrobalan has exhibited antioxidant and radical scavenging activities in animal studies (Hazra et al., 2010), and can also prevent age-induced damages by protecting against oxidative stress (Mahesh et al., 2009).

Burns: Topical application of creams containing 5% and 10% chebulic myrobalan extract has been compared with silver sulfadiazine 1% cream in a hot water-induced burn wound model in rats. Results showed that chebulic myrobalan can accelerate wound healing and is even more efficient than silver sulfadiazine (Nasiri et al., 2015).

ADVERSE REACTIONS

TPM Literature

Single use of chebulic myrobalan can harm the brain and liver and is better used with honey to prevent this effect. Due to potent astringent properties, it may harm the bowels and thus is recommended to be used with jujube fruit, Assyrian plum, almond oil, honey, sugar, or manna as corrigent. Chebulic myrobalan decoction is not recommended for use as enema due to potent astringent effect and, if necessary, the macerated solution in mixture with emollient ingredients should be used (Aghili Khorasani 1771).

Current Evidence

Administration of chebulic myrobalan in therapeutic doses is safe. Acute and subacute toxicity studies have demonstrated oral administration of chebulic myrobalan to be nontoxic (Suganthy et al., 2018). At doses up to 3 g/kg, no alterations in liver and kidney function were observed (Gardner and McGuffin, 2013). However, caution should be taken when administering to diabetic patients, as chebulic myrobalan has hypoglycemic activity and can increase insulin levels (Gardner and McGuffin, 2013) . Chebulic myrobalan can also cause constipation due to high tannin content (Gruenwald et al., 2007). An animal study in rats reported liver damage with 10–14 days of administration of a diet containing 25% chebulic myrobalan seed (Gardner and McGuffin, 2013); thus, when using the fruit, the seeds should be removed.

CONTRAINDICATIONS

TPM Literature

None.

Current Evidence

None.

PREGNANCY AND LACTATION

TPM Literature

None.

Current Evidence

Although safety has not been established, there is no evidence in literature for any adverse effect of chebulic myrobalan in pregnancy or lactation (Gardner and McGuffin, 2013).

DRUG INTERACTIONS

Chebulic myrobalan can inhibit activities of CYP2E1 and CYP2C19, and therefore, caution should be taken in concomitant use with drugs metabolized by these enzymes, such as albendazole (Wu et al., 2020).

METHOD OF ADMINISTRATION

TPM Literature

Chebulic myrobalan is mainly recommended for oral use. However, the powder is also used topically on the skin and in the mouth. Keeping the fruit in the mouth is regarded beneficial for the teeth and gingiva and also prevention of hair graying.

In oral use, the fruit should not be grinded as fine particles, but should be prepared as coarse particles. Also, it should be rubbed with almond oil to prevent probable colic caused by the plant (Aghili Khorasani 1771).

Current Evidence

Chebulic myrobalan is generally used orally. Topical administration of chebulic myrobalan as cream formulations has been used on the skin in a number of studies. Mouthwash preparations have been used in clinical trials.

DOSAGE

The dosage of orally administered chebulic myrobalan in RCTs is 250–1,000 mg of the extract or up to 3,000 mg of the fruit powder daily.
Daily amount of 3–9 g of the fruit can be orally used (Gruenwald et al., 2007).

REFERENCES

Aghili Khorasani MH 1771. *Makhzan-al-Adviah* (*The treasury of drugs*) (rewritten by Shams Ardakani MR, Rahimi R, Farjadmand F, 1st ed.). Tehran: Tehran University of Medical Sciences; 2009.

Ahmadi-Naji R, Heidarian E, Ghatreh-Samani K. Evaluation of the effects of the hydroalcoholic extract of *Terminalia chebula* fruits on diazinon-induced liver toxicity and oxidative stress in rats. Avicenna J Phytomed. 2017;7(5):454–466.

Avicenna 1025. *Al-Qanoon fi al-Tibb* (*The canon of medicine*) (rewritten by Masoudi A, ed.). Tehran: Almaei; 2015.

Banazadeh M, Mehrabani M, Banazadeh N, et al. Evaluating the effect of black myrobalan on cognitive, positive, and negative symptoms in patients with chronic schizophrenia: A randomized, double-blind, placebo-controlled trial. Phytother Res. 2022;36(1):543–550.

Choi MK, Kim HG, Han JM, et al. Hepatoprotective effect of *Terminalia chebula* against t-BHP-induced acute liver injury in C57/BL6 mice. Evid-Based Complement Alternat Med. 2015;2015:517350.

Gardner Z, McGuffin M. *Botanical safety handbook*. Boca Raton: Taylor & Francis; 2013.

Gruenwald J, Brendler T, Jaenicke C. *PDR for herbal medicines*. Montvale: Thomson Reuters; 2007.

Gupta D, Gupta RK, Bhaskar DJ, Gupta V. Comparative evaluation of *Terminalia chebula* extract mouthwash and chlorhexidine mouthwash on plaque and gingival inflammation: 4-week randomised control trial. Oral Health Prev Dent. 2015;13(1):5–12.

Hazra B, Sarkar R, Biswas S, Mandal N. Comparative study of the antioxidant and reactive oxygen species scavenging properties in the extracts of the fruits of *Terminalia chebula*, *Terminalia belerica* and *Emblica officinalis*. BMC Complement Altern Med. 2010;10(1):1–5.

Kalra P, Karwasra R, Gupta YK, et al. *Terminalia chebula* supplementation attenuates cisplatin-induced nephrotoxicity in Wistar rats through modulation of apoptotic pathway. Nat Prod Res. 2019;33(11):1641–1645.

Kim MS, Lee DY, Lee J, et al. *Terminalia chebula* extract prevents scopolamine-induced amnesia via cholinergic modulation and anti-oxidative effects in mice. BMC Complement Altern Med. 2018;18(1):1–11.

Kumar CU, Pokuri VK, Pingali U. Evaluation of the analgesic activity of standardized aqueous extract of *Terminalia chebula* in healthy human participants using hot air pain model. J Clin Diagn Res. 2015;9(5):FC01.

Kumar R, Arora R, Agarwal A, Gupta YK. Protective effect of *Terminalia chebula* against seizures, seizure-induced cognitive impairment and oxidative stress in experimental models of seizures in rats. J Ethnopharmacol. 2018;215:124–131.

Lee HS, Won NH, Kim KH, et al. Antioxidant effects of aqueous extract of *Terminalia chebula* in vivo and in vitro. Biol Pharm Bull. 2005;28(9):1639–1644.

Liu W, Mu F, Liu T, et al. Ultra performance liquid chromatography/quadrupole time-of-flight mass spectrometry-based metabonomics reveal protective effect of *Terminalia chebula* extract on ischemic stroke rats. Rejuvenation Res. 2018;21(6):541–552.

Lopez HL, Habowski SM, Sandrock JE, et al. Effects of dietary supplementation with a standardized aqueous extract of *Terminalia chebula* fruit (AyuFlex®) on joint mobility, comfort, and functional capacity in healthy overweight subjects: A randomized placebo-controlled clinical trial. BMC Complement Altern Med. 2017;17(1):1–8.

Mahesh R, Bhuvana S, Hazeena Begum VM. Effect of *Terminalia chebula* aqueous extract on oxidative stress and antioxidant status in the liver and kidney of young and aged rats. Cell Biochem Funct. 2009;27(6):358–363.

Majed F, Nafees S, Rashid S, et al. *Terminalia chebula* attenuates DMBA/croton oil-induced oxidative stress and inflammation in Swiss albino mouse skin. Toxicol Int. 2015;22(1):21.

Mani V, Sajid S, Rabbani SI, et al. Anxiolytic-like and antidepressant-like effects of ethanol extract of *Terminalia chebula* in mice. J Tradit Complement Med. 2021;11(6):493–502.

Manikandan R, Balasubramanian B, Punniyakotti P, et al. Cardio-protective effects of terminalia catappa leaves and *Terminalia chebula* fruit extract in doxorubicin-induced cardiomyopathy in rats. Biomarkers. 2022;27(5):488–495.

Mishra P, Marwah N, Agarwal N, et al. Comparison of *Punica granatum*, *Terminalia chebula*, and *Vitis vinifera* seed extracts used as mouthrinse on salivary *Streptococcus mutans* levels in children. J Contemp Dent Pract. 2019;20(8):920–927.

Nasiri E, Hosseinimehr SJ, Azadbakht M, et al. The effect of *Terminalia chebula* extract vs. silver sulfadiazine on burn wounds in rats. J Complement Integr Med. 2015;12(2):127–135.

Nayak SS, Ankola AV, Metgud SC, Bolmal U. Effectiveness of mouthrinse formulated from ethanol extract of *Terminalia chebula* fruit on salivary *Streptococcus mutans* among 12 to 15 year old school children of Belgaum city: A randomized field trial. J Indian Soc Pedod Prev Dent. 2012;30(3):231.

Nigam M, Mishra AP, Adhikari-Devkota A, et al. Fruits of *Terminalia chebula* Retz.: A review on traditional uses, bioactive chemical constituents and pharmacological activities. Phytother Res. 2020;34(10):2518–2533.

Palit M, Hegde SK, Bhat SS. Effectiveness of mouthrinse formulated from aqueous extract of *Terminalia chebula* on salivary *Streptococcus mutans* count and pH among 8-to 12-year-old school children of Karnataka: A randomized clinical trial. Int J Clin Pediatr Dent. 2016;9(4):349.

Pingali U, Sukumaran D, Nutalapati C. Effect of an aqueous extract of *Terminalia chebula* on endothelial dysfunction, systemic inflammation, and lipid profile in type 2 diabetes mellitus: A randomized double-blind, placebo-controlled clinical study. Phytother Res. 2020;34(12):3226–3235.

Pokuri VK, Kumar CU, Pingali U. A randomized, double-blind, placebo-controlled, cross-over study to evaluate analgesic activity of *Terminalia chebula* in healthy human volunteers using a mechanical pain model. J Anaesthesiol Clin Pharmacol. 2016;32(3):329.

Prasad L, Khan TH, Jahangir T, Sultana S. Abrogation of DEN/Fe-NTA induced carcinogenic response, oxidative damage and subsequent cell proliferation response by *Terminalia chebula* in kidney of Wistar rats. Pharmazie. 2007;62(10):790–797.

Prasad L, Khan TH, Jahangir T, Sultana S. Chemomodulatory effects of *Terminalia chebula* against nickel chloride induced oxidative stress and tumor promotion response in male Wistar rats. J Trace Elem Med Biol. 2006;20(4):233–239.

Randhawa M, Meyer T, Sachdev M, Chaudhuri RK. Standardized *Terminalia chebula* fruit extract: A natural ingredient that provides long-lasting antioxidant protection and reverses visible signs of pollution-induced skin damage. Clin Cosmet Investig Dermatol. 2021;14:1257–1269.

Sarkar R, Hazra B, Mandal N. Reducing power and iron chelating property of *Terminalia chebula* (Retz.) alleviates iron induced liver toxicity in mice. BMC Complement Altern Med. 2012;12(1):1–10.

Sharma P, Prakash T, Kotresha D, et al. Antiulcerogenic activity of *Terminalia chebula* fruit in experimentally induced ulcer in rats. Pharm Biol.2011;49(3):262–268.

Sheng Z, Yan X, Zhang R, et al. Assessment of the antidiarrhoeal properties of the aqueous extract and its soluble fractions of chebulae fructus (*Terminalia chebula* fruits). Pharm Biol. 2016;54(9):1847–1856.

Suchalatha S, Devi CS. Protective effect of *Terminalia chebula* against experimental myocardial injury induced by isoproterenol. Indian J Exp Biol. 2004;42(2):174–178.

Suchalatha S, Devi CS. Protective effect of *Terminalia chebula* against lysosomal enzyme alterations in isoproterenol-induced cardiac damage in rats. Exp Clin Cardiol. 2005;10(2):91–95.

Suganthy N, Muniasamy S, Archunan G. Safety assessment of methanolic extract of *Terminalia chebula* fruit, *Terminalia arjuna* bark and its bioactive constituent 7-methyl gallic acid: In vitro and in vivo studies. Regul Toxicol Pharmacol. 2018;92:347–357.

Tamhane MD, Thorat SP, Rege NN, Dahanukar SA. Effect of oral administration of *Terminalia chebula* on gastric emptying: An experimental study. J Postgrad Med. 1997;43(1):12–13.

Usharani P, Nutalapati C, Pokuri VK, et al. A randomized, double-blind, placebo-, and positive-controlled clinical pilot study to evaluate the efficacy and tolerability of standardized aqueous extracts of *Terminalia chebula* and *Terminalia bellerica* in subjects with hyperuricemia. Clin Pharmacol. 2016;8:51–59.

Wu G, Dong Z, Dong J, et al. Effects of mongolian medicine *Terminalia chebula* Retz. on 6 CYP450 enzymes in rats. Int J Clin Exp Pathol. 2020;13(12):3128–3138.

Yakaew S, Itsarasook K, Ngoenkam J, et al. Ethanol extract of *Terminalia chebula* fruit protects against UVB-induced skin damage. Pharm Biol. 2016;54(11):2701–2707.

Zeng Q, Xiong Q, Lin K, et al. *Terminalia chebula* extracts ameliorate methamphetamine-induced memory deficits via activating the ERK and Nrf2 pathway. Brain Res Bull. 2022;184:76–87.

37 *Thymus vulgaris* L., *Zataria multiflora* Boiss.

Azadeh Zarei and Mehrdad Karimi

Scientific name: *Zataria multiflora* Boiss., *Thymus vulgaris* L.
Family: Lamiaceae
Common names:

- **English:** Thyme, common thyme, garden thyme (*T. vulgaris*), Shirazi thyme (*Z. multiflora*)
- **Persian:** *'ābšan, 'ūšan, 'āvīšan*
- **Arabic:** *ṣa'ṭar*

Medicinal part(s): Leaves (Figure 37.1)
Temperament (nature): Hot and dry in the second degree
Major chemical constituents:

- ***T. vulgaris:***
  - **Volatile oil (2.5%):** Thymol (20–55%), *p*-cymene (14–45%), carvacrol (1–10%), γ-terpinene (5–10%), borneol (up to 8%), linalool (up to 8%)
  - **Hydroxycinnamic acids:** Rosmarinic acid (0.15–1.35%)
  - **Flavonoids:** Luteolin, apigenin, naringenin, eriodictyol, cirsilineol, salvigenin, cirsimaritin, thymonin, thymusin, partially present as glycosides
  - **Triterpenes:** Ursolic acid, oleanolic acid (Gruenwald et al., 2007; Williamson et al., 2013)

- ***Z. multiflora:***
  - **Volatile oil:** Thymol, carvacrol, *p*-cymene, linalool, caryophyllene, γ-terpinene, borneol
  - **Nonvolatile glycosides**: Zatariol and zataroside A as derivatives of *p*-cymene
  - **Alkanes:** *N*-nonacosane, *n*-hentriacontane, *n*-dotriacontane, *n*-tritriacontane, *n*-pentatriacontane
  - **Fatty acids:** Behenic acid, lignoceric acid, cerotic acid, montanic acid
  - **Phytosterols:** β-sitosterol, stigmasterol
  - **Triterpenes:** Betulin, betulinic acid, oleanolic acid
  - **Hydroxycinnamic acids:** Rosmarinic acid
  - **Flavonoids:** Apigenin, luteolin, 6-hydroxyluteolin (Shokri and Sharifzadeh, 2017)

THERAPEUTIC USE

TPM Literature

Pouring thyme extract in the ear is used in the treatment of hearing loss, and if it is dripped in the ear along with milk, it reduces ear pain. Consuming its fresh extract is effective in tonsillitis and mouth sores. Also, pouring its extract into the eyes is claimed to cure night blindness. Long-term intake of

DOI: 10.1201/b22971-37

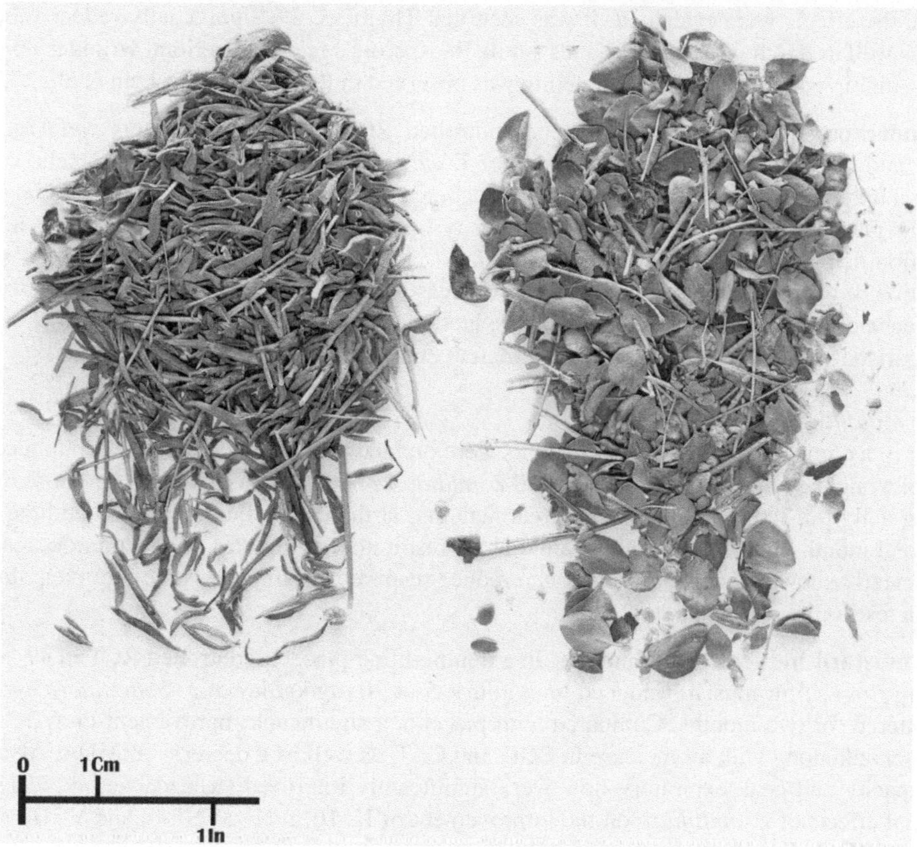

FIGURE 37.1 Garden thyme (left) and Shirazi thyme (right) aerial parts.

thyme at night before bedtime strengthens the mind, improves the color of the face, and reduces the possibility of cataracts. Using thyme combined with honey in a form that can be licked is useful for reproductive cough. Eating it together with slow-digesting food accelerates digestion and eliminates flatulence and dyspepsia. It is used to treat toothache and sore throat. Topically, its poultice with honey is effective for the treatment of painful joint swellings. Also, its poultice with olive oil is used in children's umbilical hernia. Drinking its decoction relieves tooth, bladder and uterus pain (Aghili Khorasani 1771; Avicenna 1025).

Current Evidence

Clinical Evidence

Thymus vulgaris

Facial skin wrinkles: In a double-blind, placebo-controlled RCT, 54 female volunteers were randomly divided into three groups. ThymLec gel containing aerial parts extract of *T. vulgaris* (2%) in the base containing lecithin, propanediol, water, and glycerin was topically administered to 19 women. Another group with 18 participants received a placebo gel (with a formulation having the same base of the treatment gel), and the 17 volunteers of the third group applied a commercial product containing water, propanediol, ornithine, phospholipids, and glycolipids. After 30 and

60 days, the effects were evaluated. It was seen that ThymLec 2% significantly reduced the area, length as well as depth of nasolabial lines, smile lines, crow's feet, and perioral wrinkles on day 30 and 60. Additionally, a face oval remodeling was observed in this group (Caverzan et al., 2021).

Dysmenorrhea: In a triple-blind, placebo-controlled RCT, 84 female students were randomly divided into three groups receiving 25 drops of *T. vulgaris* essential oil 2% plus placebo capsule; 200 mg ibuprofen capsules plus 25 drops of placebo essential oil; and 25 drops of essential oil placebo plus placebo capsule. Dysmenorrhea intensity was evaluated three times: before the intake of medication or placebo, 1 hour after taking each dose (for four doses) and 48 hours after starting medication. It was observed that pain severity decrease was not statistically significant between the ibuprofen and *T. vulgaris* groups, though this reduction was significant for ibuprofen and *T. vulgaris* in comparison with placebo ($p < 0.001$) (Salmalian et al., 2014).

Zataria multiflora

COPD: In a clinical study, 41 COPD patients were divided into three groups: one group received a placebo, while the other two groups received *Z. multiflora* hydroalcoholic extract at a dose of 3 and 6 mg/kg daily for 2 months. Before the treatment and at the end of the first month and the end of the second month, the patients were evaluated for respiratory symptoms and respiratory tests. The results clearly showed that *Z. multiflora* can reduce respiratory symptoms and improve pulmonary function tests (Ghorani et al., 2022).

Sulfur mustard-induced lung damage: In a double-blind placebo-controlled RCT in 47 veterans suffering from sulfur mustard-induced lung injury, 5 or 10 mg/kg/day of a *Z. multiflora* syrup was administered for two months. Compared with placebo, a significant improvement of WBC profile was observed, along with an increase in SOD and CAT, as well as a decrease in MDA. Also, force vital capacity and peak expiratory flow were significantly improved (Khazdair et al., 2018). The beneficial effects of *Z. multiflora* on the improvement of IL-10, IFN-γ, TNF-α, and VEGF are also reported (Khazdair et al., 2020).

Dysmenorrhea: In a single-blind RCT with 120 students aged 18–25 years old, it was seen that *Z. multiflora* reduced the pain intensity of dysmenorrhea. In this study there were two randomized groups: one group received four times a day 5 mL *Z. multiflora* preparation, and another group took ibuprofen 400 mg three times daily. In both groups the pain intensity was decreased without any significant difference. In addition, the two groups had similar pain duration in the first and second treatment month (Direkvand-Moghadam and Khosravi, 2012).

Bacterial vaginosis: In a study, 420 women with vaginosis due to bacterial infection, *Trichomonas vaginalis,* or both infections, were divided into six groups. In fact, all three vaginitis groups were divided into two groups, the first group received oral metronidazole and topical placebo cream, and the second group received oral metronidazole and topical *Z. multiflora* cream. This study showed that *Z. multiflora* vaginal cream is useful in reducing the symptoms of vaginitis (Abdali et al., 2015).

In another clinical trial, 90 female patients with bacterial vaginosis were divided into two groups of 45 people. In this study, the target group received *Z. multiflora* vaginal cream and the control group used metronidazole vaginal gel for five nights, and then the patients were examined and evaluated for the next 7 days based on Amsel and Gram criteria. The results showed that *Z. multiflora* vaginal cream has therapeutic effects similar to metronidazole vaginal gel and can be used as an effective and alternative treatment in bacterial vaginosis (Simbar et al., 2008).

Insulin resistance: In an RCT, the obese patients were divided into three groups: The first group received 0.75 g of *Z. multiflora* in 10 mL of oxymel, the second group received 1.5 g of *Z. multiflora* in 10 mL of oxymel, and the third group received only 10 mL of oxymel twice a day for 2 weeks. The results showed that the consumption of *Z. multiflora* with higher doses can significantly decrease the anthropometric parameters. The reduction of waist circumference and the reduction of insulin resistance were clearly observed in these patients (Abolghasemi et al., 2020).

Denture stomatitis: In an RCT conducted on 24 patients with Candida-related artificial dental stomatitis, the effect of *Z. multiflora* gel 0.1% was compared with miconazole 2% gel. Both interventions were used two times a day for 4 weeks. The results demonstrated that both groups significantly reduced palatal erythema and the number of colonies. However, *Z. multiflora* gel reduced the amount of superficial palatal erythema more effectively than miconazole (Amanlou et al., 2006).

Radiotherapy-induced oral mucositis: In an RCT on 63 patients with head and neck cancer, the effect of *Z. multiflora* mouthwash was compared with placebo for the treatment of oral mucositis, a complication caused by radiotherapy in the head and neck area. The patients gargled *Z. multiflora* mouthwash (containing 136 mg *Z. multiflora* aqueous extract) three times a day, as well as before each radiotherapy session. The results of the study showed that the severity of oral mucositis in patients who received *Z. multiflora* was nearly three times lower compared to placebo. Oral pain was also less in these patients (Aghamohammadi et al., 2018).

Preclinical Evidence

Thymus vulgaris

Lung fibrosis: Intraperitoneal administration of *T. vulgaris* aqueous extract in rats with pulmonary fibrosis induced by bleomycin showed antioxidant and antifibrotic effects in histopathological investigations in highest given doses (200 mg/kg/day) (Bahri et al., 2022).

Hepatotoxicity: Pretreatment administration of *T. vulgaris* ethanolic extract at oral dose of 500 mg/kg/day for 15 days in mice revealed hepatoprotective activity against hepatic injury due to $NaNO_2$. The extract showed decreased effect of $NaNO_2$ on AST as well as ALT levels and total proteins. Also, the effect of $NaNO_2$ on antioxidant levels was reversed (Soliman et al., 2021).

GI problems: Oral administration of *T. vulgaris* aqueous extract (100 and 200 mg/kg) in male Wistar rats with stomach ulcer (induced by oral indomethacin) and constipation (induced by intravenous vinblastine) had positive effects on delayed gastric emptying and gastrointestinal transit (Rtibi et al., 2019).

Zataria multiflora

Pain and inflammation: Intraperitoneal and subcutaneous injection of the aqueous and ethanolic extracts from the aerial part of *Z. multiflora* demonstrated central and peripheral antinociceptive activities on male and female albino mice and Wistar rats. These analgesic effects were at their maximum effect 60 and 150 minutes after injection. The extracts also showed activity against acute and chronic inflammation (Hosseinzadeh et al., 2000).

Insulin resistance: Laboratory male Wistar rats were fed a high-fructose diet for 6 weeks, and after 2 weeks of treatment with intragastric injection of *Z. multiflora* aqueous extract (1,000 mg/kg) or pioglitazone solution (10 mg/kg), blood and tissue samples were collected for analysis. This study shows the beneficial effects of *Z. multiflora* extract on insulin resistance in rats fed a high-fructose diet through the direct effect on insulin, increasing adiponectin and PPARγ protein expression (Mohammadi et al., 2014).

Memory and lung damage: After administration of paraquat aerosol eight times a day 30 minutes each time, for a total of 16 days to mice, two doses of hydroalcoholic extract (200 and 800 mg/kg/day) of *Z. multiflora* and dexamethasone (0.03 mg/kg/day) were gavaged daily for 16 days. The results showed *Z. multiflora* improved learning and memory impairment as well as lung inflammation and oxidative stress induced by inhaled paraquat (Heydari et al., 2021).

ADVERSE REACTIONS

TPM Literature

It is harmful to the lungs, and the use of vinegar can reduce this side effect (Aghili Khorasani 1771).

Current Evidence

No health hazards or side effects are known upon administration of therapeutic dosages (Gruenwald, 2007). Allergic reactions to thyme, confirmed by patch testing, have been reported. Relative to urban-dwelling control groups, respiratory ailments and sensitivity to microbial allergens were increased in thyme farmers regularly exposed to airborne thyme dust. Occupational airborne contact dermatitis caused by thyme dust was reported in some farmers during threshing of thyme (Gardner and McGuffin, 2013).

CONTRAINDICATIONS

TPM Literature

None.

Current Evidence

None.

PREGNANCY AND LACTATION

TPM Literature

It is an emmenagogue from the view of TPM and so is contraindicated during pregnancy (Aghili Khorasani 1771).

Current Evidence

Thyme (*T. vulgaris*) is known as an abortifacient and the essential oil should not be used during pregnancy. Large doses of thymol which is the major ingredient of thyme essential oil, have been associated with the abortifacient activity. Consequently, its use during pregnancy is not recommended except under the supervision of a qualified healthcare practitioner. No information on the safety of thyme during lactation was identified in the scientific or traditional literature (Gardner and McGuffin, 2013). Data on *Z. multiflora* during pregnancy and lactation is limited. Some animal studies suggest this plant may have minor developmental effects on fetus and thus, should be used with caution in pregnancy (Anvari et al., 2011).

DRUG INTERACTIONS

None.

METHOD OF ADMINISTRATION

TPM Literature

It is used orally in the form of powder and decoction. Its flower oil and extract are applied topically (Aghili Khorasani 1771).

Current Evidence

Thyme is used orally as powder, dry extract, tincture, fluid extract, decoction, and infusion (Gruenwald et al., 2007).

DOSAGE

***Thymus vulgaris*:** 1–8.4 g of dried leaf and/or flowering herb top, per day (ESCOP, 2003; Gruenwald et al., 2007).
***Zataria multiflora*:** Up to 10 mg/kg/day of the extract is used in RCTs.

REFERENCES

Abdali K, Jahed L, Amooee S, et al. Comparison of the effect of vaginal *Zataria multiflora* cream and oral metronidazole pill on results of treatments for vaginal infections including trichomoniasis and bacterial vaginosis in women of reproductive age. Biomed Res Int. 2015;2015:683640.

Abolghasemi J, Jahromi MA, Sharifi MH, et al. Effects of *Zataria oxymel* on obesity, insulin resistance and lipid profile: A randomized, controlled, triple-blind trial. J Integr Med. 2020;18(5):401–408.

Aghamohammadi A, Moslemi D, Akbari J, et al. The effectiveness of Zataria extract mouthwash for the management of radiation-induced oral mucositis in patients: A randomized placebo-controlled double-blind study. Clin Oral Investig. 2018; 22:2263–2272.

Aghili Khorasani MH 1771. *Makhzan-al-Adviah* (*The treasury of drugs*) (rewritten by Shams Ardakani MR, Rahimi R, Farjadmand F, 1st ed.). Tehran: Tehran University of Medical Sciences; 2009.

Amanlou M, Beitollahi JM, Abdollahzadeh S, Tohidast-Ekrad Z. Miconazole gel compared with *Zataria multiflora* Boiss. gel in the treatment of denture stomatitis. Phytother Res. 2006;20(11):966–969.

Anvari M, Dashti MH, Zeinali F, Hosseini-Bioki SM. The effect of thyme (Zataria multiflora Boiss.) decoction on pregnancy in rats. J Med Plants. 2011;10(38):19–25.

Avicenna 1025. *Al-Qanoon fi al-Tibb* (*The canon of medicine*) (rewritten by Masoudi A, ed.). Tehran: Almaei; 2015.

Bahri S, Mlika M, Nahdi A, et al. *Thymus vulgaris* inhibit lung fibrosis progression and oxidative stress induced by bleomycin in Wistar rats. Nutr Cancer. 2022;74(4):1420–1430.

Caverzan J, Mussi L, Sufi B, et al. A new phytocosmetic preparation from *Thymus vulgaris* stimulates adipogenesis and controls skin aging process: In vitro studies and topical effects in a double-blind placebo-controlled clinical trial. J Cosmet Dermatol. 2021;20(7):2190–2202.

Direkvand-Moghadam A, Khosravi A. The impact of a novel herbal Shirazi *Thymus vulgaris* on primary dysmenorrhea in comparison to the classical chemical Ibuprofen. J Res Med Sci. 2012;17(7):668–670.

Ebrahimzadeh H, Yamini Y, Sefidkon F, et al. Chemical composition of the essential oil and supercritical CO_2 extracts of *Zataria multiflora* Boiss. Food Chem. 2003;83(3):357–361.

ESCOP. *ESCOP monographs: The scientific foundation for herbal medicinal products*. 2nd ed. Exeter: European Scientific Cooperative on Phytotherapy and Thieme; 2003.

Gardner Z, McGuffin M. *Botanical safety handbook*. Boca Raton: Taylor & Francis; 2013.

Ghorani V, Khazdair MR, Mirsadraee M, et al. The effect of two-month treatment with *Zataria multiflora* on inflammatory cytokines, pulmonary function testes and respiratory symptoms in patients with chronic obstructive pulmonary disease (COPD). J Ethnopharmacol. 2022;293:115265.

Gruenwald J, Brendler T, Jaenicke C. *PDR for herbal medicines*. Montvale: Thomson Reuters; 2007.

Heydari M, Mokhtari-Zaer A, Amin F, et al. The effect of *Zataria multiflora* hydroalcoholic extract on memory and lung changes induced by rats that inhaled paraquat. Nutr Neurosci. 2021;24(9):674–687.

Hosseinzadeh H, Ramezani M, Salmani GA. Antinociceptive, anti-inflammatory and acute toxicity effects of *Zataria multiflora* Boiss extracts in mice and rats. J Ethnopharmacol. 2000;73(3):379–385.

Khazdair MR, Rajabi O, Balali-Mood M, et al. The effect of *Zataria multiflora* on pulmonary function tests, hematological and oxidant/antioxidant parameters in sulfur mustard exposed veterans, a randomized doubled-blind clinical trial. Environ Toxicol Pharmacol. 2018;58:180–188.

Khazdair MR, Rezaeetalab F, Rafatpanah H, Boskabady MH. The effect of *Zataria multiflora* on inflammatory cytokine and respiratory symptoms in veterans exposed to sulfur mustard. Environ Sci Pollut Res Int. 2020;27:22451–22460.

Mohammadi A, Gholamhoseinian A, Fallah H. *Zataria multiflora* increases insulin sensitivity and PPARγ gene expression in high fructose fed insulin resistant rats. Iranian J Basic Med Sci. 2014;17(4):263–270.

Rtibi K, Selmi S, Wannes D, et al. The potential of *Thymus vulgaris* aqueous extract to protect against delayed gastric emptying and colonic constipation in rats. RSC Adv. 2019;9(36):20593–20602.

Salmalian H, Saghebi R, Moghadamnia AA, et al. Comparative effect of *Thymus vulgaris* and ibuprofen on primary dysmenorrhea: A triple-blind clinical study. Caspian J Intern Med. 2014;5(2):82–88.

Shokri H, Sharifzadeh A. Zataria multiflora Boiss.: A review study on chemical composition, anti-fungal and anti-mycotoxin activities, and ultrastructural changes. J Herbmed Pharmacol. 2016;6(1):1–9.

Simbar M, Azarbad Z, Mojab F, Majd HA. A comparative study of the therapeutic effects of the *Zataria multiflora* vaginal cream and metronidazole vaginal gel on bacterial vaginosis. Phytomedicine. 2008;15(12):1025–1031.

Soliman MM, Aldhahrani A, Metwally MM. Hepatoprotective effect of *Thymus vulgaris* extract on sodium nitrite-induced changes in oxidative stress, antioxidant and inflammatory marker expression. Sci Rep. 2021;11(1):5747.

Williamson E, Driver S, Baxter K (eds.). *Stockley's herbal medicines interactions*. London: Pharmaceutical Press; 2013.

38 *Trigonella foenum-graecum* L.

Parva Namiranian and Mehrdad Karimi

Scientific name: *Trigonella foenum-graecum* L.
Family: Fabaceae
Common names:

- **English:** Fenugreek
- **Persian:** *šanbalīleh, šambalīleh*
- **Arabic:** *ḥulbah*

Medicinal part(s): Seeds, leaves (Figure 38.1)
Temperament (nature): Hot in the second degree, dry in the first or second degree
Major chemical constituents:

- Mucilage (25–45%, mannogalactans)
- Proteins (25–30%)
- **Steroid saponins (1.2–1.5%):** Trigofoenosides A to G, diosgenin, yamogenin, gitogenin, smilagenin, tigogenin, yuccagenin
- **Sterols:** β-Sitosterol, sterols that are to some extent estered (Ciftci et al., 2011)
- **Flavonoids:** Isoorientin, isovitexin, orientin and its glycosides, saponaretin, vicenin-1, vincenin-2, vitexin
- Trigonelline (Gruenwald et al., 2007)
- Fenugreekine (Mills et al., 2006)
- 4-Hydroxyisoleucine (Mills et al., 2006)

THERAPEUTIC USE

TPM Literature

External application of fenugreek decoction on the face acts as a facial cleanser and improves the skin brightness. Washing the head with its decoction is useful for hair, wet ulcers of the scalp, and acts as an antidandruff. When macerated in water, or the decoction is applied on eyes, it may be used in the form of eye drop for some eye diseases. Fenugreek clears the voice and has a good nourishing value for the lungs, meaning that it is a tonic for lung and is generally useful in respiratory diseases. Having a positive effect on the lungs and throat, it relieves cough and asthma, especially if cooked with honey, dates, or figs. A decoction of the seeds with honey acts as a mucolytic and helps the lung to expel the sticky sputum by coughing. It is mentioned that cooking fenugreek fresh plant with vinegar is useful for gastric problems including weakness and inflammation. Vinegar is added to prevent the possible abdominal colic as a side effect of the seeds. The use of fenugreek decoction as an oral formulation or enema is helpful in the treatment of inflammatory bowel disease and related colic and diarrhea. Fenugreek can dissolve phlegmatic and firm swellings, both in external (in the form of poultice) and internal use. When pounded and used in the form of flour, fenugreek reduces hot external and internal swellings if they are not inflamed, but

DOI: 10.1201/b22971-38

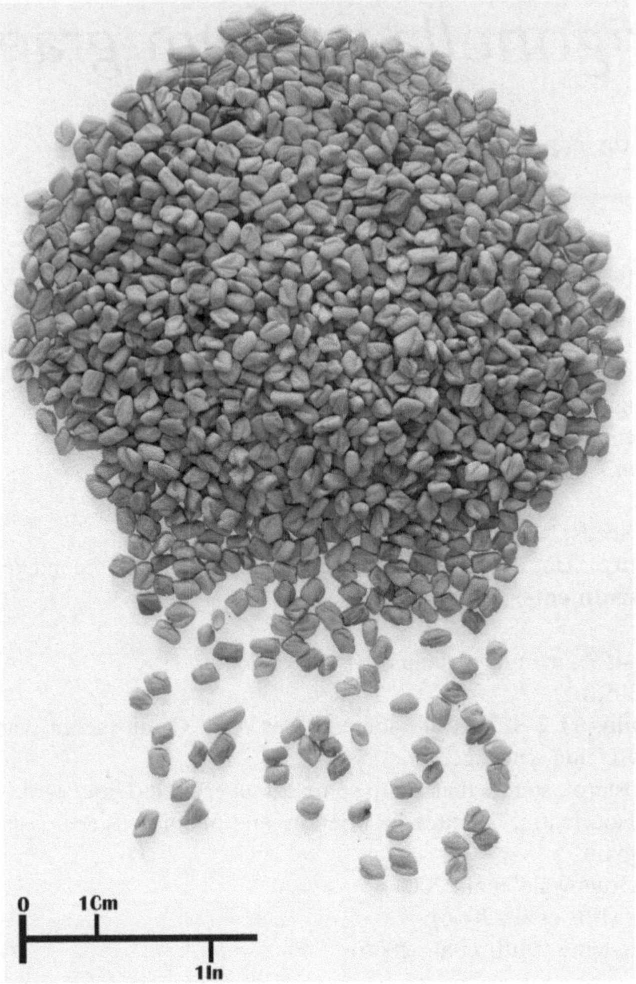

FIGURE 38.1 Fenugreek seeds.

rather with some stiffness. The plant can maturate these swellings. Topical application as a paste is recommended in a variety of problems including cold fissures, crooked nails, liver problems, inflammation of spleen and uterus, burns due to fire, hair fall, and some skin problems such as scars. Additionally, its poultice strengthens the hair.

Fenugreek decoction is beneficial for facilitating birth, either in oral intake, vaginal insert, or as a sitz bath. Sitz bath using the decoction is also recommended for uterus pain, inflammation, uterine adhesions, and cleansing the uterus from retained placenta after birth. Due to emmenagogue properties, the seeds are useful for the treatment of menstruation problems such as amenorrhea. The decoction sweetened with honey can be used as a diuretic and helps with some bladder and urinary problems. Moreover, this decoction is appropriate for dysentery and diarrhea.

It is suggested that fenugreek seed oil can be used for swellings in the anal region and its enema is useful for dysentery, abdominal pain, and colics. Moreover, its seed oil is beneficial for maturing and removing firmness and face wounds, when used topically (Aghili Khorasani 1771; Avicenna 1025).

Current Evidence

Clinical Evidence

PCOS: In a double-blind, placebo-controlled RCT, 58 oligo-anovulatory PCOS women randomly received either two capsules of 500 mg hydroalcoholic extract of fenugreek seeds plus metformin, or placebo capsules with metformin. Upon 8 weeks of treatment, ultrasound scans showed a significant decrease in polycystic appearing ovaries in the group received fenugreek (Hassanzadeh Bashtian et al., 2013). In another clinical trial on 50 patients diagnosed with PCOS who were aged 18–45 years old, fenugreek seed extract, enriched in 40% furostanolic saponins were administered as two 500 mg capsules per day for 3 months. A significant reduction of ovary volume and the number of ovarian cysts was observed in fenugreek-treated group. Moreover, 71% of patients experienced the regular menstrual cycle after completing the treatment. In comparison with the baseline values, there was a significant increase in the levels of FSH and LH (Swaroop et al., 2015).

Dysmenorrhea: In an open-labeled RCT, pain intensity of primary dysmenorrhea in 60 cases was studied. Patients were divided into three groups: 20 individuals (group A) took 3 g fenugreek seed powder two times a day within the first and third day of menstruation; Group B included 20 cases who consumed similar amount of fenugreek seed along with 15 minutes dry cupping therapy below the umbilicus on the same days of menstruation for 3 months; Group C involved 20 cases who took 500 mg mefenamic acid twice daily, on the same days of menstruation cycle. According to well validated VAS, the menstrual pain intensity was reduced 66.89%, 66.49%, and 62.88% in groups A, B, and C, respectively (Inanmdar et al., 2016). In another RCT, 51 students took 900 mg fenugreek seed powder three times a day from the first to the third day of menstruation for two cycles; and 50 students received placebo. Pain severity and duration between the two cycles significantly decreased in the fenugreek group ($p < 0.001$) (Younesy et al., 2014).

Vaginal atrophy: In a double-blind RCT, 60 postmenopausal women with vaginal atrophy were divided into two groups of 30. One group received fenugreek 5% vaginal cream and the other group received placebo. After 8 weeks and compared to the study start, the individuals consuming fenugreek vaginal cream exhibited a significant improvement in symptoms related to vaginal atrophy ($p < 0.001$) (Mazalzadeh et al., 2020). In another RCT, 30 participants received two times a week 0.5 g fenugreek vaginal cream 5%, while 0.625 mg conjugated estrogens vaginal cream was given to the 30 participants of the control group. After 12 weeks, the mean (standard error) score for atrophic vaginitis signs was in intragroup comparison statistically significant and in intergroup comparison in favor of the control group ($p = 0.001$). According to the results of this study, although total fenugreek extract can be useful for treating atrophic vaginitis signs, ultra-low-dose estrogen had better outcomes (Safary et al., 2020).

Menopausal symptoms: In a double-blind, placebo-controlled RCT, 115 women aged 40–65 years were treated with 600 mg of fenugreek seed extract or placebo. After 12 weeks, a significant reduction was observed in menopausal symptoms in the medication group compared with placebo including physical, psychosocial, vasomotor (hot flushes and night sweats), and sexual symptoms (all $p < 0.001$). In both groups the average estradiol levels were similar (Steels et al., 2017). In another double-blind, placebo-controlled RCT, 24 healthy women with perimenopausal symptoms received 250 mg fenugreek seeds hydro-ethanolic extract twice daily. The same number of women received placebo. After 42 days, the discomforts, such as vasomotor symptoms, as well as depression were reduced significantly in medication group, and a hormonal balance was attained (Khanna, 2020). Another double-blind, placebo-controlled RCT evaluated the result of using a standardized extract of fenugreek (FenuSMART™) in two groups of women, including 44 women in medication group and 44 women in placebo group. After using 1,000 mg per day of the medication for 90 days, plasma estrogens, as well as postmenopausal discomforts were studied. In the medication group, a significant increase ($p < 0.01$) in plasma estradiol (120%) and improvement of postmenopausal discomforts and quality of life was observed compared with the baseline and placebo (Shamshad Begum, 2016).

Milk production: In a double-blind, placebo-controlled RCT, 66 postpartum mothers were randomly divided into three groups: 22 mothers having three cups of fenugreek tea (each 200 mL) per day, 22 mothers receiving placebo (the same amount of apple tea), and 22 mothers as the control group. On the third day after delivery, it was seen that milk production was enhanced in the fenugreek-treated group and the mean measured breast milk volume (by electrical pump) of the mothers in the first group was significantly higher than the other two groups. Additionally, infants in the first group had a significantly faster birth weight regain in comparison to the other groups (Turkyılmaz et al., 2011).

Type 2 diabetes mellitus: In a double-blind, placebo-controlled RCT, 25 patients with type 2 diabetes mellitus were randomly divided into two groups. Hydroalcoholic extract of fenugreek seeds (1 g per day) was given to the 12 patients of the first group, while 13 patients in the other group received placebo capsules. After 2 months, there was a decrease in percent beta-cell secretion in the HOMA model derived insulin resistance of the first group. Additionally, a significant increase in insulin sensitivity percent was observed in this group. Another point was the significant decrease of serum TAG and increase of HDL-C in the first group as compared to the placebo group (Gupta et al., 2001). In an RCT on 66 prediabetic cases and 74 matched controls, 5 g fenugreek seed powder was administered twice a day before meals and the study population was followed every 3 months for 3 years. It was shown that intake of fenugreek is associated with lower conversion of prediabetes to diabetes. Additionally, there was a significant reduction in postprandial plasma glucose, FBS, and LDL-C in the fenugreek-treated group. Meanwhile, this group showed a significant serum insulin increase (Gaddam et al., 2015). A meta-analysis of 10 RCTs showed that fenugreek can significantly change FBS by –0.96 mmol/L, 2-hour post-load glucose by –2.19 mmol/L, as well as HbA1c by –0.85% compared with control interventions. This result supports the beneficial effects of fenugreek on glycemic control in diabetic patients (Neelakantan et al., 2014). Another meta-analysis on 12 studies confirms the above finding, as well (Gong et al., 2016).

Sexual desire: In a double-blind, placebo-controlled RCT, healthy men aged between 43 and 70 years old received a dose of 600 mg per day of standardized fenugreek seed extract ($n = 60$) or placebo ($n = 60$) three times daily for 12 weeks. The Aging Male Symptom score was significantly decreased in the active group compared to placebo. Moreover, compared to placebo, there was an increase in the total serum testosterone and free testosterone level, along with an improvement in sexual function (Rao et al., 2016). In another double-blind, placebo-controlled study, 60 healthy male participants aged between 25 and 52 were studied. Those who were in the active group and received two 600 mg tablets of fenugreek seed extract for 6 weeks, reported a significant increase in libido compared to the placebo group, although the serum testosterone was not increased (Steels et al., 2011).

Fenugreek may also have promising effects in women suffering from decreased libido. In a double-blind, placebo-controlled RCT, eighty 20–49-year-old healthy women complaining of low sexual arousal received 600 mg per day standardized fenugreek seed extract or placebo for 8 weeks. The sexual desire and arousal significantly increased in fenugreek group compared to placebo. Additionally, a significant increase in free testosterone and estradiol levels was found in the fenugreek group compared to the placebo group (Rao et al., 2015).

Respiratory problems: In a placebo-controlled RCT, 90 individuals were divided to three groups randomly: In one group patients received the aqueous extract of fenugreek seeds, in another one the patients received honey syrup, and the third group of patients received placebo. After 4 weeks, it was observed that the FEV1 in lung function test was improved more than 10% in patients receiving fenugreek (Emtiazy, 2018).

Preclinical Evidence

Retinal degeneration in diabetes: In a rat model of diabetes, administration of fenugreek seed hydroethanolic extract (100 and 200 mg/kg) for 24 weeks showed a significant reduction in FBS, HbA1c, and body weight, compared with negative control. Also, a significant inhibition of retinal inflammatory markers including TNF-α and IL-1β, as well as the angiogenic factors VEGF and PKC-β was reported. Fenugreek had positive modulatory effects on retinal oxidative stress via restoration of GSH, SOD, and CAT. In addition, vascular leakage was not seen when fenugreek was administered to the diabetic rats (Gupta et al., 2014).

Lung injury: Oral administration of nano-formulated fenugreek seed extract (2.5 and 5 mg/kg) in mice with gastric acid-induced acute lung injury showed significant amelioration of the lung injury in histopathological investigations in a dose dependent manner. Fenugreek was given at 0, 24, 48, and 72 h and gastric acid was applied 1 hour after it. Also, fenugreek inhibited the DNA content increase and showed a prevention in proliferation of goblet cells which were induced by gastric acid instillation alone. Thus, it was found to be useful in acute lung injury of rats (Hamad and El-Naggar, 2020).

Hepatotoxicity: In a rat model of thioacetamide-induced liver damage, daily oral administration of 2% extract (2 mL) of fenugreek seeds for 4 weeks could decrease total bilirubin, ALT, and ALP. Also, fenugreek improved CAT and SOD activity (Fatima and Masood, 2021). In another study, aged mice had a dietary intervention with fenugreek seeds (0.125 and 0.250 g per 2.5 g of diet) for 4 weeks. The improved activity of enzymatic antioxidant defense mechanisms, including SOD, Gpx, and GR, in fenugreek-treated group compared with control animals demonstrated the hepatoprotective activity of the plant (Tewari et al., 2020).

ADVERSE REACTIONS

TPM Literature

Excessive use of fenugreek is nauseating, causes headache, and is harmful for the genital organs. To prevent these adverse effects, it is better to be used with sour oxymel, aniseed, and sour-sweet pomegranate. People with hot temperament should avoid taking fenugreek leaves, unless together with chicory. Also, these people should use the decoction of fenugreek leaves with spinach leaves, purslane leaves, or parsnip to prevent possible adverse reactions (Aghili Khorasani 1771).

Current Evidence

Allergic reactions to fenugreek have been reported (Gardner and McGuffin, 2013). It should be cautiously used in patients with allergy to chickpeas due to probable cross-reactivity. Bronchospasm, asthmatic, and allergic reactions might happen due to inhalation of its seed powder (Ulbricht, 2010).

Rare cases of diarrhea, swelling of face, dizziness, numbness, fainting, hypoglycemia, hypokalemia, breathing with difficulty, higher bleeding risk, and change of thyroid hormone levels have been reported (Gardner and McGuffin, 2013).

When high amounts of fenugreek were administered to infants, either directly or through intake of mothers, smell of maple syrup was sensed. It is important to know this in order to prevent false suspicion of maple syrup urine disease (Gardner and McGuffin, 2013).

Inflammation may happen in repeated external use of fenugreek (Kargozar et al., 2017).

Animal studies of rabbits, rats, and mice showed antifertility effects and testicular toxicity in male animals. Abortifacient, antifertility, and anti-implantation properties are also reported in female animals (Ouzir et al., 2016).

CONTRAINDICATIONS

TPM Literature

None.

Current Evidence

None.

PREGNANCY AND LACTATION

TPM Literature

Fenugreek is emmenagogue and should be avoided during pregnancy (Aghili Khorasani 1771).

Current Evidence

Fenugreek is galactagogue and has potential oxytocic activity (Mills et al., 2006). Due to possible abortifacient effects, it is not recommended during pregnancy (Ulbricht, 2010; Gruenwald et al., 2007).

DRUG INTERACTIONS

Antidiabetic agents: Due to the hypoglycemic effect of fenugreek, there is a probability of interaction with hypoglycemic medications used to treat diabetes (Gruenwald et al., 2007).

Antiplatelets and anticoagulants: Fenugreek may increase the risk of bleeding in concomitant use with medications that increase bleeding risk (Ulbricht, 2010), including warfarin (Aronson, 2009).

Oral medications: Since the mucilage and fiber content of fenugreek may slow the absorption of oral medications (Mills et al., 2006), other medications should be taken 1 hour before or several hours after fenugreek consumption (Gardner and McGuffin, 2013).

METHOD OF ADMINISTRATION

TPM Literature

Fenugreek decoction is administered either orally or topically. For topical administration, the plant can be also used as a poultice or may be used in the form of eyedrop for some eye diseases. Fenugreek powder can be topically used for firm swellings. For anal region swellings and enema (in case of dysentery and abdominal pain and colics), fenugreek is used as oil. Use of the decoction as a sitz bath is recommended for uterine/vaginal problems and easing childbirth (Aghili Khorasani 1771).

CURRENT EVIDENCE

Fenugreek seed may be recommended as whole and powdered form of teas (0.5 g drug in cold water for 3 h) as well as compound preparations including capsules, poultice (50 g of powdered seeds in boiling water), and cold maceration (0.5 g of soaked drug in cold water) (Gruenwald et al., 2007).

DOSAGE

The daily internal dose is 6 g as infusion (Gruenwald et al., 2007).

REFERENCES

Aghili Khorasani MH 1771. *Makhzan-al-Adviah* (*The treasury of drugs*) (rewritten by Shams Ardakani MR, Rahimi R, Farjadmand F, 1st ed.). Tehran: Tehran University of Medical Sciences; 2009.

Aronson JK (ed.). *Meyler's side effects of herbal medicines*. San Diego: Elsevier; 2009.

Avicenna 1025. *Al-Qanoon fi al-Tibb* (*The canon of medicine*) (rewritten by Masoudi A, ed.). Tehran: Almaei; 2015.

Ciftci ON, Przybylski R, Rudzinska M, Acharya S. Characterization of fenugreek (Trigonella foenum-graecum) seed lipids. J Am Oil Chem Soc. 2011;88(10):1603–1610.

Emtiazy M, Oveidzadeh L, Habibi M, et al. Investigating the effectiveness of the *Trigonella foenum-graecum* L.(fenugreek) seeds in mild asthma: A randomized controlled trial. Allergy Asthma Clin Immunol. 2018;14(1):1–8.

Fatima SN, Masood J. Fenugreek seeds attenuate thioacetamide induced liver damage. Pak J Pharm Sci. 2021;34(3):933–942.

Gaddam A, Galla C, Thummisetti S, et al. Role of fenugreek in the prevention of type 2 diabetes mellitus in prediabetes. J Diabetes Metab Disord. 2015;14:74.

Gardner Z, McGuffin M. *Botanical safety handbook*. Boca Raton: Taylor & Francis; 2013.

Gong J, Fang K, Dong H, et al. Effect of fenugreek on hyperglycaemia and hyperlipidemia in diabetes and prediabetes: a meta-analysis. J Ethnopharmacol. 2016;194:260–268.

Gruenwald J, Brendler T, Jaenicke C. *PDR for herbal medicines*. Montvale: Thomson Reuters; 2007.

Gupta A, Gupta R, Lal B. Effect of *Trigonella foenum-graecum* (fenugreek) seeds on glycaemic control and insulin resistance in type 2 diabetes. J Assoc Physicians India. 2001;49:1057–1061.

Gupta SK, Kumar B, Nag TC, et al. Effects of *Trigonella foenum-graecum* (L.) on retinal oxidative stress, and proinflammatory and angiogenic molecular biomarkers in streptozotocin-induced diabetic rats. Mol Cell Biochem. 2014;388(1–2):1–9.

Hamad SR, El-Naggar ME. Blocking of gastric acid induced histopathological alterations, enhancing of DNA content and proliferation of goblet cells in the acute lung injury mice models by nano-fenugreek oral administration. Toxicol Mech Methods. 2020;30(2):153–158.

Hassanzadeh Bashtian M, Emami SA, Mousavifar N, et al. Evaluation of fenugreek (*Trigonella foenum-graceum* L.), effects seeds extract on insulin resistance in women with polycystic ovarian syndrome. Iran J Pharm Res. 2013;12(2):475–481.

Inanmdar W, Sultana A, Mubeen U, Rahman K. Clinical efficacy of *Trigonella foenum-graecum* (fenugreek) and dry cupping therapy on intensity of pain in patients with primary dysmenorrhea. Chin J Integr Med. 2016; 2016:1–8.

Kargozar R, Azizi H, Salari R. A review of effective herbal medicines in controlling menopausal symptoms. Electron Physician. 2017;9(11):5826–5833.

Khanna A, John F, Das S, et al. Efficacy of a novel extract of fenugreek seeds in alleviating vasomotor symptoms and depression in perimenopausal women: A randomized, double-blinded, placebo-controlled study. J Food Biochem. 2020;44(12):e13507.

Mazalzadeh F, Hekmat K, Namjouyan F, Saki A. Effect of *Trigonella foenum* (fenugreek) vaginal cream on vaginal atrophy in postmenopausal women. J Family Med Prim Care. 2020;9(6):2714–2719.

Mills E, Dugoua JJ, Perri D, Koren G. *Herbal medicines in pregnancy and lactation: An evidence-based approach*. London: CRC Press; 2006.

Neelakantan N, Narayanan M, de Souza RJ, van Dam RM. Effect of fenugreek (*Trigonella foenum-graecum* L.) intake on glycemia: A meta-analysis of clinical trials. Nutr J. 2014;13:7.

Ouzir M, El Bairi K, Amzazi S. Toxicological properties of fenugreek (*Trigonella foenum-graecum*). Food Chem Toxicol. 2016;96:145–154.

Rao A, Steels E, Beccaria G, et al. Influence of a specialized *Trigonella foenum-graecum* seed extract (libifem), on testosterone, estradiol and sexual function in healthy menstruating women: A randomized placebo-controlled study. Phytother Res. 2015;29(8):1123–1130.

Rao A, Steels E, Inder WJ, et al. Testofen, a specialised Trigonella foenum-graecum seed extract reduces age-related symptoms of androgen decrease, increases testosterone levels and improves sexual function in healthy aging males in a double-blind randomised clinical study. Aging Male. 2016;19(2):134–142.

Safary M, Hakimi S, Mobaraki-Asl N, et al. Comparison of the effects of fenugreek vaginal cream and ultra-low-dose estrogen on atrophic vaginitis. Curr Drug Deliv. 2020;17(9):815–822.

Shamshad Begum S, Jayalakshmi HK, Vidyavathi HG, et al. A novel extract of fenugreek husk (FenuSMART™) alleviates postmenopausal symptoms and helps to establish the hormonal balance: A randomized, double-blind, placebo-controlled study. Phytother Res. 2016;30(11):1775–1784.

Steels E, Rao A, Vitetta L. Physiological aspects of male libido enhanced by standardized *Trigonella foenum-graecum* extract and mineral formulation. Phytother Res. 2011;25(9):1294–1300.

Steels E, Steele ML, Harold M, Coulson S. Efficacy of a proprietary *Trigonella foenum-graecum* L. de-husked seed extract in reducing menopausal symptoms in otherwise healthy women: A double-blind, randomized, placebo-controlled study. Phytother Res. 2017;31(9):1316–1322.

Swaroop A, Jaipuriar AS, Gupta SK, et al. Efficacy of a novel fenugreek seed extract (*Trigonella foenum-graecum*, Furocyst™) in polycystic ovary syndrome (PCOS). Int J Med Sci. 2015;12(10):825–831.

Tewari D, Jóźwik A, Łysek-Gładysińska M, et al. Fenugreek (*Trigonella foenum-graecum* L.) seeds dietary supplementation regulates liver antioxidant defense systems in aging mice. Nutrients. 2020;12(9):2552.

Turkyılmaz C, Onal E, Hirfanoglu IM, et al. The effect of galactagogue herbal tea on breast milk production and short-term catch-up of birth weight in the first week of life. J Altern Complement Med. 2011;17(2):139–142.

Ulbricht CE. *Natural standard herb & supplement guide: An evidence-based reference*. St. Luis: Elsevier; 2010.

Younesy S, Amiraliakbari S, Esmaeili S, et al. Effects of fenugreek seed on the severity and systemic symptoms of dysmenorrhea. J Reprod Fertil. 2014;15(1):41–48.

39 *Viola odorata* L.

Hananeh Aliakbarzadeh and Hossein Rezaeizadeh

Scientific name: *Viola odorata* L.
Family: Violaceae
Common names:

- **English:** Sweet violet
- **Persian:** Banafsheh
- **Arabic:** Banafsaj, ferfir

Medicinal part(s): Flowers, leaves (Figure 39.1)
Temperament (nature): Cold and wet in the first degree
Major chemical constituents:

- **Volatile oil of flower (0.003%):** Parmone, isoborneol
- Mucilage (18.0%)
- **Anthocyanins (4.0%):** Cyanidin, violanin
- **Flavonoids (1.1%):** Quercetin, kaempferol, apigenin
- Saponins
- Alkaloids
- Cyclotides (Gruenwald et al., 2007; Lim, 2014)

THERAPEUTIC USE

TPM LITERATURE:

Smelling the fresh violet flower, oral intake of its infusion, intranasal use of traditional violet oil (violet soaked in sweet almond oil), or insert of a cotton ball soaked in violet oil in the anus can act as sleep aids. Inhaling fresh flower or its topical application as a poultice on forehead, as well as intranasal use of its oil relieves the headaches due to hot dystemperament. It can be used in some types of pediatric epilepsy. Its use as an eyedrop and infusion is recommended in cases of hot conjunctivitis. Violet processed with sugar (jam) or the syrup is effective in pneumonia, pleurisy, hot and dry cough, and hoarseness. Violet infusion is beneficial for dyspnea if used frequently after sweat bathing. Traditional violet oil applied inside of the navel or chest is also administrated for chronic cough. Violet is administered for allergic rhinitis, rhinosinusitis, common cold, fever, and palpitation. It quenches thirst. The infusion is laxative, especially with sugar, but is less effective with honey. Oral intake of powdered violet taken with cold water can eliminate choleric diarrhea. Also, oral intake of the infusion or topical application of violet poultice on the anus is beneficial for anal prolapse and fissure. It is also beneficial for spleen, liver and stomach diseases caused by hot dystemperament.

Violet infusion orally used or topically applied in pubic area as well as violet poultice in pubic area is helpful for soothing dysuria and urinary retention. Furthermore, its jam is diuretic and also useful for renal colic. Violet oil is beneficial in cases of hair loss, healing of skin wounds, focal itching and eczema, preserving nail health and joint stiffness. Sweet violet can be recommended for

DOI: 10.1201/b22971-39

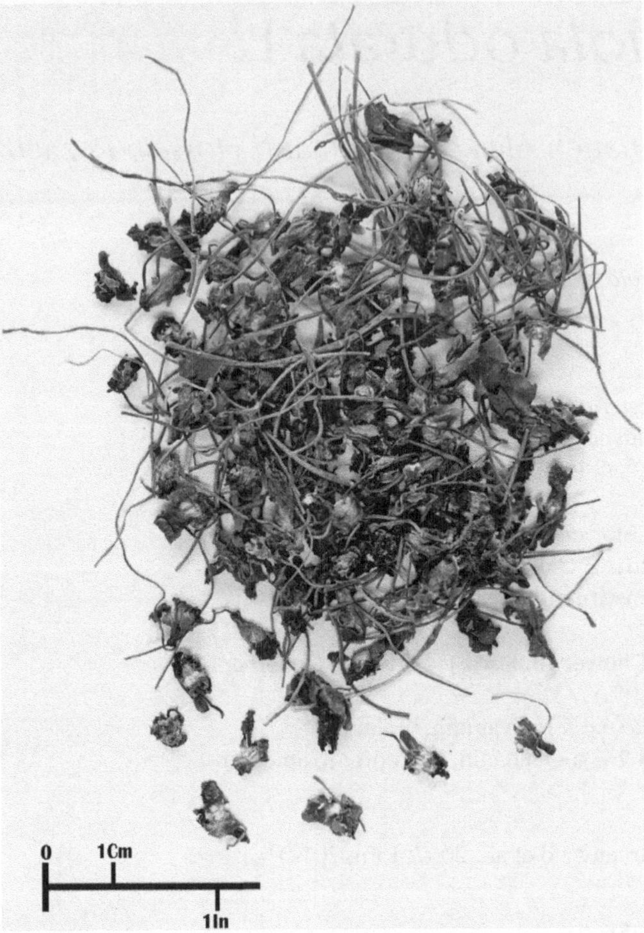

FIGURE 39.1 Sweet violet flowers.

cancer and inflammation. In addition, its fresh flowers are useful for detoxifying pollutants (Aghili Khorasani 1771; Avicenna 1025)

Current Evidence

Clinical Evidence

Allergic rhinitis: In a randomized, double-blind, placebo-controlled clinical trial including 81 patients with mild to moderate allergic rhinitis, traditional violet oil was prepared using 40 g of dried extract in 4 L of sweet almond oil and was given to patients as a nasal drop with a dose of one drop in each nostril every 12 hours for 2 weeks. The severity of the symptoms of nasal itching, sneezing, nasal congestion, rhinorrhea, itchy eyes, eye irritation, tearing, sleep quality, daily activity and fatigue based on a Rhinitis Quality of Life Questionnaire (RQLQ) were studied on days 3, 7, and 14 which revealed a significant and time-dependent improvement in the violet oil group compared to placebo (Yazdi et al., 2020).

Asthma: In a randomized, double-blind, placebo-controlled trial, 182 children, 2–12 years old, with intermittent asthma, were treated with violet syrup (12 g of dried violet flowers in 100 mL of syrup) with a dose of 2.5 mL for children 2–5 years old and 5 mL for children over 5 years old, three times a day for 5 days. Both groups received a short-acting beta-agonist as common standard treatment. The time it took for the cough to be reduced by 50% and eliminated by 100% was significantly shorter in the group received violet syrup compared with placebo group (Qasemzadeh et al., 2015).

Insomnia: In a pilot randomized, double-blind, placebo-controlled trial, 83 patients with OCD or depression suffering from insomnia were divided into two groups, depression and OCD. Both groups had received their usual treatments and then each group was divided into two subgroups of violet syrup (prepared as a concentration of 50 g/L) and placebo. Patients received 5 mL of violet syrup or placebo every 12 hours for 4 weeks. According to the Pittsburgh Sleep Quality Index, a significant improvement in insomnia of the intervention group was observed. Also in the intervention group, a significant improvement in depression based on Beck Depression Inventory-II score and OCD based on Yale-Brown Obsessive-Compulsive Scale was observed (Shayesteh et al., 2020). In another double-blind, placebo-controlled RCT, 75 patients with chronic insomnia were divided into three groups receiving either three drops of violet oil, almond oil, or placebo in each nostril every night before bed for 30 days. The violet oil was obtained using cold press of combined violet and peeled sweet almond with a 1:2 ratio. Considering Pittsburgh Sleep Quality Index and Insomnia Severity Index questionnaires, sleep rate was significantly improved in all three groups, with violet oil having a greater effect compared to two other groups. Additionally, it also profoundly affected the sleep quality, rather than the sleep quantity (Feyzabadi et al., 2018).

Uremic pruritus: In a randomized controlled trial including 44 hemodialysis patients with uremic pruritus, the healthy hand without fistula were massaged with violet oil in six sessions every other day and for 7 minutes each time by a researcher physician. The control group received an oil-free massage. Violet oil was prepared by macerating violet flowers in sweet almond oil in a ratio of 1:3. In the group of violet oil, the severity of itching and dryness of the skin significantly decreased based on VAS, but there was no significant change in the inflammatory biomarkers of the blood, IL-2, IL-4, and interferon (Ghazanfari et al., 2022).

Constipation: In a randomized, active-controlled, noninferiority clinical trial, 140 children aged 4–10 years with functional constipation diagnosis based on Rome III criteria were compared in two groups of violet syrup and PEG. Violet syrup (concentration of 1 kg of dried plant in 6 L of water with a little sugar) was given to children at a dose of 5 mL, three times a day and PEG 40% was given at a dose of 1 mg/kg/day for 4 weeks. Both groups found a significant improvement in all criteria compared to baseline mode with no significant difference between the two groups. In the violet syrup group, patients experienced fewer side effects including abdominal pain, loose stool, nausea, vomiting, and unpleasant taste (Tavassoli et al., 2021).

Dry eye: In a double-blind, placebo-controlled RCT, 105 patients aged 18–60 years with dry eye were divided into three groups: traditional violet almond oil, almond oil, and placebo. Patients used two drops in each nostril three times a day for 4 weeks. A significant improvement in Schirmer's score, tear breakup time and ocular Surface Disease Index was observed in the violet oil group compared to the other two groups; however, they had no effect on the Oxford staining grade (Saffar Shahroodi et al., 2019).

Fever: In a triple-blinded, placebo-controlled RCT on 41 of children with cancer, fever and neutropenia, 20 drops of traditional violet oil was rubbed around the umbilicus and underarm temperature was measured at 30, 60, and 240 minutes after the intervention. The mean temperature after 30 minutes was significantly lower in the violet oil group. Also, a significantly fewer number of patients needed to take paracetamol in the intervention group (Tafazoli et al., 2020).

Repellency effect: The volunteer human arm was rubbed with the extract and exposed to three insects, the yellow fever mosquito, *Aedes aegypti* (Linnaeus), the malaria vector, *Anopheles stephensi* (Liston), and the filariasis and encephalitis vector, *Culex quinquefasciatus* (Say). Out of 41 tested essential oils, violet essential oil at 20% concentration was able to 100% prevent insect bites for 8 hours. This activity was similar or higher than the positive controls, N, N-diethyl-m-toluamide and 1-piperidinecarboxylic acid, 2-(2-hydroxyethyl)-1-methylpropylester, both in case of protection period and percentage of repellency (Amer et al., 2006).

Preclinical Evidence

Anticancer effect: In 4T1 breast cancer mouse model, oral 50, 150, and 250 mg/kg of violet hydroethanolic extract for 21 days significantly reduced tumor size and cell viability, serum LDH along with decreased liver and lung metastasis. Also, immunohistochemistry evaluation showed that the extract prevented cell proliferation, but had no effect on angiogenesis. The highest dose also led to induction of apoptosis (increasing Bax/Bcl-2 ratio) and increased tumor tissue CAT, but CAT and SOD activities decreased in tumor tissue at a dose of 50 mg/kg. No linear correlation was observed between tumor size and serum carcinoembryonic antigen and cancer antigen 15-3 (Alipanah et al., 2018). In mice with 4-nitroquinoline-1-oxide (4-NQO)-induced tongue dysplasia, violet syrup (5 and 15 mg/kg) was administered three times a week for 12 weeks to prevent dysplasia. In comparison to negative control, violet syrup could reduce the severity of hyperplasia and hyperkeratosis in a dose-dependent manner. Also, the body weight of mice treated with violet extracts were significantly improved compared with the groups receiving 4-NQO (Helli et al., 2016).

ADVERSE REACTIONS

TPM Literature

Excessive consumption of sweet violet results in weakness, anxiety and inquietude, nausea, and epigastric discomfort, which can be prevented if taken with aniseed.

Smelling the fresh violet flower scent can cause allergic rhinitis, which can be ameliorated by oregano and wallflower (*Erysimum cheiri* (L.) Crantz) (Aghili Khorasani 1771).

Current Evidence

There is no side effect reported if used properly in appropriate therapeutic doses (Gruenwald et al., 2007; Gardner and McGuffin, 2013). Consuming syrup equivalent to 2.5 g of dry plant per day for 1 month had no side effects.

Dyspnea, circulatory disturbances, nervousness, and gastritis have been reported from high dose consumption (Duke, 2002).

CONTRAINDICATIONS

TPM Literature

None.

Current Evidence

None.

PREGNANCY AND LACTATION

TPM Literature

It is contraindicated during pregnancy.

Current Evidence

None.

DRUG INTERACTIONS

None.

METHOD OF ADMINISTRATION

TPM Literature

It is orally used as infusion, syrup, or dried powdered plant. The plant should not be boiled directly on fire since the therapeutic effects could be lost due to high temperature or long-term heating.

Filtered infusion, poultice, or its traditional oil are topically used. Intranasal use of its traditional oil or inhalation of the flower scent is used in the treatment of rhinosinusitis and head/brain disorders (Aghili Khorasani 1771).

The violet oil is prepared by maceration of violet flower in sweet almond oil or sesame oil for at least 40 days under sunlight. It can also be prepared by adding violet flower to almond kernel or sesame seeds while being cold-pressed for oil extraction.

Current Evidence

Violet is administered as decoction, infusion, and syrup. Its traditional oil can be used intranasally or topically.

DOSAGE

Average daily dose: 3 g of the plant as an infusion 1–3 times daily (European Medical Agency, 2010), or one teaspoonful of the plant twice daily as infusion (Gruenwald et al., 2007).

REFERENCES

Aghili Khorasani MH 1771. *Makhzan-al-Adviah* (*The treasury of drugs*) (rewritten by Shams Ardakani MR, Rahimi R, Farjadmand F, 1st ed.). Tehran: Tehran University of Medical Sciences; 2009.

Alipanah H, Bigdeli MR, Esmaeili MA. Inhibitory effect of *Viola odorata* extract on tumor growth and metastasis in 4T1 breast cancer model. Iran J Pharm Res. 2018;17(1):276–291.

Amer A, Mehlhorn H. Repellency effect of forty-one essential oils against Aedes, Anopheles, and Culex mosquitoes. Parasitol Res. 2006;99:478–490.

Avicenna 1025. *Al-Qanoon fi al-Tibb* (*The canon of medicine*) (rewritten by Masoudi A, ed.). Tehran: Almaei; 2015.

Duke JA, Bogenschutz-Godwin MJ, duCellier J, Duke P-AK. *Handbook of medicinal herbs*. 2nd ed. Boca Raton: Taylor & Francis; 2002.

European Medical Agency. *Community herbal monograph on Viola tricolor L. and/or subspecies Viola arvensis Murray (Gaud) and Viola vulgaris Koch (Oborny), herba cum flore*. EMA/HMPC/131734/2009. London: Committee on Herbal Medicinal Products.

Feyzabadi Z, Rezaeitalab F, Badiee S, et al. Efficacy of violet oil, a traditional Iranian formula, in patients with chronic insomnia: A randomized, double-blind, placebo-controlled study. J Ethnopharmacol. 2018;214:22–28.

Gardner Z, McGuffin M. *Botanical safety handbook*. Boca Raton: Taylor & Francis; 2013.

Gharebaghi R, Heidary F. Effects of *Viola odorata* as an add-on therapy on insomnia in patients with obsession or depression: A pilot randomized double-blind placebo-controlled trial. J Altern Complement Med. 2020;26(5):398–408.

Ghazanfari SM, Mirmoosavi SJ, Jamali J, et al. Inflammatory bio-marker changes in hemodialysis patients with pruritus receiving violet oil: A randomized controlled trial. J Herb Med. 2022;32:100538.

Gruenwald J, Brendler T, Jaenicke C. *PDR for herbal medicines*. Montvale: Thomson Reuters; 2007.

Helli S, Damghani H, Mohajeri D, et al. Evaluation of the effect of two different systemic doses of *Viola odorata* on prevention of induced tongue dysplasia in rats. J Dent. 2016;17(3):185–192.

Lim TK. *Edible medicinal and non-medicinal plants*. New York: Springer; 2014.

Qasemzadeh MJ, Sharifi H, Hamedanian M, et al. The effect of *Viola odorata* flower syrup on the cough of children with asthma: A double-blind, randomized controlled trial. Evid-Based Complement Altern Med. 2015;20(4):287–291.

Saffar Shahroodi A, Nejabat M, Nimrouzi M, et al. Effects of intranasal administration of violet oil in dry eye disease. Clin Exp Optom. 2019;102(6):576–582.

Shayesteh M, Vaez-Mahdavi MR, Shams J, et al. The effect of *Viola Odorata* L. oil for fever in children: A randomized triple-blinded placebo-controlled clinical trial. Curr Drug Discov Technol. 2020;17(5):696–703.

Tafazoli V, Shahriari M, Heydari M, et al. The Effect of Viola Odorata L. Oil for Fever in Children: A Randomized Triple-blinded Placebo-controlled Clinical Trial. Curr Drug Discov Technol. 2020;17(5):696–703.

Tavassoli S, Eftekhari K, Karimi M, et al. Effectiveness of viola flower syrup compared with polyethylene glycol in children with functional constipation: A randomized, active-controlled clinical trial. Evid-Based Complement Altern Med. 2021;2021.

Yazdi N, Kardooni M, Namjuyan F, et al. Efficacy of sweet violet (*Viola odorata*) flower oil on the symptoms of adults with allergic rhinitis: A double-blind randomized placebo-controlled clinical trial. Complement Ther Med. 2020;51:102408.

40 *Vitex agnus-castus* L.

Rezvan Ghaderpanah and Ehsan Amiri-Ardekani

Scientific name: *Vitex agnus-castus* L.
Family: Lamiaceae
Common names:

- **English:** Agnus-castus, Chaste tree, chasteberry, Abraham's balm, lilac chaste tree, monk's pepper
- **Persian:** *panǧ-angošt, fanǧ-angošt, felfel-e kūhī*
- **Arabic:** *'aṯlaq, ḏū ḫamsat al-awrāq, ḏū ḫamsat al-aǧniḥa, ḥabb al-fiqd, ḥabb al-nasl*

Medicinal part(s): Fruit (berry) (Figure 40.1)
Temperament (nature): Hot and dry in the second degree
Major chemical constituents

- **Essential oil (0.8–2%):** Limonene, 1,8-cineol, α-pinene, β-pinene, and sabinene
- **Iridoid glycosides:** Aucubin, agnoside, agnusoside, agnucastoside A/B
- **Flavonoids:** Casticin, kaempferol, quercetagetin, orientin, penduletin, luteolin, artemetin, vitexin, isovitexin
- **Diterpenes:** Vitexilactone, vitexlactam, viteagnusin I, rotundifuran, and 6-β,7-β diacetoxy-13-hydroxylabda-8,14-diene
- **Fatty acids:** Oleic acid, linolenic acid, palmitic acid, and stearic acid (Boujbiha et al., 2023; Gruenwald et al., 2007; World Health Organization, 2009)

THERAPEUTIC USE

TPM Literature

Chasteberry is an astringent and is useful to treat obstructions in brain and therefore, is recommended for psychosis and headaches due to inflammation of meninges layers or the brain itself, both in oral and topical use as a poultice. It reduced palpitations which are caused due to the phlegmatic or melancholic dystemperament upon oral consumption. It also reduces flatulence. Additionally, it is helpful against obstructions of liver and spleen. Chasteberry is recommended for amenorrhea and uterine inflammation via different routes of administration including vaginal insert, fumigation, and sitz bath. It is both a galactagogue and an emmenagogue. It is also suggested to stop bleeding from hemorrhoids and anal fisher. Chaste tree reduces libido in male in oral use and even in chronic close topical contact with the plant parts. The leaves, if being heated, can be used as a plaster to cover testis in case of cold-tempered inflammation and hydrocele. Chaste tree is also mentioned to be an insect repellent (Aghili Khorasani 1771).

DOI: 10.1201/b22971-40

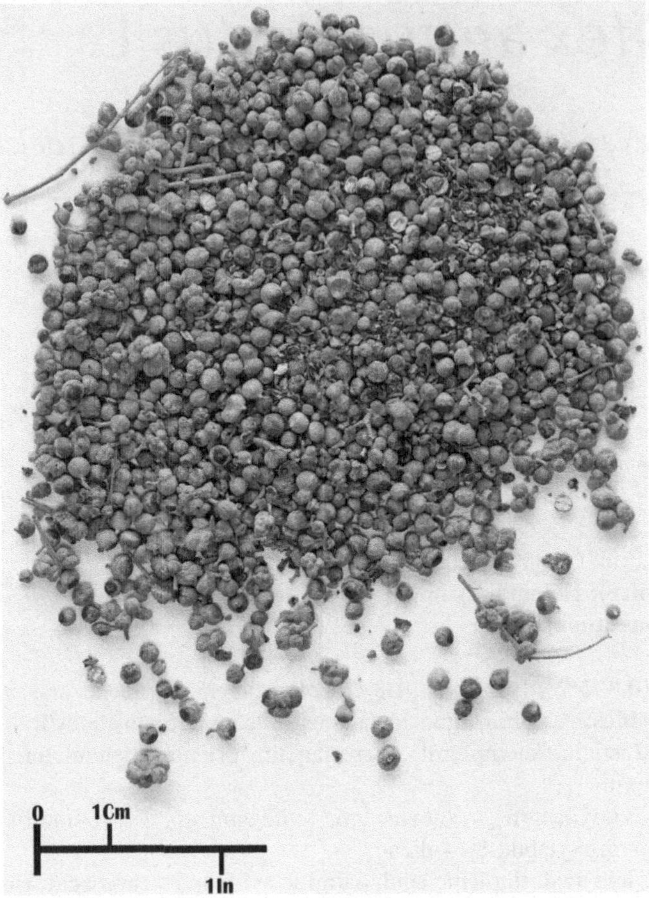

FIGURE 40.1 Chasteberry fruits.

Current Evidence

Clinical Evidence

PMS and PMDD: In an RCT comparing the effect of chasteberry with fluoxetine in 41 patients with PMS, herbal intervention showed a nearly similar efficacy to fluoxetine. It was suggested that chasteberry is a better option to control the physical PMS symptoms; while fluoxetine better controls psychological symptoms (Van Die et al., 2013). According to a meta-analysis including three RCTs, chasteberry is more than twice as likely to induce a relief in the symptoms vs. placebo and thus, is recommended for mild to moderate PMS at a daily dose of 30–40 mg (Csupor et al., 2019). Another systematic review on the use of chasteberry to treat PMS/PMDD symptoms which included eight RCTs found that this plant within a dose range of 3.2–40 mg per day of the commercial extracts is a safe and effective option to consider (Cerqueira et al., 2017). Also, a meta-analysis including 14 RCTs reported that in general, chasteberry preparations have significant beneficial effects on the improvement of PMS symptoms; however, the heterogeneity of the reported data and high risk of bias makes future studies necessary (Verkaik et al., 2017).

Cyclic mastalgia: In a systematic review and meta-analysis of 17 RCTs and eight nonrandomized clinical trials, chasteberry could significantly decrease breast pain and prolactin level with a dosage of 20–40 mg per day and a mean treatment period of 3 months. While six of the studies included in the quantitative analysis showed a moderate effect size in favor of chasteberry vs. placebo; seven studies showed this plant to be noninferior to conventional gold standards such as dopamine agonists, NSAIDs, SSRIs, and OCPs (Ooi et al., 2020).

Hyperprolactinemia: In a placebo-controlled RCT in 52 women with latent hyperprolactinemia and luteal phase defects, 20 mg daily intake of chasteberry capsules for 3 months could significantly decrease prolactin level and normalize luteal phase length, along with restoration of luteal progesterone synthesis (Milewicz et al., 1993). In another RCT in 105 women with hyperprolactinemia, patients were randomized to receive bromocriptine (2.5–7.5 mg daily), dostinex (0.25 mg, 2–4 times per week), or chasteberry tablet (equal to 3.3 mg of acubin, 2–4 times daily) for four menstrual cycles. Chasteberry caused a significant reduction of endometrial thickness vs. the other two groups. Also, this plant could reduce prolactin and increase estradiol, progesterone, and LH, without any significant change in FSH (Haerifar et al., 2020).

Sexual function: A double-blind, placebo-controlled RCT in 102 women of reproductive age showed that administration of chasteberry tablet (3.2–4.8 mg daily) for 16 weeks makes a significant improvement in the overall assessment of sexual function (Dalil Heirati et al., 2021).

Menopause: In a double-blind RCT in 52 menopausal women, participants were treated with 30 mg per day of chasteberry tablet or placebo for 8 weeks. Accordingly, chasteberry caused a significant improvement in total menopausal disorder, vasomotor dysfunction, and anxiety vs. placebo; while no difference was observed in sexual dysfunction, depression, and somatic complications (Naseri et al., 2019).

Sleep disturbances: In an open-label, placebo-controlled RCT in 20 healthy men, chasteberry hydroethanolic extract was administered with three doses of 120, 240, and 360 mg per day for 14 days. A dose-dependent elevation of melatonin serum concentration was observed in subjects which suggest the possible effect of this plant for sleep disturbances without any effect of melatonin circadian rhythm; however, as the study subjects were healthy cases, this hypothesis should be evaluated in future studies in individuals with insomnia (Dericks-Tan et al., 2003).

Preclinical Evidence

Sex hormones: In the STZ-induced type 2 diabetes in female rats, oral administration of chasteberry hydroethanolic extract (100–400 mg/kg) for 7 days could significantly restore the reduced levels of FHS, LH, estrogen, and progesterone vs. negative control (Soleymanzadeh et al., 2020). Another animal study in ovariectomized female mice showed that chasteberry hydroethanolic extract (0.6 and 1.2 g/kg) could increase the level of estrogen and progesterone, as well as the weight of uterine. Additionally, the extract increased the ovarian weight in normal mice. No significant change was observed regarding FSH in normal or ovariectomized animal; while LH and prolactin were significantly reduced only in ovariectomized mice (Ibrahim et al., 2008). In another animal study, 30-day i.p. injection of chasteberry hydroethanolic extract (56–465 mg/kg) to male mice significantly decreased LH and testosterone levels. Also, coadministration of the extract with haloperidol could prevent haloperidol-induced elevation of these hormones (Nasri et al., 2007). In D-galactose-induced aging model in female mice, oral administration of 1,200 mg/kg of chasteberry hydroethanolic extract for 7 days could successfully reverse elevations of LH, FSH, body weight, and MDA. The extract also increased SOD, CAT, and estrogen levels in animals (Ahangarpour et al., 2016).

Seizure: In amygdala-kindling model of seizure in mice, hydroethanolic extract of chasteberry (60–180 mg/kg) could significantly increase after discharge threshold and decrease duration of seizure in a dose-dependent manner (Saberi et al., 2008).

Insect repellent: In a study using mice, jirds, cats, dogs, and human arm (for mosquitoes), repellency effect of a topical preparation containing 1–3% concentration of chaste tree seeds CO_2

extract was assessed. The extract showed significant repellent activity against rodent ticks, cat fleas (*Ctenocephalides felis*), females *Culex quinquefasciatus*, *Anopheles stephensi*, *Aedes aegypti*, and *Stomoxys calcitrans* (Mehlhorn et al., 2005). There are also reports on the larvicidal effects of chaste tree essential oil against *Spilosoma obliqua* (Tandon et al., 2008) and *Aedes aegypti* (Ricarte et al., 2020).

ADVERSE REACTIONS

TPM Literature

Chaste tree may cause headache and be harmful for kidneys. It is recommended to be taken with gum Arabic to reduce the side effects. Use of chaste tree in men may cause erectile dysfunction and decrease in libido (Aghili Khorasani 1771).

Current Evidence

It is generally safe and well tolerated within recommended dosage. Mild and reversible GI symptoms such as nausea and vomiting, menstruation disturbances, headache, as well as allergic skin reactions have been reported for chasteberry (Gardner and McGuffin, 2013; Daniele et al., 2005).

CONTRAINDICATIONS

TPM Literature

Long-term use in men should be avoided because of erectile dysfunction, loss of libido, and infertility (Aghili Khorasani 1771).

Current Evidence

It should be avoided in patients with hormone-sensitive cancers and women undergoing *in vitro* fertilization (Ulbricht, 2010).

PREGNANCY AND LACTATION

TPM Literature

Due to emmenagogue properties, chasteberry should be avoided during pregnancy (Aghili Khorasani 1771).

Current Evidence

Due to the possible uterine stimulatory effects, chaste tree and its products should be avoided during pregnancy.

The use of chasteberry products as galactagogue is popular, and current evidence considers side effects due to this plant to be unlikely in nursing infants (Gardner and McGuffin, 2013).

DRUG INTERACTIONS

Dopamine agonists and antagonists: Due to dopaminergic activity via interaction with D2 receptors, chaste tree products may interact with either dopamine agonists or dopamine antagonists. It is possible to increase the effects of dopamine agonists such as bromocriptine and apomorphine and reduce the effects of dopamine antagonists including antipsychotics as well as some antiemetics like metoclopramide and prochlorperazine (Williamson et al., 2013).

Estrogenic drugs: Due to the effects of chaste tree products on sex hormone levels, there is a possibility of herb–drug interaction with OCPs, birth control pills, hormone replacement therapy, or any other hormonal drugs (Ulbricht, 2010).

METHOD OF ADMINISTRATION

TPM Literature

Chasteberry and leaves can be used orally or as vaginal insert, topical solution, or sitz bath (Aghili Khorasani 1771).

Current Evidence

Chasteberry is usually taken as commercial tablets or drops.

DOSAGE

Adults (18 years and older): The typical daily dosage is 800 mg of dried fruit or 20 mg dried extract. In RCTs, up to 40 mg daily dose of commercial products has been used. There is not enough data to suggest a dosage of chasteberry for children (younger than 18 years) (HMPC, 2018).

REFERENCES

Aghili Khorasani MH 1771. *Makhzan-al-Adviah* (*The treasury of drugs*) (rewritten by Shams Ardakani MR, Rahimi R, Farjadmand F, 1st ed.). Tehran: Tehran University of Medical Sciences; 2009.

Ahangarpour A, Najimi SA, Farbood Y. Effects of *Vitex agnus-castus* fruit on sex hormones and antioxidant indices in a D-galactose-induced aging female mouse model. J Chin Med Assoc. 2016;79(11):589–596.

Baxter K, Preston CL (eds.). *Stockley's drug interactions*. London: Pharmaceutical Press; 2013.

Cerqueira RO, Frey BN, Leclerc E, Brietzke E. *Vitex agnus castus* for premenstrual syndrome and premenstrual dysphoric disorder: A systematic review. Arch Womens Ment Health. 2017;20(6):713–719.

Committee on Herbal Medicinal Products (HMPC). *European Union herbal monograph on Vitex agnus-castus L., fructus*. EMA/HMPC/606742/2017. Amsterdam: HPMC; 2018.

Csupor D, Lantos T, Hegyi P, et al. *Vitex agnus-castus* in premenstrual syndrome: A meta-analysis of double-blind randomised controlled trials. Complement Ther Med. 2019;47:102190.

Dalil Heirati SF, Ozgoli G, KabodMehri R, et al. The 4-month effect of *Vitex agnus-castus* plant on sexual function of women of reproductive age: A clinical trial. J Edu Health Promot. 2021;10:294.

Daniele C, Coon JT, Pittler MH, Ernst E. *Vitex agnus castus*: A systematic review of adverse events. Drug Saf. 2005;28:319–332.

Dericks-Tan JS, Schwinn P, Hildt C. Dose-dependent stimulation of melatonin secretion after administration of *Agnus castus*. Exp Clin Endocrinol Diabetes. 2003;111(1):44–46.

Gardner Z, McGuffin M. *Botanical safety handbook*. Boca Raton: Taylor & Francis; 2013.

Gruenwald J, Brendler T, Jaenicke C. *PDR for herbal medicines*. Montvale: Thomson Reuters; 2007.

Haerifar N, Vaezi G, Samani ZG, Lak SS. The effect of *Vitex agnus castus* extract on the blood level of prolactin, sex hormones levels, and the histological effects on the endometrial tissue in hyperprolactinemic women. Crescent J Med Biol Sci. 2020;7(4):545–550.

Ibrahim NA, Shalaby AS, Farag RS, et al. Gynecological efficacy and chemical investigation of *Vitex agnus-castus* L. fruits growing in Egypt. Nat Prod Res. 2008;22(6):537–546.

Mehlhorn H, Schmahl G, Schmidt J. Extract of the seeds of the plant *Vitex agnus castus* proven to be highly efficacious as a repellent against ticks, fleas, mosquitoes and biting flies. Parasitol Res. 2005;95:363–365.

Milewicz A, Gejdel E, Sworen H, et al. *Vitex agnus castus* extract in the treatment of luteal phase defects due to latent hyperprolactinemia: Results of a randomized placebo-controlled double-blind study. Arzneimittelforschung. 1993;43(7):752–756.

Naseri R, Farnia V, Yazdchi K, et al. Comparison of *Vitex agnus-castus* extracts with placebo in reducing menopausal symptoms: A randomized double-blind study. Korean J Fam Med. 2019;40(6):362–367.

Nasri S, Oryan S, Rohani AH, Amin GR. The effects of *Vitex agnus castus* extract and its interaction with dopaminergic system on LH and testosterone in male mice. Pak J Biol Sci. 2007;10(14):2300–2307.

Ooi SL, Watts S, McClean R, Pak SC. *Vitex agnus-castus* for the treatment of cyclic mastalgia: A systematic review and meta-analysis. J Womens Health. 2020;29(2):262–278.

Ricarte LP, Bezerra GP, Romero NR, et al. Chemical composition and biological activities of the essential oils from *Vitex-agnus castus*, Ocimum campechianum and Ocimum carnosum. An Acad Bras Cienc. 2020;92(1):e20180569.

Saberi M, Rezvanizadeh A, Bakhtiarian A. The antiepileptic activity of *Vitex agnus* castus extract on amygdala kindled seizures in male rats. Neurosci Lett. 2008;441(2):193–196.

Soleymanzadeh F, Mahmoodi M, Shahidi S. Effect of *Vitex agnus-castus* ethanolic extract on sex hormones in streptozotocin-induced diabetic rats. J Family Reprod Health. 2020;14(2):102–105.

Tandon S, Mittal AK, Pant AK. Insect growth regulatory activity of *Vitex trifolia* and *Vitex agnus-castus* essential oils against *Spilosoma obliqua*. Fitoterapia. 2008;79(4):283–286.

Ulbricht CE. *Natural standard herb & supplement guide: An evidence-based reference*. St. Luis: Elsevier; 2010.

Van Die MD, Burger HG, Teede HJ, Bone KM. *Vitex agnus-castus* extracts for female reproductive disorders: A systematic review of clinical trials. Planta Med. 2013;79(07):562–575.

Verkaik S, Kamperman AM, Van Westrhenen R, Schulte PF. The treatment of premenstrual syndrome with preparations of Vitex agnus castus: A systematic review and meta-analysis. Am J Obstet Gynecol. 2017;217(2):150–166.

Williamson E, Driver S, Baxter K (eds.). *Stockley's herbal medicines interactions*. London: Pharmaceutical Press; 2013.

World Health Organization. *WHO monographs on selected medicinal plants*, vol. 4. Geneva: World Health Organization; 2009.

41 *Zingiber officinale* Roscoe

Ghazaleh Mosleh and Meysam Zaeri

Scientific name: *Zingiber officinale* Roscoe
Family: Zingiberaceae
Common names:

- **English:** Ginger
- **Persian:** *zanğabīl, zanğafīl, zanğabīr, zangabīl*
- **Arabic:** *zanğabīl*

Medicinal part(s): Rhizome and root (Figure 41.1)
Temperament (nature): Hot in the third degree and dry in the first degree (dried ginger is hot in the third degree and dry in the second degree)
Major chemical constituents:

- **Essential oil (2.5–3%):** α-curcumene, α-zingiberene, β-sesquiphellandrene, geranial, neral, and β-bisabolene
- **Pungent principles:** Gingerols and shogaols
- **Diarylheptanoids:** Gingerenone A and B
- **Other constituents:** Diterpenes, diarylheptenones, gingesulphonic acid, monoacyl digalactosyl glycerols (Gruenwald et al., 2007; Khare, 2007)

THERAPEUTIC USE

TPM Literature

The powder is recommended for some ocular diseases. Oral intake of ginger is considered a potent memory enhancer, digestion promoter, stomach and liver tonic, carminative, anthelmintic, and laxative. It is a potent cleanser of body from thick phlegm humor, especially in GI tract and nervous system. Ginger is a potent aphrodisiac, especially when eaten with egg yolk. It is also prescribed to treat palsy, obstructive jaundice, urinary incontinence induced by cold dystemperament, and diarrhea due to indigestion. Ginger paste is topically used for hemorrhoids and reinforcement of body organs. Fresh ginger paste is suggested for alopecia, anti-inflammatory, and analgesic purposes. In addition, topical administration of dried powder or fresh juice of ginger can relieve joint pain (Aghili Khorasani 1771; Avicenna 1025).

Current Evidence

Clinical Evidence

Nausea and vomiting: A systematic review and meta-analysis on 18 articles with 301 participants showed that a ginger supplement (≤1 g per day for >3 days) decreases acute vomiting by 60% and fatigue by 80%. This review claims that ginger supplementation can be a beneficial choice to reduce chemotherapy-induced vomiting and fatigue (Crichton et al., 2019). A meta-analysis including 363

DOI: 10.1201/b22971-41

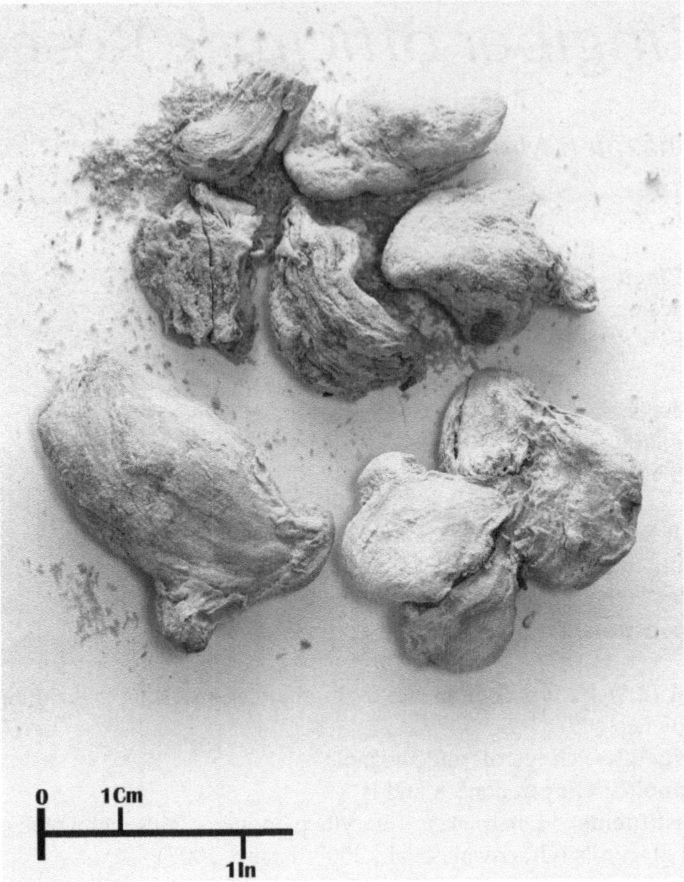

FIGURE 41.1 Ginger rhizomes.

patients in five RCTs indicated that at least a fixed dose of 1 g ginger effectively reduces postoperative nausea and vomiting (Chaiyakunapruk et al., 2006). A systematic review and meta-analysis of 14 RCTs including 1,506 patients showed that ginger could reduce nausea at 2, 6, and 12 h after the operation, but there were no significant changes in the incidence rates of postoperative vomiting and nausea (Lu et al., 2022). A systematic review and meta-analysis of 10 RCTs with 918 patients suggested that ginger (≥1,000–2,000 mg) can be a safe and well-tolerated alternative to decrease the severity of postoperative nausea and vomiting (Tóth et al., 2018). Another meta-analysis of 10 studies revealed that 0.5–2 g per day of ginger could decrease acute chemotherapy-induced nausea and vomiting (Chang and Peng, 2019). In a study on 15 patients with advanced cancer, taking 1.650 g of ginger per day for 14 days improved nausea, dysmotility, and reflux conditions (Bhargava et al., 2020). A systematic review of nine RCTs suggested that ginger may decrease nausea in the acute chemotherapy phase in breast cancer patients; the most considerable effect was seen with doses of 0.5 and 1 g of ginger (Saneei Totmaj et al., 2019). Nevertheless, a systematic review and meta-analysis conducted on five RCTs and 872 cancerous patients showed that ginger and control groups do not significantly differ in the incidence and severity of acute nausea and vomiting in patients with cancer. Four of the studies indicated that 0.5–3.5 g of ginger daily could relieve acute nausea and vomiting. Though, another study reported no significant effects on nausea or vomiting by daily consumption of 1 g ginger. Besides, a study has reported increased severity of nausea by daily indication of 2 g ginger (Lee and Oh, 2013).

Migraine headache: A systematic review and meta-analysis on three RCTs, including 227 patients suffering from migraine, showed that ginger is a safe and effective choice for treating migraine patients having pain assessed at 2 h (Chen and Cai, 2021). However, a double-blind, placebo-controlled RCT in 107 patients with migraine reported ginger capsules with a dose of 0.2 g (three times per day for 3 months) to have no significant prophylactic effect on the number of migraine attacks, severe pain days, and migraine duration (Martins et al., 2020).

Dysmenorrhea: A systematic review of 12 RCTs and three quasi-experimental studies showed that both oral administration (250–500 mg ginger capsule, 3–4 times a day) and topical application (rubbing 3–4 drops of ginger oil daily for 15 minutes) have positive effects on reducing pain and inflammation of dysmenorrhea, especially during the first 3 days of the menstrual cycle, possibly due to reduction of cyclooxygenase activity and GI leukotrienes (Mozafari et al., 2018). A systematic review and meta-analysis of seven RCTs showed a significant effect of 0.75–2 g of ginger powder in the first 3–4 days of the menstrual cycle in reducing dysmenorrheal pain in participants having primary dysmenorrhea (Daily et al., 2015). Another systematic review and meta-analysis of six RCTs showed that oral ginger could be a promising treatment for menstrual pain. Ginger and mefenamic acid (as an NSAID) were similar in this regard (Chen et al., 2016).

Heavy menstrual bleeding: In a placebo-controlled RCT on 92 high school girls with menorrhagia, patients were treated with 250 mg capsules of ginger powder, three times daily, from the day before the beginning of menstrual bleeding for 4 days, and for three consecutive menstrual cycles. Compared with placebo, ginger treatment caused a significant decrease in blood loss (Kashefi et al., 2015). Also, another RCT in 102 cases with menorrhagia showed that 300 mg ginger powder or frankincense capsules, three times daily, along with ibuprofen, causes a significant reduction in the amount and duration of menstruation vs. placebo (Eshaghian et al., 2019).

Muscle pain after prolonged exercise: A systematic review of seven studies found that taking 2 g per day of ginger for at least 5 days could reduce muscle pain of prolonged exercise and inflammation of cardiorespiratory exercise (Wilson, 2015). In a double-blind, placebo-controlled RCT on 74 volunteers consuming 2 g of either raw or heated ginger for 11 days, it was demonstrated that ginger results in a moderate to large decrease in postexercise muscle pain (Black et al., 2010). A study was done to assess the effects of the preexercise ginger supplement on muscle damage among 20 participants consuming 4 g of ginger for 5 days. This study concluded that ginger supplements may accelerate recovery of muscle strength after severe exercise, but do not affect muscle damage indicators (Matsumura et al., 2015).

Osteoarthritis: A meta-analysis on five placebo-controlled trials having 593 patients showed that oral ginger (0.5–1 g per day) was effective and safe for osteoarthritis treatment (Bartels et al., 2015). However, in a systematic review and meta-analysis of four RCTs, there was not sufficient evidence to support the benefits of oral ginger for relieving pain in knee osteoarthritis (Araya-Quintanilla et al., 2020).

Inflammation and oxidative stress: A systematic review and meta-analysis of 16 RCTs comprising 1,010 participants indicated that ginger supplementation reduces CRP, hs-CRP, and TNF-α (Morvaridzadeh et al., 2020). According to another meta-analysis of 14 RCTs, ginger significantly decreased CRP, IL-6, and TNF-α and increased TAC (Askari et al., 2020). A meta-analysis of 25 RCTs indicated that ginger supplementation significantly affects inflammatory and oxidative stress markers, including CRP, IL-6, TNF-α, PGE2, TAC, and LPO (Jalali et al., 2020). Another meta-analysis on nine studies indicated a significant, but nondose-dependent, decrease in serum CRP after ginger supplementation. In addition, HDL-C and TAG were significantly improved (Mazidi et al., 2016). In a meta-analysis including 11 RCTs, ginger showed an increasing effect on Gpx and decreasing effect on LPO, especially using ≤1 g per day of ginger and duration of fewer than 12 weeks. No significant change was observed in TAC, but there was an increasing trend in high doses of ginger and a duration of more than 12 weeks (Sheikhhossein et al., 2021).

Type 2 diabetes mellitus: A systematic review and meta-analysis on 10 RCTs considering 490 diabetic patients showed that ginger has a beneficial effect on glucose and insulin sensitivity. A significant reduction of FBS, and an improvement in lipid profile were observed (Zhu et al., 2018). A pooled meta-analysis on 10 RCTs found that ginger supplementation causes a significant reduction in FBS and blood pressure in patients with type 2 diabetes mellitus, but there were no significant changes in lipid profiles. Also, the effect of ginger on HbA1C was only significant in patients under 50 years old (Ebrahimzadeh et al., 2022). Another meta-analysis on eight RCTs including 454 type 2 diabetic patients showed that ginger consumption (1.6–4 g daily) improves HbA1C, but there was no significant difference in FBS (Huang et al., 2019). A meta-analysis on nine RCTs involving diabetic and hyperlipidemic patients revealed that ginger supplementation significantly decreases FBS, TC, and TAG, and increases HDL-C. However, the changes were related to the patients' clinical conditions (Jafarnejad et al., 2017).

Obesity: A meta-analysis of 20 studies showed that ginger decreases BMI significantly, and the relation between ginger and energy metabolism can have beneficial effects on obesity (Macit et al., 2019). A systematic review and meta-analysis of 14 RCTs with 473 subjects indicated that ginger supplementation significantly decreases body weight, hip ratio, FBS, and insulin resistance and significantly increases HDL-C levels. Ginger had no considerable effect on BMI, insulin, and TAG (Maharlouei et al., 2019).

Colitis: A placebo-controlled RCT was done to assess the effects ginger on oxidative stress in patients with mild to moderate ulcerative colitis. Forty-six patients consumed 2 g per day of dried ginger for 12 weeks. The results showed that ginger reduces MDA significantly after 6 and 12 weeks, but it did not affect total antioxidant capacity. It improved the severity of the disease in the 12th week. In addition, ginger could increase patients' quality of life after 12 weeks. This study concluded that ginger could be a reasonable choice to improve the treatment of patients with ulcerative colitis (Nikkhah-Bodaghi et al., 2019). In addition, a double-blind RCT was done to evaluate the effect of ginger supplementation on 44 patients with active ulcerative colitis. The study showed that consuming 3 g per day of ginger capsules for 12 weeks has promising results for ulcerative colitis (Shayesteh et al., 2020).

Cardiovascular outcomes: A systematic review and meta-analysis of 12 RCTs (586 patients) suggested that ginger supplementation reduces TAG and LDL-C (low dose of ginger [≤2 g per day] had much lowering effect). According to the review, ginger has no significant impact on TC and HDL-C. Overall, this review claimed that ginger has a favorable impact on TAG and LDL-C (Pourmasoumi et al., 2018). A systematic review and meta-analysis on six RCTs (345 participants) showed that ginger supplement reduces SBP and DBP, particularly for patients with a mean age of fewer than 50 years, follow-up duration of fewer than 8 weeks, and ginger doses more than 3 g per day (Hasani et al., 2019). According to a systematic literature review on 10 studies (eight clinical trials and two observational studies), the evidence for ginger to affect platelet aggregation and coagulation was equivocal. So further study is needed regarding the beneficial effects of ginger platelet aggregation and coagulation (Marx et al., 2015).

Semen quality: A systematic review of 35 original articles summarized the link between ginger active compounds with semen quality. Results showed that ginger improves semen quality and different sperm parameters and increases gonadal hormones and nitric oxide production (Banihani, 2019).

Preclinical Evidence

Liver disease: In a study on rats, ginger ethanolic extract had protective effects on CCl_4 and acetaminophen-induced liver damage. Based on histopathologic examinations, the study indicates that ginger rhizome could be beneficial to prevent liver injury caused by chemicals (Yemitan and Izegbu, 2006). A study assessed the hepatoprotective property of ginger ethanolic extract (0.25 and 0.5 g/kg for 14 days) in rats. It reduced thioacetamide-induced hepatotoxicity and showed antiproliferative activity on Hep-G2 cells (Abdulaziz Bardi et al., 2013). A systematic review and meta-analysis on 18 preclinical and clinical studies showed that ginger might reduce several clinical aspects of NAFLD such as TC, TAG, MDA, FBS, and CAT. In this review, several mechanisms are mentioned for ginger, including insulin-sensitizing effects, expression of antioxidant enzymes, reducing oxygen species, and antihyperlipidemic effects (Samadi et al., 2022).

Neurological problems: A review showed that ginger and its constituents, like 6-gingerol and 6-shogaol are effective for age-related neurological problems (neuropathological problems of the central nervous system, such as oxidative stress and protein misfolding) by modulating cell death and cell survival molecules. This review concluded that ginger active ingredients have a therapeutic potential in managing age-related neurological problems (Choi et al., 2018). A review of preclinical studies about Alzheimer's disease showed that ginger and its active ingredients (gingerol, shogaol, and borneol) have a significant role in improving and decreasing memory dysfunctions in preclinical studies on Alzheimer's disease (Talebi et al., 2021). A study on 48 mice showed that ginger rhizome (0.5% for 8 weeks) improves mechanical and thermal allodynia and improves cognitive problems, anxiety, and depression. Moreover, ginger decreases the response of proinflammatory mediators. This study suggests that ginger enhances the antinociceptive effect of paracetamol and improves cognitive problems associated with chronic pain (Montserrat-de la Paz et al., 2018).

GI motility problems: A study investigated the effects of oral administration of ginger extract or 6-gingerol on small intestine contractility. Ginger extract (0.01, 0.02, and 0.1 g/kg/day) or 6-gingerol (0.002 g/kg/day) were given to rats orally for 7 days. Contractions were reduced in small intestine in rats receiving ginger extract or 6-gingerol. There were no considerable changes in intestine histology. The results showed that ginger could be applied for GI motility problems (Chatturong et al., 2018).

Arthritis: A study was done to evaluate the effect of ginger rhizomes extract on collagen-induced arthritis in rats. Results showed that intraperitoneal ginger in doses higher than 0.05 g/kg/day for 26 days could decrease disease incidence, joint swelling, cartilage decomposition, IL-1β, IL-2, IL-6, and TNF-α. Ginger extract at the dose of 0.2 g/kg/day was better than 0.002 g/kg/day of indomethacin at most parameters. This study claims that ginger extract can be a beneficial alternative to NSAIDs for managing rheumatoid arthritis (Fouda and Berika, 2009).

Metabolic syndrome, inflammation, and oxidative stress: In a study on high-fat diet-induced hyperlipidemia in mice, taking 0.25 and 0.5 g/kg of aqueous ginger extract once daily orally for 12 weeks improved lipid profile and antioxidant capacity, revealing that ginger could treat hyperlipidemia and cardiovascular problems in the animals (Bekkouch et al., 2019). A study on rats showed that ginger (oral 0.05 g daily for 6 weeks) decreases CRP, homocysteine, and cathepsin G levels. The results suggested that ginger could reduce heart structural problems in diabetic rats (Ilkhanizadeh et al., 2016). A study compared the effects of garlic, ginger, and turmeric on metabolic syndrome and oxidative stress in diabetic rats. The results showed that 0.2 g/kg of the garlic bulb, ginger rhizome, and turmeric rhizome for 28 days alleviate metabolic syndrome (hyperglycemia and dyslipidemia) by increasing insulin, antioxidant defense system, and decreasing lipid peroxidation; however, garlic was more effective than ginger and turmeric in this regard (Madkor et al., 2011).

Skin damage: A study showed that water extract of ginger, gingerol, and shogaol decreases cytokine production, leukocyte infiltration, and blood vessels dilation due to UVB radiation in mice's skin. This study suggested that ginger has a potential anti-inflammatory property for the skin against UVB harms (Guahk et al., 2010).

Semen quality: A meta-analysis was done on 21 studies to assess the effects of *Z. officinale* on health conditions and production factors in chickens. Ginger administration improved semen quality, body weight gain, and feed conversion ratio. In conclusion, the study revealed enhanced performance in chickens due to ginger administration (Ogbuewu and Mbajiorgu, 2020).

ADVERSE REACTIONS

TPM Literature

It is harmful to the throat, and honey or almond oil can ameliorate its damage (Aghili Khorasani 1771).

Current Evidence

Few adverse reactions have been reported with low doses of ginger. The most common side effects include triggering stomach and intestine discomforts. Bad taste or irritation in the mouth, belching, bloating, nausea, and heartburn have been associated especially with ginger powder. It is thought that mild gastric upset symptoms induced by ginger may be attenuated by the consumption of ginger capsules instead of powder. Several reports indicate that swallowing fresh ginger without enough chewing can lead to intestinal blockage (Ulbricht, 2010). A systematic search on 100 published reports, including 1,073 patients taking ginger, showed that 3.3% of patients had slight side effects (GI symptoms and sleepiness). It is worth mentioning that ginger's maximum daily dose of 6 g has few side effects (Betz et al., 2005). GI problems, nosebleeds, sore throat, and kidney inflammation are occasionally associated with excessive doses of ginger. One study on pregnant participants with a daily intake of 1.95 g ginger indicated that 12% of the women experienced heartburn (Gardner and McGuffin, 2013). In addition, allergic contact dermatitis may occur, especially in spice factory workers (Gardner and McGuffin, 2013; Ulbricht, 2010).

Conjunctivitis is considered a rare adverse effect associated with ginger (Ulbricht, 2010). Some studies reveal ginger's probable decreasing or increasing effects on blood pressure, although there is limited scientific data. Theoretically, ginger can induce arrhythmia, despite the lack of clinical evidence. Furthermore, it may prevent the coagulation process by preventing platelet clumping, in theory. One study on gingerol and its derivatives demonstrated stronger antiplatelet properties than aspirin. It is a concern that ginger supplements may increase the risk of bleeding if taken in patients who undergo surgery or take anticoagulant/antiplatelet drugs (Ulbricht, 2010). According to a case report study, a woman got subacute thyroiditis after ginger consumption (Sanavi and Afshar, 2010). In addition, traditionally, high doses of ginger were considered to lower blood sugar levels. However, scientific information is lacking in this case. Also, there is a lack of studies on the safety of prolonged use of ginger supplements (Ulbricht, 2010).

CONTRAINDICATIONS

TPM Literature

None.

Current Evidence

Ginger supplements should be used cautiously under the supervision of an healthcare provider in patients with active gallstone problems (Gardner and McGuffin, 2013; Ulbricht, 2010, Mills et al., 2006), gastric ulcers, blocked intestines, or inflammatory bowel disease (Mills et al., 2006). In addition, people with allergies to ginger and its chemical constituents, or other herbs of the Zingiberaceae family, should avoid ginger supplements (Ulbricht, 2010).

PREGNANCY AND LACTATION

TPM LITERATURE

None.

CURRENT EVIDENCE

According to a systematic review and meta-analysis of 12 RCTs including 1,278 pregnant participants, ginger was harmless and significantly effective in preventing nausea (lower dosage <1.5 g per day); however, it did not produce beneficial effects to reduce vomiting episodes during pregnancy (Viljoen et al., 2014). According to a systematic literature review of RCTs with 675 pregnant participants, no significant adverse effects were reported after ginger consumption. In general, the therapy duration of studies has been limited to 4 days, but some other studies continued for 2–3 weeks. In addition, the most common dose was 1 g divided into smaller doses. Several clinical studies on pregnant women, including over 900 participants with the daily dose of 1–2 g ginger, did not observe any adverse outcomes (Gardner and McGuffin, 2013; Aronson, 2009). On the other hand, some authors recommend that no more than 1 g of dry weight per day should be taken by pregnant women because ginger can increase uterus discharge during menstruation, and it may lead to a higher risk of abortion, bleeding, or fetal mutations (Ulbricht, 2010). Powerful scientific data indicate that using ginger up to 1.5 g of dry weight per day has minimal risk in pregnancy and spontaneous abortion. Also, scientific evidence reveals that ginger consumption is not associated with major malformations (Mills et al., 2006). Based on the literature, daily intake of 1 g of fresh ginger for 4 days is reported to be a safe and effective treatment for nausea and vomiting during pregnancy (Stanisiere et al., 2018).

A systematic review of five RCTs found that ginger could increase the volume of human milk in mothers that had vaginal births but not cesarian sections (Dilokthornsakul et al., 2022). There is a lack of information in the scientific literature on the safety of ginger in lactation (Gardner and McGuffin, 2013).

DRUG INTERACTIONS

Antihypertensives: Nifedipine, a calcium channel blocker which is typically administrated for hypertension treatment, has synergistic antiplatelet effects with ginger (Gardner and McGuffin, 2013; Mills et al., 2006; Williamson et al., 2013). This effect was stronger in normal blood pressure people than in patients with hypertension (Williamson et al., 2013).

Cardiovascular drugs: Ginger may interfere with heart medications such as beta-blockers and digoxin (Ulbricht, 2010; Mills et al., 2006). Also, taking large amounts of calcium with ginger may increase the risk of arrhythmia (Ulbricht, 2010).

Anticoagulants and antiplatelets: In theory, ginger may increase the effects of oral anticoagulants (Ulbricht, 2010; Mills et al., 2006; Aronson, 2009). Isolated cases have reported the synergistic effect of ginger with warfarin and related anticoagulant drugs (Williamson et al., 2013). In contrast, some pharmacological evidence does not confirm this theory (Williamson et al., 2013; Gardner and McGuffin, 2013).

Acid-inhibiting drugs: According to available literature, stomach acid production may be increased after the intake of ginger. Thus, it theoretically may oppose the antacid effects. On the other hand, some animal studies report the protecting effects of ginger on the stomach (Mills et al., 2006; Ulbricht, 2010).

Antidiabetic drugs: In theory, ginger can reduce blood sugar levels. So, the interaction of ginger with oral diabetes medications or insulin is probable. Caution must be taken when supplements or herbs affecting blood sugar are prescribed (Ulbricht, 2010; Mills et al., 2006).

Others: Barbiturates may interact with ginger (Mills et al., 2006). Furthermore, taking excessive amounts of ginger may have synergistic effects with medications that cause drowsiness or slow thinking. In theory, bleeding risk may be increased when ginger and NSAIDS are taken together (Ulbricht, 2010). Also, two suspected drug interactions with celecoxib and phenprocoumon were reported in previous case reports, but the type of products or doses were not identified (Gardner and McGuffin, 2013). On the other hand, coadministration of tacrolimus and ginger have shown increasing effects on tacrolimus bioavailability in human and animal models via inhibiting the PGP efflux pump and/or CYP450 system (Abushammala, 2021).

METHOD OF ADMINISTRATION

TPM Literature

The comminuted rhizome, decoction, or jam is indicated orally. For topical administration, ginger powder can be applied to the eyes or rubbed on the skin to treat several disorders. Furthermore, fresh juice, oil, or the poultice made from dried or fresh plant material is topically administered (Aghili Khorasani 1771).

Current Evidence

Fresh or dried root may be recommended as powder, capsules, liquid extract, tablets, tea, and tincture (Ulbricht, 2010).

DOSAGE

Adults (≥18 years): A large number of studies indicate that the maximum daily dose is 4 g. Many publications and experts suggest the oral daily dose of 1–5g of powder, tablets, capsules, or fresh ginger, taken in divided doses.
Children (<18 years): There is insufficient scientific data in this case (Ulbricht, 2010).

REFERENCES

Abdulaziz Bardi D, Halabi MF, Abdullah NA, et al. *In vivo* evaluation of ethanolic extract of *Zingiber officinale* rhizomes for its protective effect against liver cirrhosis. Biomed Res Int. 2013;2013:918460.

Abushammala I. Tacrolimus and herbs interactions: A review. Pharmazie. 2021;76(10):468–472.

Aghili Khorasani MH 1771. *Makhzan-al-Adviah* (*The treasury of drugs*) (rewritten by Shams Ardakani MR, Rahimi R, Farjadmand F, 1st ed.). Tehran: Tehran University of Medical Sciences; 2009.

Araya-Quintanilla F, Gutierrez-Espinoza H, Munoz-Yanez MJ, et al. Effectiveness of ginger on pain and function in knee osteoarthritis: A PRISMA systematic review and meta-analysis. Pain Physician. 2020;23(2):E151–161.

Aronson JK. *Meyler's side effects of herbal medicines*. Amsterdam: Elsevier; 2009.

Askari G, Aghajani M, Salehi M, et al. The effects of ginger supplementation on biomarkers of inflammation and oxidative stress in adults: A systematic review and meta-analysis of randomized controlled trials. J Herb Med. 2020;22(1):100364.

Avicenna 1025. *Al-Qanoon fi al-Tibb* (*The canon of medicine*) (rewritten by Masoudi A, ed.). Tehran: Almaei; 2015.

Banihani SA. Effect of ginger (*Zingiber officinale*) on semen quality. Andrologia. 2019;51(6):e13296.

Bartels EM, Folmer VN, Bliddal H, et al. Efficacy and safety of ginger in osteoarthritis patients: A meta-analysis of randomized placebo-controlled trials. Osteoarthritis Cartilage. 2015;23(1):13–21.

Bekkouch O, Harnafi M, Touiss I, et al. *In vitro* antioxidant and *in vivo* lipid-lowering properties of *Zingiber officinale* crude aqueous extract and methanolic fraction: A follow-up study. Evid-Based Complement Alternat Med. 2019;2019:9734390.

Betz O, Kranke P, Geldner G, et al. Ist ingwer ein klinisch relevantes antiemetikum? eine systematische übersicht randomisierter kontrollierter studien (Is ginger a clinically relevant antiemetic? A systematic review of randomized controlled trials). Forsch Komplementarmed Klass Naturheilkd. 2005;12(1):14–23.

Bhargava R, Chasen M, Elten M, et al. The effect of ginger (*Zingiber officinale* Roscoe) in patients with advanced cancer. Support Care Cancer. 2020;28(7):3279–3286.

Black CD, Herring MP, Hurley DJ, et al. Ginger (*Zingiber officinale*) reduces muscle pain caused by eccentric exercise. J Pain. 2010;11(9):894–903.

Chaiyakunapruk N, Kitikannakorn N, Nathisuwan S, et al. The efficacy of ginger for the prevention of postoperative nausea and vomiting: a meta-analysis. Am J Obstet Gynecol. 2006;194(1):95–99.

Chang WP, Peng YX. Does the oral administration of ginger reduce chemotherapy-induced nausea and vomiting? A meta-analysis of 10 randomized controlled trials. Cancer Nurs. 2019;42(6):E14–23.

Chatturong U, Kajsongkram T, Tunsophon S, et al. Ginger extract and [6]-gingerol inhibit contraction of rat entire small intestine. J Evid-Based Integr Med. 2018;23(1):2515690X18774273.

Chen CX, Barrett B, Kwekkeboom KL. Efficacy of oral ginger (*Zingiber officinale*) for dysmenorrhea: A systematic review and meta-analysis. Evid-Based Complement Alternat Med. 2016;2016:6295737.

Chen L, Cai Z. The efficacy of ginger for the treatment of migraine: A meta-analysis of randomized controlled studies. Am J Emerg Med. 2021;46:567–571.

Choi JG, Kim SY, Jeong M, et al. Pharmacotherapeutic potential of ginger and its compounds in age-related neurological disorders. Pharmacol Ther. 2018;182(1):56–69.

Crichton M, Marshall S, Marx W, et al. Efficacy of ginger (*Zingiber officinale*) in ameliorating chemotherapy-induced nausea and vomiting and chemotherapy-related outcomes: A systematic review update and meta-analysis. J Acad Nutr Diet. 2019;119(12):2055–2068.

Daily JW, Zhang X, Kim DS, et al. Efficacy of ginger for alleviating the symptoms of primary dysmenorrhea: A systematic review and meta-analysis of randomized clinical trials. Pain Med. 2015;16(12):2243–2255.

Dilokthornsakul W, Rinta A, Dhippayom T, et al. Efficacy and safety of ginger regarding human milk volume and related clinical outcomes: A systematic review of randomized controlled trials. Complement Med Res. 2022;29(1):67–73.

Ebrahimzadeh A, Ebrahimzadeh A, Mirghazanfari SM, et al. The effect of ginger supplementation on metabolic profiles in patients with type 2 diabetes mellitus: A systematic review and meta-analysis of randomized controlled trials. Complement Ther Med. 2022;65(1):102802.

Eshaghian R, Mazaheri M, Ghanadian M, Rouholamin S, Feizi A, Babaeian M. The effect of frankincense (*Boswellia serrata*, oleoresin) and ginger (*Zingiber officinale*, rhizoma) on heavy menstrual bleeding: A randomized, placebo-controlled, clinical trial. Complement Ther Med. 2019;42:42–47.

Fouda AM, Berika MY. Evaluation of the effect of hydroalcoholic extract of *Zingiber officinale* rhizomes in rat collagen-induced arthritis. Basic Clin Pharmacol Toxicol. 2009;104(3):262–271.

Gardner Z, McGuffin M. *Botanical safety handbook*. Boca Raton: Taylor & Francis; 2013.

Gruenwald J, Brendler T, Jaenicke C. *PDR for herbal medicines*. Montvale: Thomson Reuters; 2007.

Guahk GH, Ha SK, Jung HS, et al. *Zingiber officinale* protects HaCaT cells and C57BL/6 mice from ultraviolet B-induced inflammation. J Med Food. 2010;13(3):673–680.

Hasani H, Arab A, Hadi A, et al. Does ginger supplementation lower blood pressure? A systematic review and meta-analysis of clinical trials. Phytother Res. 2019;33(6):1639–1647.

Helalizadeh M, Hatami E, Labbafi M, et al. Effect of ginger supplement on lipid peroxidation induced by exercise: A metaanalysis study. J Med Plant. 2020;19(74):25–38.

Huang FY, Deng T, Meng LX, et al. Dietary ginger as a traditional therapy for blood sugar control in patients with type 2 diabetes mellitus: A systematic review and meta-analysis. Medicine (Baltimore). 2019;98(13):e15054.

Ilkhanizadeh B, Shirpoor A, Khadem Ansari MH, et al. Protective effects of ginger (*Zingiber officinale*) extract against diabetes-induced heart abnormality in rats. Diabetes Metab J. 2016;40(1):46–53.

Jafarnejad S, Keshavarz SA, Mahbubi S, et al. Effect of ginger (*Zingiber officinale*) on blood glucose and lipid concentrations in diabetic and hyperlipidemic subjects: A meta-analysis of randomized controlled trials. J Funct Foods. 2017;29(1): 127–134.

Jalali M, Mahmoodi M, Moosavian SP, et al. The effects of ginger supplementation on markers of inflammatory and oxidative stress: A systematic review and meta-analysis of clinical trials. Phytother Res. 2020;34(8):1723–1733.

Kashefi F, Khajehei M, Alavinia M, Golmakani E, Asili J. Effect of ginger (*Zingiber officinale*) on heavy menstrual bleeding: A placebo-controlled, randomized clinical trial. Phytother Res. 2015;29(1):114–119.

Khare CP. *Indian medicinal plants: An illustrated dictionary*. New Delhi: Springer; 2007.

Lee J, Oh H. Ginger as an antiemetic modality for chemotherapy-induced nausea and vomiting: A systematic review and meta-analysis. Oncol Nurs Forum. 2013;40(2):163–170.

Lu C, Chen X, Yan X, et al. The preventive and relieving effects of ginger on postoperative nausea and vomiting: A systematic review and meta-analysis of randomized controlled trials. Int J Nurs Stud. 2022;125:104094.

Macit MS, Sözlü S, Kocaadam B, et al. Evaluation of ginger (*Zingiber officinale* Roscoe) on energy metabolism and obesity: Systematic review and meta-analysis. Food Rev Int. 2019;35(7):685–706.

Madkor HR, Mansour SW, Ramadan G. Modulatory effects of garlic, ginger, turmeric and their mixture on hyperglycaemia, dyslipidaemia and oxidative stress in streptozotocin-nicotinamide diabetic rats. Br J Nutr. 2011;105(8):1210–1217.

Maharlouei N, Tabrizi R, Lankarani KB, et al. The effects of ginger intake on weight loss and metabolic profiles among overweight and obese subjects: A systematic review and meta-analysis of randomized controlled trials. Crit Rev Food Sci Nutr. 2019;59(11):1753–1766.

Martins LB, Rodrigues AMDS, Monteze NM, et al. Double-blind placebo-controlled randomized clinical trial of ginger (*Zingiber officinale Rosc.*) in the prophylactic treatment of migraine. Cephalalgia. 2020;40(1):88–95.

Marx W, McKavanagh D, McCarthy AL, et al. The effect of ginger (*Zingiber officinale*) on platelet aggregation: A systematic literature review. PLoS One. 2015;10(10):e0141119.

Matsumura MD, Zavorsky GS, Smoliga JM. The effects of pre-exercise ginger supplementation on muscle damage and delayed onset muscle soreness. Phytother Res. 2015;29(6):887–893.

Mazidi M, Gao HK, Rezaie P, et al. The effect of ginger supplementation on serum C-reactive protein, lipid profile and glycaemia: A systematic review and meta-analysis. Food Nutr Res. 2016;60(1):32613.

Mills E, Dugoua JJ, Perri D, Koren G. *Herbal medicines in pregnancy and lactation: An evidence-based approach*. Toronto: Taylor & Francis; 2006.

Montserrat-de la Paz S, Garcia-Gimenez MD, Quilez AM, et al. Ginger rhizome enhances the anti-inflammatory and anti-nociceptive effects of paracetamol in an experimental mouse model of fibromyalgia. Inflammopharmacology. 2018;26(4):1093–1101.

Morvaridzadeh M, Fazelian S, Agah S, et al. Effect of ginger (*Zingiber officinale*) on inflammatory markers: A systematic review and meta-analysis of randomized controlled trials. Cytokine. 2020;135:155224.

Mozafari S, Naz MSG, Ozgoli G. Effect of ginger on primary dysmenorrhea: A systematic review of clinical trials and quasi-experimental studies in the world. Iran J Obstet Gynecol Infertil. 2018;21(1):86–93.

Nikkhah-Bodaghi M, Maleki I, Agah S, et al. *Zingiber officinale* and oxidative stress in patients with ulcerative colitis: A randomized, placebo-controlled, clinical trial. Complement Ther Med. 2019;43(1):1–6.

Ogbuewu IP, Mbajiorgu CA. Meta-analysis of the effect of ginger (*Zingiber officinale*) on health status, production indices and semen quality in chickens. Agric Res. 2020;9(4):640–651.

Pourmasoumi M, Hadi A, Rafie N, et al. The effect of ginger supplementation on lipid profile: A systematic review and meta-analysis of clinical trials. Phytomedicine. 2018;43:28–36.

Samadi M, Moradinazar M, Khosravy T, et al. A systematic review and meta-analysis of preclinical and clinical studies on the efficacy of ginger for the treatment of fatty liver disease. Phytother Res. 2022;36(3):1182–1193.

Sanavi S, Afshar R. Subacute thyroiditis following ginger (*Zingiber officinale*) consumption. Int J Ayurveda Res. 2010;1(1):47–48.

Saneei Totmaj A, Emamat H, Jarrahi F, et al. The effect of ginger (*Zingiber officinale*) on chemotherapy-induced nausea and vomiting in breast cancer patients: A systematic literature review of randomized controlled trials. Phytother Res. 2019;33(8):1957–1965.

Shayesteh F, Haidari F, Shayesteh AA, et al. Ginger in patients with active ulcerative colitis: A study protocol for a randomized controlled trial. Trials. 2020;21(1):278.

Sheikhhossein F, Borazjani M, Jafari A, et al. Effects of ginger supplementation on biomarkers of oxidative stress: A systematic review and meta-analysis of randomized controlled trials. Clin Nutr ESPEN. 2021;45(1):111–119.

Stanisiere J, Mousset PY, Lafay S. How safe is ginger rhizome for decreasing nausea and vomiting in women during early pregnancy? Foods. 2018;7(4):50.

Talebi M, İlgün S, Ebrahimi V, et al. *Zingiber officinale* ameliorates Alzheimer's disease and cognitive impairments: Lessons from preclinical studies. Biomed Pharmacother. 2021;133:111088.

Tóth B, Lantos T, Hegyi P, et al. Ginger (*Zingiber officinale*): An alternative for the prevention of postoperative nausea and vomiting. A meta-analysis. Phytomedicine. 2018;50:8–18.

Ulbricht CE. *Mosby's natural standard herb & supplement guide*. St. Luis: Elsevier; 2010.

Viljoen E, Visser J, Koen N, et al. A systematic review and meta-analysis of the effect and safety of ginger in the treatment of pregnancy-associated nausea and vomiting. Nutr J. 2014;13:20.

Williamson E, Driver S, Baxter K (eds.). *Stockley's herbal medicines interactions*. London: Pharmaceutical Press; 2013.

Wilson PB. Ginger (*Zingiber officinale*) as an analgesic and ergogenic aid in sport: A systemic review. J Strength Cond Res. 2015;29(10):2980–2995.

Yemitan OK, Izegbu MC. Protective effects of *Zingiber officinale* (Zingiberaceae) against carbon tetrachloride and acetaminophen-induced hepatotoxicity in rats. Phytother Res. 2006;20(11):997–1002.

Zhu J, Chen H, Song Z, et al. Effects of ginger (*Zingiber officinale* Roscoe) on type 2 diabetes mellitus and components of the metabolic syndrome: A systematic review and meta-analysis of randomized controlled trials. Evid-Based Complement Alternat Med. 2018;2018:5692962.

42 *Ziziphus jujuba* Mill.

Zahra Sobhani

Scientific name: *Ziziphus jujuba* Mill.
Family: Rhamnaceae
Common names:

- **English:** Jujube, jujube date, Ziziphus, Indian jujube, Chinese date
- **Persian:** *'annāb, 'onnāb*
- **Arabic:** *'unnāb*

Medicinal part(s): Fruit, leaves (Figure 42.1)
Temperament (nature): Cold in the first degree, moderately dry, or slightly wet
Major chemical constituents:

- **Triterpene saponins:** Zyzyphus saponins, jujuboside-B
- Mucilage
- Tannins
- **Flavonoids:** Naringenin-6,8-di-C-glucosides
- **Alkaloids:** Oxonuciferine, nornuciferine, cyclopeptide alkaloids, daechualkaloid-A
- **Triterpenes:** Betulinic acid, betulonic acid, maslinic acid, alphitolic acid, oleanolic acid
- Hydroxycoumarins
- **Sugars:** Saccharose, glucose, fructose, galactose
- **Alpha hydroxy acids:** Malic acid, tartaric acid (Liu et al., 2021; Gruenwald et al., 2007)

THERAPEUTIC USE

TPM Literature

Topical application of macerated jujube powder (with or without seeds) on the eyes can alleviate inflammation and swelling. Oral administration of jujube fruit decoction is beneficial for respiratory system disorders including cough, throat roughness, asthma, laryngitis, chest pain, and hoarseness due to hot dystemperament. Interestingly, the dried fruit is more suitable for these indications than the fresh fruits. Ripe jujube fruit is laxative; whereas its unripe fruit is astringent and is used to treat diarrhea. Oral consumption of whole jujube fruit powder (pulp and seed) is useful for intestinal ulcers. Jujube fruit decoction is recommended for liver diseases. In addition, it can relieve the feeling of thirst caused by liver diseases due to hot dystemperament. Also, jujube fruit is prescribed for urinary system diseases. The fruit of jujube is applied as an anti-inflammatory agent. Topical application of its pulp or whole fruit can treat edema and rash.

Chewing fresh *Z. jujuba* leaves numbs the tongue and it is suggested before taking bad-tasting medicine. Topical application of dried *Z. jujuba* leaves or bark powder is recommended for chronic and hard-to-heal wounds. Oral consumption of leaves decoction sweetened with sugar, relieves itching of the body (Aghili Khorasani 1771; Avicenna 1025).

DOI: 10.1201/b22971-42

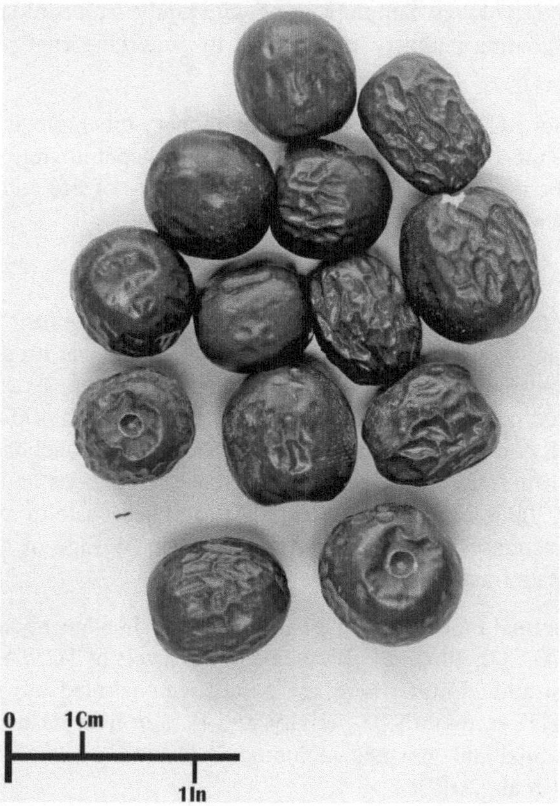

FIGURE 42.1 Jujube fruits.

Current Evidence

Clinical Evidence

Type 2 diabetes mellitus: In an RCT in 116 diabetic patients, jujube fruit infusion (three times daily, 10 g before each meal for 12 weeks) could significantly reduce TC, TAG, LDL-C, LDL-C/HDL-C ratio, and HbA1c (Yazdanpanah et al., 2017).

The effect of dried *Z. jujuba* fruit on cardiometabolic factors in patients with type 2 diabetes mellitus was determined during a randomized controlled trial. The FBS, LDL-C, HDL-C, TC, IL-6, and hs-CRP were all measured at the beginning and end of the trial. Daily consumption of 30 g of *Z. jujuba* for 12 weeks markedly lowered LDL-C, TAG, FBS, whereas HDL-C plasma concentration and IL-6 were not affected. It was also shown that at the end of week 12, hs-CRP decreased considerably in the *Z. jujuba* group by 24.46% from baseline, although this decrease was not statistically considerable compared with the control group (Farhadnejad et al., 2022).

Dyslipidemia: In a triple-blind, placebo-controlled RCT in 86 adolescents with obesity, daily administration of jujube fruit (5 g three times per day) for 1 month caused a significant reduction of TC and LDL-C in comparison to control; though, no significant change was observed in other lipid parameters and BMI (Sabzghabaee et al., 2013).

Immunomodulatory effects: A survey investigated the immunomodulatory effects of 7 days jujube fruit supplementation (0.5 g/kg body weight) in 14 young healthy volunteers. In this research, immune fluctuations have been induced with a session of circuit resistance exercise. Acute exercise could promote apoptotic signaling in human neutrophils by increasing the expression of calpain, caspase-3, and the ([Ca^{2+}]i) pathway. Supplementing with jujube fruit could prevent these alterations and reduce cell death signaling pathway, presumably by supplying energy to neutrophils (Tayebi et al., 2021).

Hepatotoxicity: In a pilot RCT in 17 patients with pulmonary tuberculosis, 4-week administration of jujube fruit syrup (10 mL daily) was shown to reduce the hepatotoxicity due to antituberculosis drugs. In addition, jujube fruit syrup could enhance the quality of life and reduce the intensity of cough in tuberculosis patients (Maddahi et al., 2022).

Preclinical Evidence

Hypertension: The administration of hydroalcoholic extract of jujube fruit for 28 days at doses 100 and 200 mg/kg significantly decreased the elevation of mean arterial pressure and SBP in angiotensin II-induced hypertension in mice. Also, pretreatment with jujube extract at a dose of 200 mg/kg significantly decreased the heart rate. However, pretreatment with 400 mg/kg of jujube extract increased SBP and MAP compared with negative control group (Mohebbati et al., 2017). Another study in agreement with the previous one indicated that the aqueous and ethyl acetate fractions of jujube fruit (150 and 300 mg/kg) reduce SBP, MAP, and heart rate in rats via the NO pathway. Furthermore, stronger responses were recorded with a lower dosage of aqueous fractions and a higher dose of ethyl acetate fractions (Mohebbati et al., 2020).

Hepatotoxicity: In an animal model of alcohol-induced liver damage, aqueous extract of *Z. jujuba* cv. Jinsixiaozao fruit (100, 200, 400 mg/kg) lowered blood levels of TC, TAG, AST, LDH, and ALT after 1 month of administration. Furthermore, the extract demonstrated anti-inflammatory properties by decreasing NF-κB, TNF-α, total iNOS activity, and IL-6 in liver tissue. A significant enhancement in the activity of antioxidant enzymes, including SOD and Gpx, as well as a reduction of MDA were also observed (Liu et al., 2017).

Another study demonstrated that oral administration of jujube polysaccharides (200, 400, 800 mg/kg) to mice with CCl_4-induced hepatotoxicity for 7 days significantly decreased the level of AST and ALT (Yue et al., 2014).

Nephrotoxicity: Oral administration of jujube fruit methanolic extract (1,500, 3,000 mg/kg) for 8 days could protect rats against cisplatin-induced nephrotoxicity, evidenced by significant reduction of BUN, ALT, AST, and MDA (Tanideh et al., 2020).

Inflammation: In an animal model of carrageenan-induced paw edema, ethanolic extract of jujube fruit (600, 1,200, and 1,600 mg/kg, orally) revealed anti-inflammatory effects via inhibition of the volume and thickness of both paws in comparison to control group (Mesaik et al., 2018).

Immune system disorders: Four weeks of treatment with 150, 300, or 600 mg/kg of *Z. jujuba* cv. *Pozao* polysaccharides enhanced peripheral immunity and intestinal barrier function in mice with cyclophosphamide-induced hypoimmunity. The plant enhanced lymphocyte proliferation in the spleen and elevated immunoglobulins and cytokines in the intestinal mucosa and serum. In addition, jujube dose-dependently modulated the expressions of tight junction protein and regulated gut microbiota (Han et al., 2020).

Diarrhea: In an animal study, the effect of hydroalcoholic extract of jujube fruit (400, 800, 1,200 mg/kg) on acute diarrhea induced by castor oil and *Escherichia coli* in a mouse model was investigated. The results revealed that jujube extract was able to inhibit diarrhea by 67% only at a dose of 1,200 mg/kg, while loperamide was 100% effective in inhibiting diarrhea. In comparison to the control group, the high dosage of the extract (1,200 mg/kg) considerably decreased both the frequency of defecation and the quantity of water in the stool. Therefore, jujube fruit hydroalcoholic extract may be effective for avoiding diarrhea-related dehydration and electrolyte imbalances (Mesaik et al., 2018).

ADVERSE REACTIONS

TPM Literature

Jujube fruit is slowly digested and can produce flatulence, especially in people with wet-tempered stomachs. In these cases, it should be prescribed with sugar, currant, or rose water.

It is mentioned that high consumption of *Z. jujuba* can reduce the amount of semen and libido. In these cases, it should be prescribed with honey and aphrodisiac medicines (Aghili Khorasani 1771).

Current Evidence

No adverse health effects have been observed as a result of proper administration of approved therapeutic doses (Gruenwald et al., 2007); however, there are some reports of allergic reactions to jujube fruit and its latex. Especially, the seeds of *Z. jujuba* var. *spinosa* are known to cause allergic reactions, including shortness of breath, dizziness, vomiting, urticaria, pruritus, numbness of the mouth and lips, nausea, pallor, and cold sweat (Gardner and MacGuffin, 2013).

CONTRAINDICATIONS

TPM Literature

None.

Current Evidence

None.

PREGNANCY AND LACTATION

TPM Literature

None.

Current Evidence

There is no evidence available in scientific or traditional literature regarding the safety of jujube fruit during pregnancy or lactation. On the other hand, jujube seeds, owing to their stimulating effect on the uterus, should be taken with caution and under the guidance of a physician during pregnancy. In addition, the safety of consuming *Z. jujuba* fruits and seeds during breastfeeding has not been conclusively proven (Gardner and McGuffin, 2013).

DRUG INTERACTIONS

Drugs metabolized by cytochrome P450: Jujube affects the activity of cytochrome P450 enzyme CYP 1A2. A study has revealed that administration of jujube aqueous extract (1 g/kg) and hydroalcoholic extract (3.6 g/kg) for 10 days decreased the blood concentration of phenacetin (probe substrate for CYP1A2) (Jing et al., 2015). Therefore, when *Z. jujuba* is administered alongside cytochrome-metabolizing medications, necessary precautions should be considered.

Venlafaxine: In a case report, the simultaneous consumption of jujube seeds (0.5 g per day) and venlafaxine (37.5 mg per day) caused an acute serotonin response and anaphylactic symptoms (Gardner and McGuffin, 2013).

Antidiabetic agents: Jujube fruit might decrease blood sugar levels and has moderate interactions with antidiabetic medications. Consequently, accurate monitoring of blood sugar levels is recommended (Yazdanpanah et al., 2016).

METHOD OF ADMINISTRATION

TPM Literature

For oral use, jujube fruit may be used as a decoction or macerated extract. Topical application of pulp or whole fruit powder as a poultice is recommended for edema and rash. In the same way, leaf powder is prescribed topically for wound healing. Chewing its leaves is recommended to numb the tongue and leaf syrup is prescribed for itching (Aghili Khorasani 1771).

Current Evidence

It may be recommended as powder, infusion, decoction, or different kinds of extracts for oral and topical administration.

DOSAGE

Based on clinical studies, up to 30 g of dried jujube fruit can be used daily without side effects (Yazdanpanah et al., 2017; Farhadnejad et al., 2022).

REFERENCES

Aghili Khorasani MH 1771. *Makhzan-al-Adviah* (*The treasury of drugs*) (rewritten by Shams Ardakani MR, Rahimi R, Farjadmand F, 1st ed.). Tehran: Tehran University of Medical Sciences; 2009.

Avicenna 1025. *Al-Qanoon fi al-Tibb* (*The canon of medicine*) (rewritten by Masoudi A, ed.). Tehran: Almaei; 2015.

Farhadnejad H, Asghari G, Hedayati M, et al. Effect of *Ziziphus jujube* on cardiometabolic factors and systemic inflammation in type 2 diabetic patients: A randomized controlled trial. Clin Nutr ESPEN. 2022; 49:53–60.

Gardner Z, McGuffin M. *Botanical safety handbook*. Boca Raton: Taylor & Francis; 2013.

Gruenwald J, Brendler T, Jaenicke C. *PDR for herbal medicines*. Montvale: Thomson Reuters; 2007.

Han X, Bai B, Zhou Q, et al. Dietary supplementation with polysaccharides from *Ziziphus jujuba* cv. Pozao intervenes in immune response via regulating peripheral immunity and intestinal barrier function in cyclophosphamide-induced mice. Food Funct. 2020;11(7):5992–6006.

Jing XY, Peng YR, Wang XM, Duan JA. Effects of *Ziziphus jujuba* fruit extracts on cytochrome P450 (CYP1A2) activity in rats. Chin J Nat Med. 2015;13(8):588–594.

Liu N, Yang M, Huang W, et al. Composition, antioxidant activities and hepatoprotective effects of the water extract of *Ziziphus jujuba* cv. Jinsixiaozao. RSC Advances. 2017;7(11):6511–6522.

Liu SJ, Lv YP, Tang ZS, et al. Ziziphus jujuba Mill., a plant used as medicinal food: a review of its phytochemistry, pharmacology, quality control and future research. Phytochem Rev. 2021;20:507–541.

Maddahi SZ, Jokar A, Kamalinejad M, Behnampur N. The efficacy of jujube syrup on the prevention of drug-induced hepatotoxicity in pulmonary tuberculosis patients: A pilot randomized double-blind placebo-controlled clinical trial. Pharmacol Res Perspect. 2022;10(1):e00902.

Mesaik AM, Poh HW, Bin OY, et al. In vivo anti-inflammatory, anti-bacterial and anti-diarrhoeal activity of *Ziziphus Jujuba* fruit extract. Open Access Maced J Med Sci. 2018;6(5):757–766.

Mohebbati R, Kamkar-Del Y, Shafei MN. Effect of aqueous and ethyl acetate fractions of *Ziziphus jujuba* Mill extract on cardiovascular responses in hypertensive rats. Malays J Med Sci. 2020;27(3):43–52.

Mohebbati R, Rahimi M, Bavarsad K, Shafei M. Long-term administration of *Ziziphus jujuba* extract attenuates cardiovascular responses in hypertensive rats induced by angiotensinii. Anc Sci Life. 2017;37(2):68–73.

Sabzghabaee AM, Khayam I, Kelishadi R, et al. Effect of *Zizyphus jujuba* fruits on dyslipidemia in obese adolescents: A triple-masked randomized controlled clinical trial. Med Arch. 2013;67(3):156–159.

Tanideh N, Zarifi F, Rafiee S, et al. *Ziziphus jujube* protects against cisplatin-induced nephrotoxicity in rats. Comp Clin Path. 2020;29(2):321–326.

Tayebi SM, Krüger K, Ebrahimi F, et al. Supplementation with *Ziziphus jujuba* suppresses apoptosis signals in neutrophils after acute exercise. Montenegrin J Sports Sci Med. 2021;10(2):31–39.

Yazdanpanah Z, Ghadiri-Anari A, Mehrjardi AV, et al. Effect of *Ziziphus jujube* fruit infusion on lipid profiles, glycaemic index and antioxidant status in type 2 diabetic patients: A randomized controlled clinical trial. Phytother Res. 2017;31(5):755–762.

Yazdanpanah Z, Ghadiri-Anari A, Vahidi Mehrjardi A, et al. Evaluation of glycemic control in women with type 2 diabetes mellitus treated with Ziziphus fruit. Iran J Diabetes Obes. 2016;8(1):10–15.

Yue Y, Wu S, Zhang H, et al. Characterization and hepatoprotective effect of polysaccharides from *Ziziphus jujuba* Mill. var. spinosa (Bunge) Hu ex HF Chou sarcocarp. Food Chem Toxicol. 2014;74:76–84.

Index

D

E

F

G